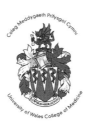

Biopsy Pathology of the Endometrium

Second Edition

C.H. Buckley

MD, FRCPath
Honorary Consultant Gynaecological Pathologist,
St Mary's Hospital, Manchester

and

H. Fox

MD, FRCPath, FRCOG
Emeritus Professor of Reproductive Pathology,
Department of Pathological Sciences,
University of Manchester

A
ARNOLD

A member of the Hodder Headline Group
LONDON   NEW YORK   NEW DELHI

First published in Great Britain in 1989 by Chapman and Hall
This edition published in 2002 by
Arnold, a member of the Hodder Headline Group,
338 Euston Road, London NW1 3BH

http://www.arnoldpublishers.com

Distributed in the United States of America by
Oxford University Press Inc.,
198 Madison Avenue, New York, NY10016
Oxford is a registered trademark of Oxford University Press

Whilst the advice and information in this book are believed to be true and
accurate at the date of going to press, neither the author[s] nor the publisher
can accept any legal responsibility or liability for any errors or omissions
that may be made. In particular (but without limiting the generality of the
preceding disclaimer) every effort has been made to check drug dosages;
however it is still possible that errors have been missed. Furthermore,
dosage schedules are constantly being revised and new side-effects
recognized. For these reasons the reader is strongly urged to consult the
drug companies' printed instructions before administering any of the drugs
recommended in this book.

British Library Cataloguing in Publication Data
A catalogue record for this book is available from the British Library

Library of Congress Cataloging-in-Publication Data
A catalog record for this book is available from the Library of Congress

ISBN 0 340 80706 7 (hb)

1 2 3 4 5 6 7 8 9 10

Commissioning Editor: Georgina Bentliff
Project Editor: Michael Lax/Tim Wale
Production Editor: Anke Ueberberg
Production Controller: Iain McWilliams

Typeset in 9.5/12.5 Stones Serif by Charon Tec Pvt. Ltd, Chennai, India
Printed and bound in Italy by Giunti

Contents

Preface to the second edition

The aim and scope of this second edition remain identical to those of the first edition. There have, however, been considerable advances in our knowledge and understanding of endometrial pathology during the last 11 years and we have tried to incorporate these in this new edition.

C.H. Buckley
H. Fox
Manchester 2001

Preface to the first edition

This volume is entitled *Biopsy Pathology of the Endometrium*. It is not intended to be a complete text on endometrial pathology and is strictly confined in content to the histological findings in endometrial tissue obtained by biopsy. We have chosen our illustrations from biopsy, rather than hysterectomy, specimens, as far as possible, achieving this aim in over 95 per cent of the figures. Our only deviation from this rule has been in Chapter 2 in which we have utilized hysterectomy specimens to illustrate the morphological aspects of the endometrium during the normal menstrual cycle. Because, however, of our awareness that these cyclical changes, as seen in biopsy specimens, differ in many subtle ways from those apparent in intact uteri the changes described in Chapter 2 have to be contrasted with those discussed in Chapter 3, in which the cyclical endometrial changes, as seen in biopsy specimens, are considered.

Endometrial biopsies are often equated with 'curettings' and we have therefore interpreted our remit rather widely to include all specimens that may be received in the laboratory under this general heading. Thus, we have included chapters on abortion material and on gestational trophoblastic disease, neither of which should, in the strict sense, appear in a text on endometrial biopsies. In doing this, however, we have accepted the reality of the day-to-day situation in most histopathological laboratories, in which 'curettings' are grouped together as a single entity irrespective of whether they are truly endometrial biopsies or not.

We have attempted, throughout this volume, to stress the necessity for close co-operation between the pathologist and the gynaecologist. The gynaecologist must supply the pathologist with all the relevant clinical information required for an intelligent approach to the interpretation of endometrial biopsies. In return, the pathologist must extract from endometrial biopsies the maximum of information and convey this to the gynaecologist in clear terms.

C.H. Buckley
H. Fox

Acknowledgements

We are deeply indebted to Linda Chawner for her invaluable help in the preparation of the additional illustrations. We are also indebted to Richard Kempson of Stanford University for kindly supplying us with Figures 8.10 and 10.12, to Robert Young of Harvard University for supplying us with Figure 12.3 and to Professor F.J. Paradinas for providing Figure 14.8. We are also grateful to our colleagues who continue to show us so many of their interesting cases and who have acted as a stimulus to the preparation of this second edition.

1 Sampling the endometrium

The term 'biopsy' is used to describe a tissue sample taken for pathological examination from a living person. Endometrial biopsy is undertaken to identify pathological processes within the endometrium to obtain, indirectly, information about ovarian function and to assess the endometrial response to ovarian or exogenous hormones. The biopsy may be obtained from the endometrium without cervical dilatation using a curette, by aspiration, by endometrial wash or by endometrial brush, as well as by cervical dilatation and curettage. Endometrial wash and brush samples provide material that is really only suitable for cytological examination and are outside the remit of this text.

1.1 TECHNIQUES OF ENDOMETRIAL SAMPLING

Endometrial biopsy may now be combined with transvaginal ultrasonography and it is recognized that, in the postmenopausal patient, the thicker the endometrium the greater the chance of identifying a pathological process in the subsequent biopsy (Giusa-Chiferi *et al.*, 1996; Guner *et al.*, 1996).

1.1.1 Dilatation of the cervix with uterine curettage

The traditional method of removing endometrium for pathological examination is by dilating the cervix and methodically scraping tissue from the anterior and posterior walls of the corpus with a curette. Many operators prefer to pass a pair of sponge forceps into the cavity prior to curettage as a means of identifying and removing polyps from within the cavity. Curettage provides an adequate, minimally traumatized sample of endometrium, which is generally easy to orientate and provides information about the functionalis and, in many cases, about the basalis. It usually provides sufficient material for several techniques to be carried out on the same specimen, for example, microbiological

1

examination, cryostat and routine paraffin-processed sections, and electron microscopy.

Curettage is most appropriate when a pathological process is suspected, for example in the diagnosis of hyperplasia or carcinoma, but it also provides an excellent sample for the assessment of the endometrial response to hormonal stimulation. In some cases, such as after miscarriage, curettage is undertaken for therapeutic rather than diagnostic purposes: the resulting sample is, however, usually treated as a biopsy.

The technique may be refined in the investigation of neoplastic lesions by the process of fractional curettage in which first the endocervical canal and then the corpus uteri is sampled in order to identify the origin of a tumour and determine the extent of its spread within the uterine cavity. Great care is required with this procedure if the samples are to represent accurately and separately the endometrium and endocervix without cross-contamination.

The drawbacks to dilatation and curettage (D & C) relate to the damage which may be inflicted on the cervix (during the dilatation) and the basalis, particularly when the endometrium is curetted in the post-partum period or when it is inflamed (see Asherman's syndrome, Section 15.1.1.2). It has, therefore, wherever possible, been replaced by endometrial sampling and hysteroscopic, directed biopsy – techniques that are less traumatic, particularly for the investigation of infertility.

1.1.2 Single curettage

The technique of taking a single strip of endometrium from the anterior or posterior uterine wall without cervical dilatation is particularly suitable for the examination of the endometrium in patients with infertility. It causes minimal cervical and endometrial damage but allows, in the well-orientated sample, for an accurate assessment of the state of the endometrium as hormone-induced changes usually develop relatively uniformly throughout the endometrium (Johannisson *et al.*, 1982). It causes so little disturbance to the endometrium that a repeat biopsy can be carried out in the same cycle. Single curettage is not suitable for the exclusion of pathological processes, their detection with this technique being often a matter purely of chance, particularly when the disease process is focal.

1.1.3 Aspiration, washes and endometrial brush techniques

Aspiration and endometrial wash techniques can be useful for the identification of a pathological process that may affect the entire endometrium and in which recognition of the abnormality does not depend upon the integrity of the tissue. However, in our experience, they are of very limited value for the interpretation of functional abnormalities. Aspiration procedures are increasingly being used because it is unnecessary to carry out prior cervical dilatation, an anaesthetic is not required and they may be used as outpatient techniques for diagnosis or triage purposes.

The specimens tend to be small, are often fragmented (Fig. 1.1) and may therefore be very difficult to orientate and are, in some cases, more suitable for examination by cytopathological than histopathological techniques. However, they provide a convenient, outpatient procedure for the identification of gross endometrial pathology and are a moderately reliable means of correctly diagnosing carcinoma. The diagnosis on a specimen obtained by a Pipelle sampler, for example, agrees with that obtained from a subsequent curettage specimen or hysterectomy in approximately 90 per cent of cases (Goldchmit *et al.*, 1993; Ben Baruch *et al.*, 1994). It may, however, fail to identify carcinoma when the lesion is limited to a polyp or is very small (Guido *et al.*, 1995). Some have found that the technique provides insufficient

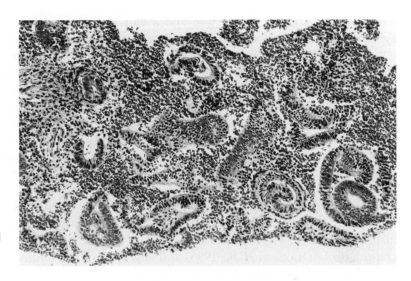

Figure 1.1 The fragmented tissue frequently seen in an aspiration biopsy. The inadequacy of this type of sample for detection of functional abnormalities is clearly apparent. Haematoxylin and eosin.

material for evaluation in as many as 25 per cent of cases compared with approximately 10 per cent after a D & C (Antoni *et al.*, 1997). It may also fail to identify the cause of abnormal uterine bleeding when this is due to the presence of an endometrial polyp or submucous 'fibroid' (Gordon and Westgate, 1999). For these reasons, the technique is often combined with an ultrasound examination of the endometrium, the result of which should be imparted to the histopathologist. It is also considered unwise to assume that a sample inadequate for histological evaluation, in a woman with postmenopausal bleeding, correlates simply with endometrial atrophy and the absence of endometrial pathology (Farrell *et al.*, 1999): there may be a pathological lesion in as many as 20 per cent of such cases.

1.1.4 Hysteroscopic directed biopsies

It has been our experience that, in the hands of a skilled operator, hysteroscopically directed biopsies are useful when there is a visible lesion, such as a small polyp, but that the absence of a visible abnormality does not exclude the possibility of disease. Loverro *et al.* (1996)

found that the positive predictive value of hysteroscopic biopsies of visible lesions in the endometrium is about 60 per cent, while the sensitivity and specificity of the endoscopic procedure in diagnosing endometrial hyperplasia is 98 per cent and 95 per cent, respectively, and the negative predictive value is 99 per cent. They also found that the positive predictive value was higher in postmenopausal patients than in women at reproductive age (72 per cent compared with 58 per cent). Ben Yehuda *et al.* (1998) found that hysteroscopic examination does not improve on the sensitivity of D & C in the detection of endometrial hyperplasia and carcinoma, while Spiewankiewic *et al.* (1995) found that hysteroscopic directed biopsy identified focal endometrial hyperplasia or carcinoma in 12.9 per cent of women with abnormal uterine bleeding in whom dilatation and curettage had been unsuccessful.

1.1.5 Transcervical endometrial resection specimens

Transcervical endometrial resection produces specimens that frequently suffer from heat damage and may be difficult to orientate and interpret. They comprise pieces of myometrium

3

with attached basal endometrium and a variable amount of functional endometrium. The quantity and appearance of the latter depends upon the pre-resection use of hormone therapy, such as goserelin and danazol (Garry *et al.*, 1996) given to diminish endometrial growth. The functional endometrium is, consequently, frequently shallow, the stroma compact and the glands narrow and inactive. The difficulty experienced in orientating these biopsies may make it difficult to say with confidence whether adenomyosis is present or not. It is important that the specimen obtained should be examined histologically in its entirety, as unsuspected carcinoma (Colafranceschi *et al.*, 1996) and endometrial stromal sarcoma have occasionally been unexpectedly identified in such specimens even when preceded by hysteroscopy. Ablation may also be subsequently complicated by the development of carcinoma (Margolis *et al.*, 1995; Valle and Baggish, 1998).

1.2   FIXATION OF ENDOMETRIAL BIOPSIES

In the majority of cases, only fixed, paraffin-processed material will be examined and biopsies for this purpose should be placed in fixative as rapidly as possible after removal to prevent drying and autolysis. Of the fixatives in current use, Bouin's solution gives, in our view, the best results although there are many who prefer buffered formalin solution. A comparison between tissues prepared after fixation in the two fluids is illustrated in Figs 1.2 and 1.3.

Bouin's solution fixes small biopsies rapidly with excellent preservation of cell detail and tissues can be processed within 2 h of their removal. It is, however, poorly penetrating and buffered formalin is preferred for larger pieces of tissue, such as bulky polyps. To the pathologist accustomed to interpreting formalin-fixed tissue, it is necessary to adjust to the characteristic appearance of Bouin-fixed tissue, in which the preservation of larger quantities of deeply staining intercellular fluid imparts an apparently increased density to the tissues. In the majority of cases, Bouin's fixative does not hinder immunohistochemistry and in many instances, the more rapid fixation enhances the value of this technique.

Formalin fixes tissues more slowly and, as a consequence, tissues are less well preserved, mitoses more difficult to identify, nuclear chromatin patterns less clearly seen and interstitial fluids lost to a greater degree than in tissues fixed by Bouin's solution.

1.3   PROCESSING AND STAINING TECHNIQUES

1.3.1   Paraffin processing

Most endometrial biopsies are paraffin-processed and sections, cut at 4–5 microns (micrometres), are stained with haematoxylin and eosin. Some pathologists also like to examine a connective tissue stain such as van Gieson but it is not our practice to do so routinely.

Periodic acid–Schiff reagent (PAS)/Alcian blue stains with and without prior digestion by diastase are useful for the identification of glycogen, histiocytes (in inflammatory processes) and mucin in both neoplasms and metaplastic foci. Gram stains for bacilli, Ziehl-Neelsen stains for acid-/alcohol-fast bacilli and von Kossa stain for calcium are also useful in their place (see Chapter 7). A reticulin stain may be helpful in distinguishing connective tissue-supported epithelial bridges, which are found in hyperplasia, from unsupported epithelial bridges, which suggest the presence carcinoma. The range of stains used in the routine reporting of endometrial biopsies is, however, very small.

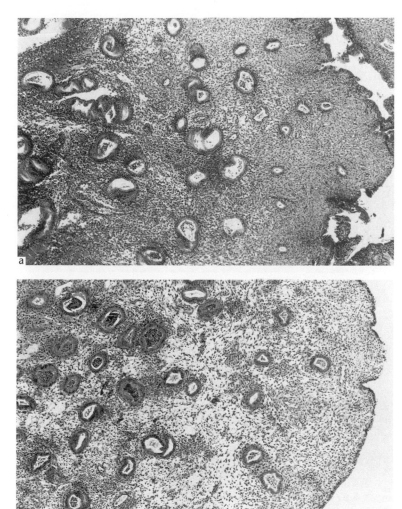

Figure 1.2 **(a)** Secretory endometrium with mild, active, non-specific, chronic inflammation, fixed in Bouin's fluid: biopsy from an IUCD user. **(b)** Part of the same tissue fixed in formalin. Glandular preservation is similar in the two samples but note the apparent patchy distribution of the predecidua and the virtual absence of a compacta in the formalin fixed tissue, and the prominent compacta and extensive predecidualization in the Bouin-fixed sample. Haematoxylin and eosin stain used on (a) and (b).

1.3.2   Frozen sectioning

Frozen sections, stained with haematoxylin and eosin, may be carried out as a prelude to hysterectomy, when they are used to determine whether there is a non-neoplastic endometrial condition for which simple hysterectomy alone will suffice, or if there is an endometrial neoplasm that necessitates hysterectomy and bilateral salpingo-oophorectomy with nodal dissection. The use of pre-hysterectomy frozen section has the advantage of obviating the need for two anaesthetics, with their attendant morbidity. It should be appreciated, however, that many of the features by which we recognize the phases of the endometrial cycle in paraffin-processed tissues are artefacts and that these will not be apparent in frozen material. A comparison between frozen material and the same specimen after Bouin's fixation and paraffin processing is shown in Figs 1.4 and 1.5.

5

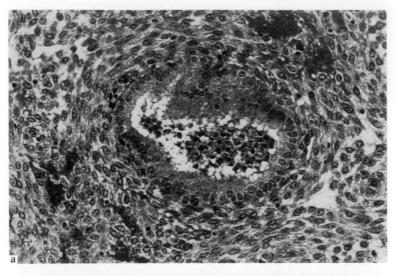

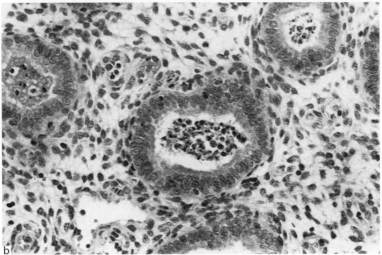

Figure 1.3 **(a)** A portion of the tissue shown in Fig. 1.2a (Bouin fixed). **(b)** A portion of the tissue shown in Fig. 1.2b (formalin fixed). Note the better nuclear and cytoplasmic preservation, the ease with which the cellular detail can be identified and the presence of darkly staining intercellular stromal fluid in the specimen fixed in Bouin's solution.

There are, however, a number of immunohistochemical techniques that require frozen rather than fixed tissues and some monoclonal antibodies will give satisfactory results only on frozen material.

1.3.3 Electron microscopy

It has been our experience that electron microscopy is seldom required in the diagnosis of routine endometrial samples. Its use appears to be limited to the recognition of the occasional poorly differentiated neoplasm and even here, its contribution is minimal. In general, more useful information is obtained from the judicious and more economical use of immunohistochemical techniques. It is not proposed, therefore, to describe the electron optic appearance of the normal endometrium or the pathological processes that affect it because it is our belief that knowledge of these will seldom be required.

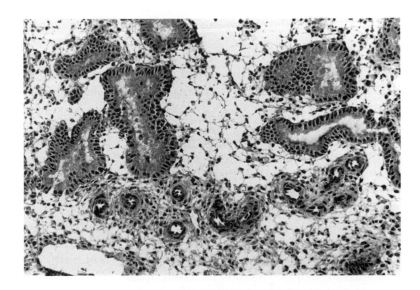

Figure 1.4 Cryostat section of a late secretory endometrium. Haematoxylin and eosin.

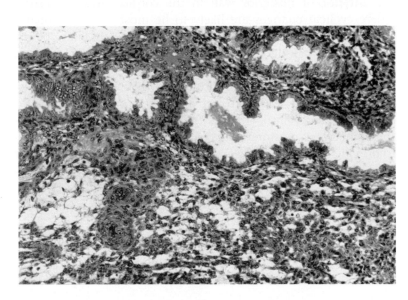

Figure 1.5 Paraffin-processed, wax-embedded, haematoxylin and eosin section of the same tissue as that seen in Fig. 1.4. Note that the serrated configuration of the glands usually considered typical of the late secretory phase is absent from the frozen material but that the spiral arteries and their surrounding cuff of predecidua are similar in the two sections.

1.3.4 Immunohistochemistry

Immunohistochemical examination of the endometrium is undertaken most frequently for the identification of neoplastic conditions. Both frozen material and paraffin-processed tissue is suitable for the purpose. The techniques are adequately described in standard texts on the subject and will not be described in detail here.

1.4 TIMING AND SITING OF ENDOMETRIAL BIOPSIES

In order to obtain the maximum information from an endometrial biopsy, it is important for the clinician first to provide accurate and complete clinical details and second for the sample to be taken at the optimum time and from the

7

appropriate site in the uterus. The request form should provide (at least) the date of the last menstrual period and preferably the date of ovulation or basal temperature change, together with information concerning the use of any steroid hormones, mode of contraception, use of any drugs known to interfere with the normal secretion of trophic hormones, details of any endocrinological disease, and such aspects of the past medical history as are required to explain the need for the examination. The menstrual history is essential and should be insisted upon.

1.4.1 Site of the endometrial biopsy

Endometrial biopsies should be taken from the anterior or posterior wall in the corpus where cyclical changes are likely to be most adequately developed. The tissue of the uterine isthmus fails to undergo cyclical changes and a common error of the inexperienced surgeon is to sample the endometrium too low down in the cavity. Basal endometrium also fails to show normal cyclical changes and therefore the immediately postmenstrual biopsy may fail to provide a representative sample.

In addition to operator errors, there are naturally occurring phenomena that may result in the removal of an unrepresentative sample. For example, the endometrium overlying a submucous leiomyoma is frequently shallow, may contain fewer than normal glands and, in extreme cases, may be represented by only a single layer of columnar epithelium with a little underlying stroma (Fig. 1.6) (Patterson-Keels *et al.*, 1994). The tissue in this area may also be ulcerated or focally inflamed. In the patient wearing an intrauterine contraceptive device (IUCD), removal of tissue from the contact site may give a false impression of infection, irregular ripening or scarring.

1.4.2 Timing of the endometrial biopsy

It may be impossible, in the presence of endometrial lesions that produce abnormal bleeding, to select accurately the time at which to take the biopsy. However, this may have little adverse effect on the detection of those pathological processes (e.g. hyperplasias and neoplasms) that may be identified at any time, whether the patient is actively bleeding or not.

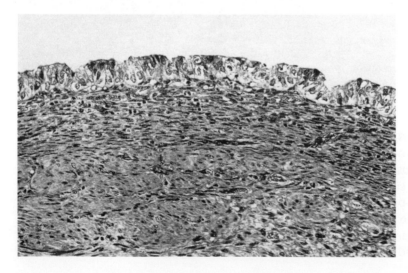

Figure 1.6 The shallow endometrium covering the surface of a submucous leiomyoma. Glands are absent and the surface epithelium is separated from the myometrium by only a wisp of endometrial stroma. Haematoxylin and eosin.

If a pathological process is suspected, there is little to gain and a great deal to lose by postponing the biopsy and, indeed, waiting for the bleeding to cease may result in complete loss of the abnormal endometrium and thus hinder diagnosis (Dallenbach-Hellweg, 1987). However, the appearances of cyclical hormone-related conditions and inflammatory processes vary according to the stage of the cycle and careful timing of such biopsies is required.

The best time for observing cyclical changes in the endometrium is between the 7th and 11th post-ovulatory days. At this stage, it is possible to assess both the adequacy of the secretory change and its uniformity. It should also be possible to identify an inflammatory process if one is present, although tuberculosis may be difficult or impossible to recognize until the 12th to 13th post-ovulatory day.

In the 2 days prior to menstruation, inflammatory changes, with the exception of tuberculosis, are difficult to identify with certainty in haematoxylin and eosin stained sections because they are masked by the physiological stromal cellular infiltrate that accompanies the late secretory phase. This is, however, the optimum time for identifying tuberculosis but as acid-/alcohol-fast bacilli are notoriously difficult to identify in endometrium, and as morphologically well-developed tubercles are an unusual finding, it is essential for simultaneous microbiological studies to be carried out.

The sample, which to the histopathologist is the most difficult to interpret, and hence the least satisfactory, is the menstrual sample. It may only be possible, at best, to determine whether bleeding has occurred from a secretory endometrium, and is therefore actually menstrual, or whether bleeding is the result of hormonal withdrawal in a non-secretory endometrium. Its most useful purpose is for microbiological studies.

1.5 REPORTING ENDOMETRIAL BIOPSIES

It is important that all endometrial biopsies are reported in the full knowledge, not only of the clinical symptoms and the reason for the biopsy, but also with knowledge of any hormones that have been used by the patient in the recent past. These may include, for example, hormone replacement therapy, contraceptive hormones and therapeutic gestagens.

The following comments are not meant to be a comprehensive guide to the reporting of endometrial biopsies but are intended to provide guidelines and suggestions for the reporting of both adequate biopsies and the increasingly diminutive biopsies that stem from endometrial samplers.

In some samples, no endometrial tissue will be found and such specimens can simply be reported as unsatisfactory.

In the normal postmenopausal patient, however, it is more usual to receive a sample consisting mainly of blood that contains short, isolated strips of inactive epithelium of endometrial (Fig. 1.7), and sometimes of endocervical type. In some samples, it may be possible only to exclude cytological atypia and to comment on the absence of mitotic activity. The gynaecologist should be alerted to the fact that morphological abnormalities cannot be excluded and that, although the biopsy is consistent with the postmenopausal state, caution should be exercised in assuming that there is no lesion in women that continue to bleed. It is not our practice, however, to describe such specimens as unsatisfactory.

It is usually possible to identify those samples that have been taken from endometria that have been subject to oestrogenic stimulation even in the absence of mitotic activity and evidence of hyperplasia. Endometrial surface cells tend to be tall (rather than cubo-columnar)

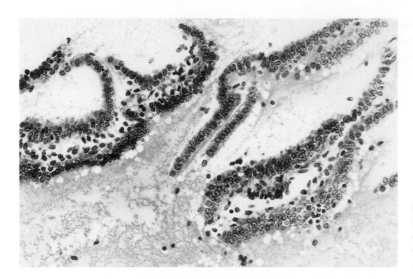

Figure 1.7 Isolated strips of inactive, cuboidal epithelium of endometrial type that is typical of the postmenopausal state. Haematoxylin and eosin.

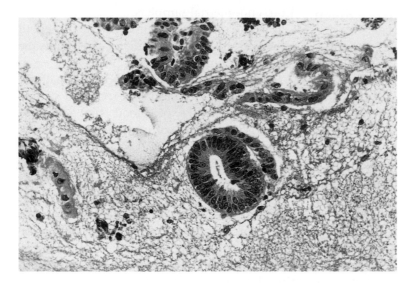

Figure 1.8 A postmenopausal sample of endometrium in which there is no obvious proliferative activity but in which the glandular epithelium is columnar and pseudostratified. Haematoxylin and eosin.

and ciliated. Glandular epithelium in such cases may be plump and pseudostratified (Fig. 1.8). In the absence of mitotic activity, we would report these as inactive but with evidence of a degree of oestrogenic stimulation, albeit at low level. The implication is that the patient is not yet postmenopausal or has a non-physiological oestrogen source.

In our experience, samples from women in the reproductive years and those from women whose endometrium has been subject to abnormal oestrogenic stimulation are, whatever the method of sampling, usually sufficiently voluminous to confirm the normality of the tissue (Fig. 1.9) or to identify morphological (Fig. 1.10) and cytological abnormalities. It has been argued

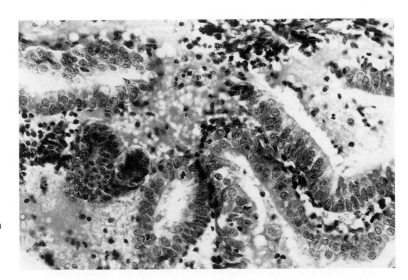

Figure 1.9 A small sample of proliferative endometrium: there is a mitosis in the gland in the centre of the field. Haematoxylin and eosin stain.

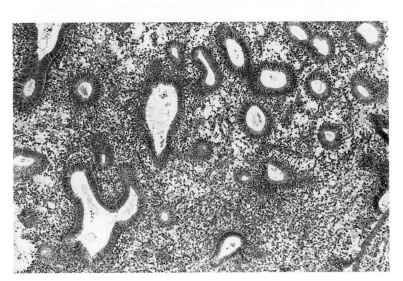

Figure 1.10 An endometrium that has been subject to uninterrupted oestrogenic stimulation resulting in the development of a disordered proliferation (see Chapter 5). Haematoxylin and eosin.

that a sample that is too small to evaluate adequately has, by virtue of its small size, come from an inactive or atrophic endometrium. This view depends upon the reliance that can be placed on the skill of the person taking the sample and the pathologist's ability to exclude oestrogen-induced changes.

In biopsies taken during the reproductive years, it is our practice to make a statement describing the activity of the tissue (for example proliferative or mid-secretory) and, for samples in the secretory phase, the approximate day of the cycle with which the sample is consistent. It is usual to comment upon the uniformity of secretory changes and its adequacy. All pathological processes or non-physiological features should be described. Negative findings, such as the absence of hyperplasia or neoplasia, are as

11

important to the gynaecologist as are the positive findings, if the clinician is to be certain that the pathologist has excluded these possibilities.

REFERENCES

Antoni, J., Folch, E., Costa, J., Foradada, C.M., Cayuela, E., Combalia, N., Rue, M. (1997) Comparison of cytospat and Pipelle endometrial biopsy instruments. *Eur. J. Obstet. Gynecol. Reprod. Biol.* **72**, 57–61.

Ben-Baruch, G., Seidman, D.S., Schiff, E., Moran, O., Menczer, J. (1994) Outpatient endometrial sampling with the Pipelle curette. *Gynecol. Obstet. Invest.* **37**, 260–2.

Ben-Yehuda, O.M., Kim, Y.B., Leuchter, R.S. (1998) Does hysteroscopy improve upon the sensitivity of dilatation and curettage in the diagnosis of endometrial hyperplasia or carcinoma? *Gynecol. Oncol.* **68**, 4–7.

Colafranceschi, M., Bettocchi, S., Mencaglia, L., van Herendael, B.J. (1996) Missed hysteroscopic detection of uterine carcinoma before endometrial resection: report of three cases. *Gynecol. Oncol.* **62**, 298–300.

Dallenbach-Hellweg, G. (1987) Functional disturbances of the endometrium. In: Fox, H. (ed.), *Haines and Taylor Obstetrical and Gynaecological Pathology*, 3rd edn. Edinburgh: Churchill Livingstone, 320–39.

Farrell, T., Jones, N., Owen, P., Baird, A. (1999) The significance of an 'insufficient' Pipelle sample in the investigation of post-menopausal bleeding. *Acta Obstet. Gynecol. Scand.* **78**, 810–12.

Garry, R., Khair, A., Mooney, P., Stuart, M. (1996) A comparison of goserelin and danazol as endometrial thinning agents prior to endometrial laser ablation. *Br. J. Obstet. Gynaecol.* **103**, 339–44.

Giusa-Chiferi, M.G., Goncalves, W.J., Baracat, E.C., de-Albuquerque-Neto, L.C., Bortoletto, C.C., de-Lima, G.R. (1996) Transvaginal ultrasound, uterine biopsy and hysteroscopy for postmenopausal bleeding. *Int. J. Gynaecol. Obstet.* **55**, 39–44.

Gordon, S.J., Westgate, J. (1999) The incidence and management of failed Pipelle sampling in a general outpatient clinic. *Aust. N.Z. J. Obstet. Gynaecol.* **39**, 115–18.

Goldchmit, R., Katz, Z., Blickstein, I., Caspi, B., Dgani, R. (1993) The accuracy of endometrial Pipelle sampling with and without sonographic measurement of endometrial thickness. *Obstet. Gynecol.* **82**, 727–30.

Guido, R.S., Kanbour, S.-A., Rulin, M.C., Christopherson, W.A. (1995) Pipelle endometrial sampling. Sensitivity in the detection of endometrial cancer. *J. Reprod. Med.* **40**, 553–5.

Guner, H., Tiras, M.B., Karabacak, O., Sarikaya, H., Erdem, M., Yildirim, M. (1996) Endometrial assessment by vaginal ultrasonography might reduce endometrial sampling in patients with postmenopausal bleeding: a prospective study. *Aust. N.Z. J. Obstet. Gynaecol.* **36**, 175–8.

Johannisson, E., Parker, R.A., Landgren, B.M., Diczfalusy, C. (1982) Morphometric analysis of the human endometrium in relation to peripheral hormone levels. *Fertil. Steril.* **38**, 564–71.

Loverro, G., Bettocchi, S., Cormio, G., Nicolardi, V., Porreca, M.R., Pansini, N., Selvaggi, L. (1996) Diagnostic accuracy of hysteroscopy in endometrial hyperplasia. *Maturitas* **25**, 187–91.

Margolis, M.T., Thoen, L.D., Boike, G.M., Mercer, L.J., Keith, L.G. (1995) Asymptomatic endometrial carcinoma after endometrial ablation. *Int. J. Gynaecol. Obstet.* **51**, 255–8.

Patterson-Keels, L.M., Selvaggi, S.M., Haefner, H.K., Randolph Jr, J.F. (1994) Morphologic assessment of endometrium overlying submucosal leiomyomas. *J. Reprod. Med.* **39**, 579–84.

Spiewankiewicz, B., Stelmachow, J., Sawicki, W., Kietlinska, Z. (1995) Hysteroscopy with selective endometrial sampling after unsuccessful dilatation and curettage in diagnosis of symptomatic endometrial cancer and endometrial hyperplasias. *Eur. J. Gynaecol. Oncol.* **16**, 26–29.

Valle, R.F., Baggish, M.S. (1998) Endometrial carcinoma after endometrial ablation: high-risk factors predicting its occurrence. *Am. J. Obstet. Gynecol.* **179**, 569–72.

2 The anatomy and histology of the endometrium

The uterine cavity is approximately triangular in coronal section with the apex below at the internal os and the base of the triangle at the fundus of the uterus. In sagittal section, it is slit-like because the anterior and posterior walls are almost in contact (Williams and Warwick, 1980). The length of the cavity varies, measuring up to 5.0 cm in the reproductive years and often less than 2.0 cm in the postmenopausal years.

2.1 THE NORMAL ENDOMETRIUM

The endometrium forms the lining of the corpus uteri from the uterine isthmus below to the commencement of the interstitial segments of the Fallopian tubes in the uterine cornua, on each side of the fundus, above. It is characterized by its striking sensitivity to ovarian hormones, its lability and its remarkable regenerative capacity. It undergoes regular cyclical changes, in response to the recurrent hormonal changes of the ovulatory cycle, during the reproductive years and provides a dormant mucous membrane for the uterus prior to the menarche and after the menopause.

The endometrium is composed of simple, tubular glands set in a cellular, vascular stroma (Fig. 2.1). There are two components, a basal layer, or basalis, which does not respond to hormonal stimulation under normal circumstances, and a changing, more superficial layer, the functionalis, which responds to the hormonal changes of the normal ovulatory cycle, and which is regularly shed and regenerated during the reproductive years. There is no sharp line of demarcation between the functionalis and basalis and the junction between the basal endometrium and myometrium is rather irregular and ill defined (Fig. 2.2). The depth of the functionalis varies throughout the menstrual cycle, reaching its maximum in the late proliferative or mid secretory phase and being least in the immediate postmenstrual phase: it is absent in the premenarchal and postmenopausal state.

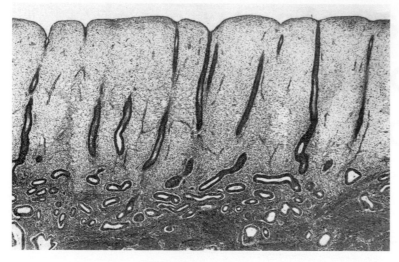

Figure 2.1 Early proliferative phase endometrium, day 8 of cycle. Straight, narrow tubular glands are set in a fragile immature cellular stroma in which there are only thin-walled blood vessels. The stroma of the basalis is more densely cellular than that of the functionalis but there is no sharp line of demarcation between these two zones or between the basalis and underlying myometrium. Haematoxylin and eosin.

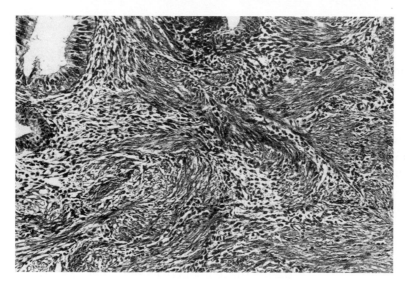

Figure 2.2 The ill-defined junction between the basalis and the myometrium. The smaller, randomly distributed, more darkly staining cells of the endometrial stroma are seen in the upper part of the field and the myometrium, with interweaving bundles of large, elongated smooth muscle cells with copious pale cytoplasm lie below. Haematoxylin and eosin.

In the uterine cornua, there is a transition to tubal mucosa, which may be abrupt or gradual, and in a proportion of women the endometrium extends for some way into the interstitial segments of the Fallopian tubes.

In the uterine isthmus, the cellular endometrial stroma is gradually replaced by a less cellular, more fibrous connective tissue resembling that of the cervix and epithelium of both endometrial and endocervical type is seen (Fig. 2.3).

2.1.1 Basal endometrium

The stroma in basal endometrium is more densely cellular than in the functionalis and nucleocytoplasmic ratios are high: thus, on

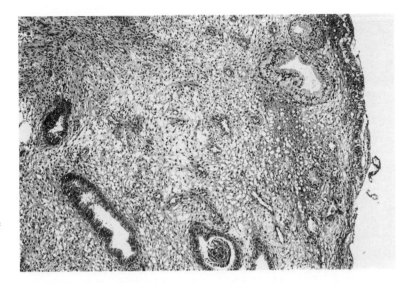

Figure 2.3 The uterine isthmus. Glands lined by epithelium of endometrial type lie to the left and the crypts, to the right, are lined by mucus-secreting epithelium of endocervical type. Mucus-secreting epithelium also covers the surface of the tissue: the stroma is more fibrous than in the uterine body. Haematoxylin and eosin.

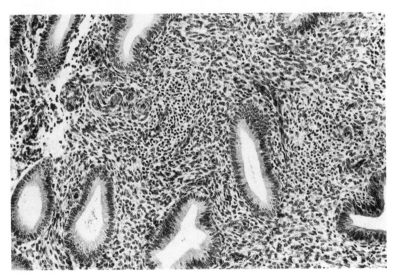

Figure 2.4 Basal endometrium. The stroma is densely cellular and contains small lymphoid aggregates: these are normally seen in the basalis. The glands are narrow and lined by a tall, columnar epithelium. Haematoxylin and eosin.

microscopic examination, the tissue is generally basophilic. A scattering of lymphocytes and lymphoid aggregates is common and constitutes part of the normal structure; thick-walled arteries are present (Figs 2.4 and 2.5). At its deep border, the basalis blends with the myometrium and there is a narrow zone in which endometrial stromal cells and smooth muscle are intermingled (Fig. 2.2).

The glands, which are often less evenly distributed in the basalis than in the functional layers (Fig. 2.5) and are, without it assuming any significance, mildly irregular, are lined by a columnar epithelium with tall, closely packed narrow cells with elongated, parallel-sided or rather cigar-shaped nuclei orientated at right angles to the basement membrane (Fig. 3.6): a minor degree of pseudostratification may be

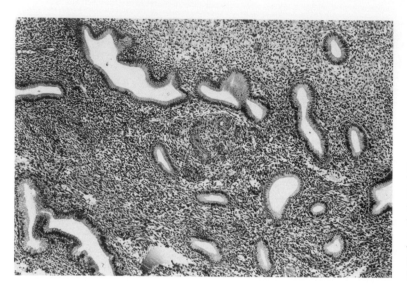

Figure 2.5 Basal endometrium. The basal glands are more irregularly dispersed and more variable in size and shape than in the functionalis: thick-walled muscular arteries, which do not vary throughout the cycle, are seen in the centre of the field. Haematoxylin and eosin.

seen. The appearance of the basalis is more or less constant throughout the normal cycle.

2.1.2 Isthmic endometrium

In the upper part of the isthmus, the stroma is similar to that in the corpus uteri but becomes progressively more fibrous, less cellular and more eosinophilic (in haematoxylin and eosin stained sections) as the proportion of collagen gradually increases, so that in the lower isthmus it comes to resemble the fibrous stroma of the endocervix. Thin-walled venous and capillary channels are present and, depending on whether it is upper or lower isthmus, the surface epithelium is of endometrial or endocervical type, respectively. In the isthmus, the glands are more widely spaced than in the true endometrium, are often a little dilated and are lined by epithelium of endometrial type, which is either unresponsive to normal hormonal stimulation or lags behind that of the corpus (Fig. 2.6) (Hendrickson and Kempson, 1980).

2.1.3 Functional endometrium

The functionalis is the superficial layer of the endometrium, which normally develops only during the reproductive years, its structure and activity accurately reflecting the pattern of ovarian hormone secretion. It may also grow under the influence of abnormal endogenous or exogenous oestrogens (see Chapter 5). During the reproductive cycle, the functionalis undergoes regular growth and maturation that terminates, in the absence of pregnancy, in its being shed, on average, every 28 days.

It is customary, in the UK, to speak of the reproductive cycle as commencing on the first day of menstruation but in some countries, the day of ovulation is regarded as the start of the cycle. It is, of course, much easier to be certain of the date of the last menstrual period than of the date of ovulation, except in those few patients in whom hormone levels are being monitored.

The cyclical changes in the functionalis may be described either in terms of the predominant endometrial morphological features or, alternatively, in terms of the ovarian cyclical hormone secretion. Thus, one speaks of the proliferative or follicular phase of the cycle, corresponding to the phase of ovarian follicular growth prior to ovulation, and of the secretory or luteal (post-ovulatory) phase after

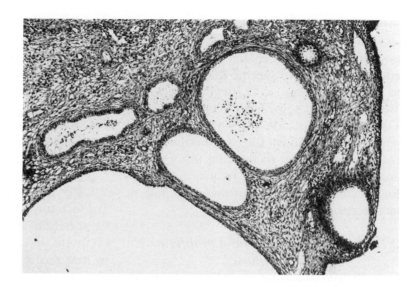

Figure 2.6 The uterine isthmus. The glands, which are lined by epithelium of endometrial type, are cystically dilated and there is no evidence of cyclical changes. Haematoxylin and eosin.

ovulation has occurred. In the normal cycle, the post-ovulatory phase is remarkably constant, lasting 14 days. Variations in cycle length are usually caused by alterations in the follicular or proliferative phase of the cycle, which may vary from 8 to 20 days.

During the phase of ovarian follicular growth, in response to pituitary follicle stimulating hormone, oestradiol, the most potent of the ovarian oestrogens, and oestrone, a weaker and less important oestrogen, are secreted by the granulosa and thecal cells of the developing follicle. Secretion reaches a peak just before ovulation, declines briefly in the early post-ovulatory phase and then increases again, to a rather lesser extent, owing to oestrogen secretion by the corpus luteum. It finally falls to resting levels in the immediate premenstrual phase as the corpus luteum degenerates. During the initial phase of follicular growth, oestrogen is responsible for the coordinated growth of the endometrial glands, stroma and vasculature, and for the induction of progesterone receptors and, during the second, minor peak, for the oedema that characterizes the mid-secretory phase.

Following ovulation, the ovarian follicle develops into the mature corpus luteum and this coincides with a rapid rise in progesterone secretion, although the first detectable increase occurs in response to the mid-cycle luteinizing hormone (LH) peak that immediately precedes ovulation. Progesterone levels reach a peak 3–4 days after ovulation, but are usually sufficient to induce changes in the endometrium within 24–36 h of ovulation. They remain high until 2 or 3 days before the end of the cycle and then, in the absence of pregnancy, as the corpus luteum degenerates, decline rapidly. Progesterone is responsible for the development, in the endometrium, of the glandular secretory changes, which become apparent 24–36 h after ovulation, for stromal maturation or decidualization and for the differentiation of the spiral arteries, which proceeds throughout the post-ovulatory phase.

2.1.4 The phases of the endometrial cycle

During the proliferative phase of the cycle, the appearance of the endometrium does not differ sufficiently from day to day for the precise stage of the cycle to be identified. However, following ovulation, the changes in the secretory endometrium are so specific that it is possible to identify the duration of the phase to within 1 or 2 days, and some would claim, to within 1 day (Noyes *et al.*, 1950). Consequently, even when precise dating of the endometrium is not required, it is usual to describe the secretory endometrium in terms of its major morphological changes, as being in the early, mid- or late-secretory phase.

2.1.4.1 Postmenstrual and proliferative (follicular) phase

Immediately following menstruation, which lasts, on average, 5 days, the uterus is lined only by basal endometrium and the residuum of the deeper part of the functionalis. Regrowth commences, even in the absence of hormonal stimulation, on days 3–4, the first evidence being a healing of the surface epithelium (Fig. 2.7). Subsequently, between days 5 and 14 of the 'typical' 28-day cycle (the proliferative or follicular phase) there is synchronous stromal, glandular and vascular growth and the endometrium increases in depth until the time of ovulation, on the 14th day of the cycle.

In the early part of the proliferative phase the glands are straight and tubular and the stroma immature (Fig. 2.1). Later in the phase, from day 10, glandular growth outstrips that of the stroma, the glands thus become progressively more convoluted (Fig. 2.8), and stromal oedema may develop.

2.1.4.2 Secretory phase

The secretory phase is characterized by glandular secretion and stromal maturation, which occur in response to progesterone produced by the post-ovulatory corpus luteum. These changes occur only when progesterone receptors are present in the endometrium and the development of these, in turn, depends upon there having been adequate oestrogen secretion in the follicular phase (progesterone receptors are oestrogen induced).

The secretory phase is divided into three stages: the early secretory phase lasts from the 2nd to 4th post-ovulatory day, the mid-secretory phase extends from the 5th to 9th post-ovulatory day and the late secretory phase lasts from the 10th to 14th post-ovulatory day.

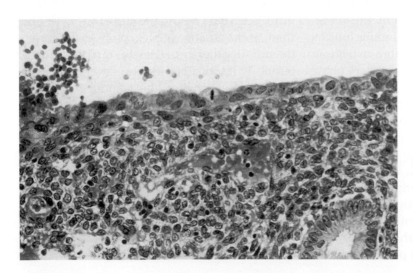

Figure 2.7 Basal endometrium in the late menstrual phase (day 4 of the cycle). Regeneration of the surface epithelium is characterized by focal immaturity, loss of cellular polarity, mild pleomorphism and the presence of mitotic figures. Haematoxylin and eosin.

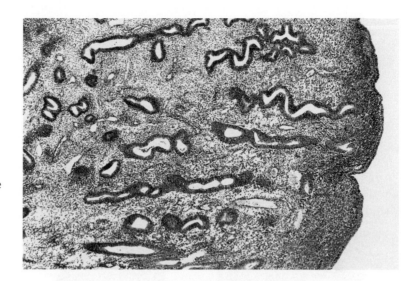

Figure 2.8 Late proliferative phase endometrium, 12th day of cycle. The glands remain simple tubular and parallel-sided but are rather tortuous and mildly convoluted: there is slight stromal oedema. Haematoxylin and eosin.

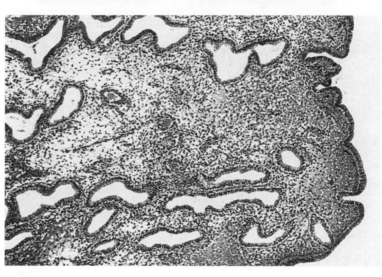

Figure 2.9 Endometrium in transition from proliferative to early secretory phase (2nd to 3rd post-ovulatory day). The glands retain the rather tortuous appearance of the late proliferative phase (Fig. 2.8) but there are vacuoles in the infranuclear cytoplasm of some of the cells in the glandular epithelium. Haematoxylin and eosin.

Secretion is not apparent in the glands until 36–48 h after ovulation, this being sometimes known as the interval phase. After the interval, in response to the rising progesterone levels, first, secretory changes become apparent in the glandular epithelium and, later, predecidual changes occur in the stroma.

- *Early secretory phase:* The glandular morphology of the early secretory phase is similar

to that of the late proliferative phase and the first presumptive evidence of ovulation is the appearance, in the glandular epithelium, of subnuclear vacuoles (Figs 2.9 and 3.13). These normally appear on the 16th day of the cycle (2nd post-ovulatory day). They are initially few in number and irregularly distributed throughout the sample, but within 12 h they become more uniform and can be detected in most glands; they reach a peak

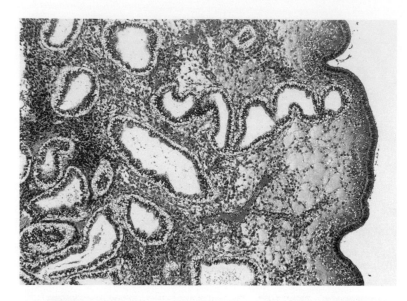

Figure 2.10 Early secretory endometrium, 4th post-ovulatory day. Prominent subnuclear vacuoles are uniformly distributed throughout the glandular epithelium and the stroma is mildly oedematous. A minor degree of glandular luminal distension is now apparent. Haematoxylin and eosin.

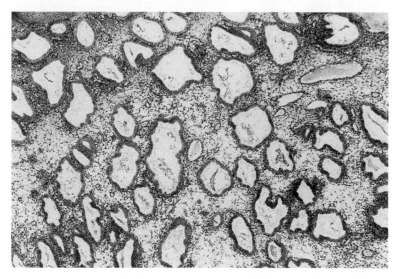

Figure 2.11 Mid-secretory endometrium, 7th to 8th post-ovulatory day. Glandular secretion has reached a peak, the lumina are distended and the glands appear somewhat angulated in cross-section: stromal oedema is marked and spiral arteries are inconspicuous. Haematoxylin and eosin.

between days 17 and 18 of the cycle (3rd to 4th post-ovulatory day) (Figs 2.10 and 3.15). It can be assumed that ovulation has occurred only when vacuoles are uniformly distributed in at least 50 per cent of the glands.

- *Mid-secretory phase:* Between days 19 and 23 of the cycle (5th to 9th post-ovulatory day) secretion of the glandular epithelial contents

occurs, reaching a peak on day 21 (7th post-ovulatory day). It is at this stage of the cycle that the most satisfactory biopsy for the assessment of secretory activity is obtained (Figs 2.11 and 3.16). Stromal oedema, which is first apparent in the early secretory phase, reaches a peak on days 22–23 and by day 23 spiral artery differentiation is apparent

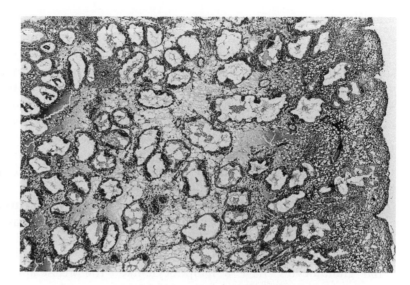

Figure 2.12 Endometrium in transition from mid to late secretory phase, 10th post-ovulatory day. Secretion is past its peak and minor glandular serrations are apparent: stromal oedema is still prominent and spiral arteries are visible, each with a narrow cuff of predecidua. Haematoxylin and eosin.

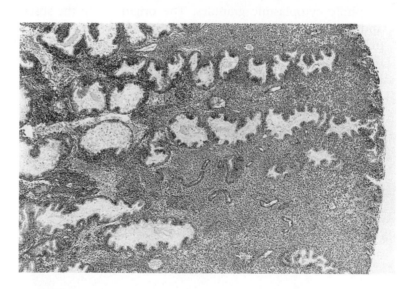

Figure 2.13 Late secretory endometrium, 12th post-ovulatory day. Glandular secretion is exhausted and stromal oedema has been lost, as a consequence, the glands have collapsed and appear serrated: a wide cuff of decidualized cells surrounds the spiral arteries, which are well muscularized, and a band of decidua lies immediately deep to the surface epithelium. Haematoxylin and eosin.

(Fig. 2.12). The vessels proliferate, pericytes widen, myofibrils differentiate and at the same time, perivascular stromal cells become more conspicuous, their cytoplasm increasing in quantity and eosinophilia; these predecidual cells first become apparent on day 23 (9th post-ovulatory day).

- *The late-secretory phase:* This phase (days 24–28 of the cycle; 10th to 14th post-ovulatory day) is characterized by exhaustion of glandular secretory activity, the glands becoming serrated and tortuous, and a general reduction in endometrial height owing to regression of the stromal oedema (Figs 2.13 and 3.18).

21

Predecidual change develops in those stromal cells, which form a cuff around the spiral arteries and a compact layer below the surface epithelium (Figs 2.14, 3.19 and 3.20). Except for the cuff of predecidua around the spiral arteries, the stroma in the mid zone of the functionalis shows little predecidual change and hence appears less opaque or solid on histological examination; this is the spongy layer. A stromal infiltrate composed predominantly of granulated lymphocytes, but also containing the occasional polymorphonuclear leucocytic cluster, characterizes the immediate premenstrual stroma (Fig. 3.21). Granulated lymphocytes or 'endometrial granulocytes' have a lymphocyte-like nucleus and a variable number of phloxinophilic cytoplasmic granules. The origin and function of these cells has been much debated but it is now clear that they are granulated lymphocytes and it is possible that they play a role in the immunological interaction between maternal and fetal tissues during pregnancy (Bulmer *et al.*, 1987).

2.1.4.3 *Menstrual phase*

Evidence of the onset of menstruation is apparent by day 28 of the cycle, before the patient has noticed any bleeding (Fig. 2.15). Over the next 24 h, a plane of separation becomes apparent (Fig. 2.16), through the spongy layer, which leads to the separation of the superficial endometrium (Fig. 2.17) from the basal; a variable amount of functional endometrium remains attached to the basalis (Fig. 2.18).

2.1.5 **Postmenopausal**

As ovulation ceases at the time of the menopause and oestrogen secretion diminishes, endometrial growth is no longer stimulated, though the precise appearance of the endometrium is somewhat variable.

In the absence of oestrogen there is no functionalis and the uterus is lined only by a shallow basalis (Fig. 2.19) similar in appearance to that seen in the reproductive years. The stroma is cellular and the small, narrow, tubular glands are lined by a cuboidal epithelium of indeterminate type. The line of demarcation between the

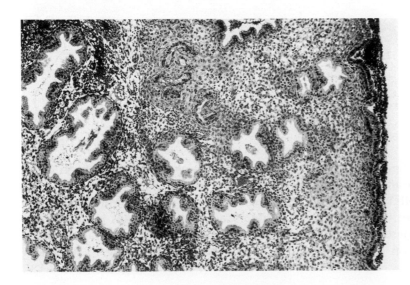

Figure 2.14 Late secretory endometrium, 13th to 14th post-ovulatory day. The glandular outline is so markedly serrated that the epithelium appears tufted where tangential cutting has occurred. A cuff of decidua surrounds the spiral artery, which is well muscularized and tortuous, and a compact layer has differentiated. Haematoxylin and eosin.

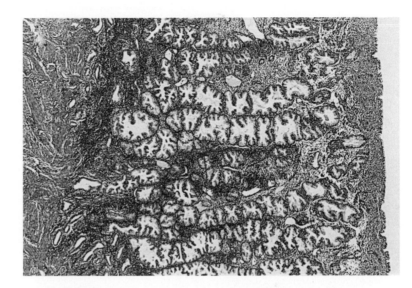

Figure 2.15 Early menstrual endometrium, day 1 of the cycle. Glandular serration is greatly exaggerated compared with that seen in Fig. 2.14, approximately 48 h earlier in the cycle. There is disruption of the stroma immediately deep to the compacta with aggregation of stromal cells and interstitial haemorrhage. Haematoxylin and eosin.

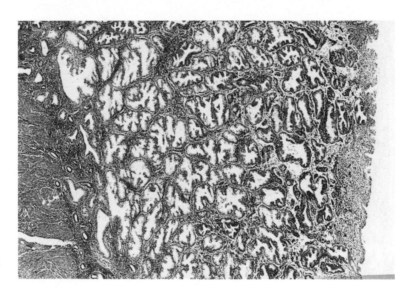

Figure 2.16 Menstrual endometrium, day 2 of the cycle. Stromal aggregation is more pronounced, disruption of the stromal skeleton has occurred, and there is separation of the glands and stroma. Haematoxylin and eosin.

myometrium and endometrium often becomes more coarsely irregular than in the reproductive years and it may be difficult to distinguish endometrial stroma from myometrium (Fig. 2.20). Several years after the menopause the stroma may have become fibrous and the typical stromal cellularity diminished.

Alternatively, and often some years after the menopause, the endometrial glands may become cystically dilated and lined by a single layer of flattened cuboidal epithelium of indeterminate type. The stroma is often partly or sometimes predominantly fibrous (Fig. 2.21). This is the picture of so-called 'senile cystic

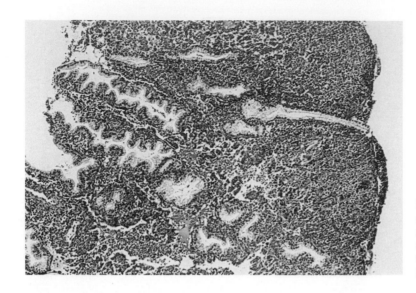

Figure 2.17 Menstrual endometrium. Fragments of superficial endometrium as they appear shed in a curettage sample taken on the first day of bleeding. Haematoxylin and eosin.

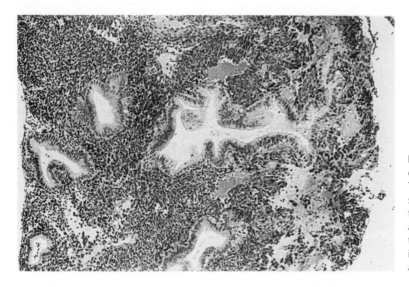

Figure 2.18 Menstrual endometrium, day 4 of the cycle. The compacta and underlying spongy layer have been shed and the uterus is lined only by basal and residual secretory endometrium: the ragged endometrial surface is seen to the right. Haematoxylin and eosin.

atrophy' and it is not unusual for the cystic areas to become somewhat polypoidal. The cystic dilatation of the atrophic glands is probably a result of blockage of the gland necks by fibrous tissue. This appearance has previously often been classed as a form of postmenopausal hyperplasia but the atrophic, inactive appearance convincingly negates any concept of a proliferative process. It is also of note that the incidence of cystic change in the endometrium is highest in women who are many years past their menopause and least in those whose menopause was relatively recent: this clearly indicates that senile cystic atrophy is not, as has frequently been

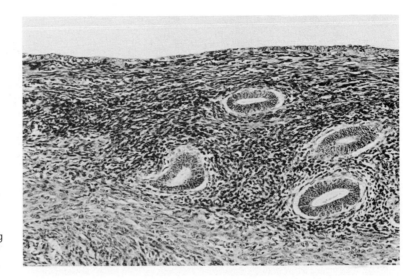

Figure 2.19 Postmenopausal endometrium. The uterus is lined by a shallow endometrium with compact stroma and scanty, tubular glands lined by epithelium exhibiting mild stratification and having scanty cytoplasm. Haematoxylin and eosin.

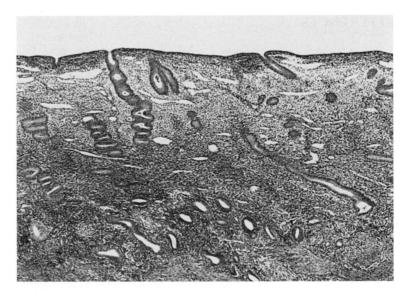

Figure 2.20 Postmenopausal endometrium. The uterus is lined by an inactive endometrium but a shallow, relatively translucent, functional layer is seen. Note the irregularity of the endometrial–myometrial junction and the blending of the basal and functional layers. Haematoxylin and eosin.

claimed, a residuum of a regressed perimenopausal endometrial hyperplasia.

If, following the menopause, reduction of oestrogen occurs to a lesser degree, or more slowly, the endometrial glands may be lined by a mildly pseudostratified columnar epithelium in which mitoses may be seen for some time (up to 2 years) after the clinical menopause (Fig. 2.20). A shallow layer of functionalis can also be seen as a very thin, superficial layer of less densely cellular stroma in which straight tubular glands are seen: mitoses are not seen in the stroma.

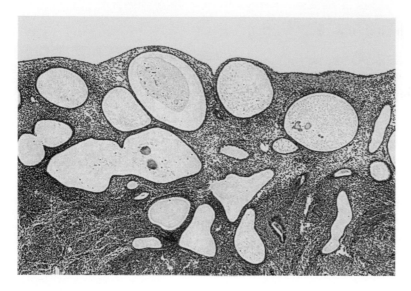

Figure 2.21 Postmenopausal endometrium, senile cystic change. The endometrium is shallow and the stroma compact but the glands, even those in the basalis, are cystically dilated. Haematoxylin and eosin.

REFERENCES

Bulmer, J.N., Hollings, D., Ritson, A. (1987) Immuno-cytochemical evidence that endometrial stromal granulocytes are granulated lymphocytes. *J. Pathol.* **155**, 281–7.

Hendrickson, M.R., Kempson, R.L. (1980) *Surgical Pathology of the Uterine Corpus*. Philadelphia, London, Toronto: W.B. Saunders.

Noyes, R.N., Hertig, A.T., Rock, J. (1950) Dating the endometrial biopsy. *Fertil. Steril.* **1**, 3–11.

Williams, P.L., Warwick, R. (eds) (1980), *Gray's Anatomy*, 36th Edn. Edinburgh: Churchill Livingstone, **798**, 1428–31.

3   The normal endometrium, as seen in biopsy material

Endometrial samples from normal women in the reproductive years vary in their content according to the mode of sampling and, often, according to the purpose for which they are intended. The size and adequacy of the sample, therefore, depends not so much upon the quantity of endometrium present in the corpus as on clinical practices and we would regard it as unwise to draw any conclusions about endometrial volume from a biopsy specimen.

The quality of the sample will also vary according to the type of fixative used and the time interval between removal of the specimen and placing it in fixative (see Chapter 1). These are factors over which the pathologist may have limited control but which must, of necessity, be taken into account when interpreting endometrial biopsies.

The tissues in an endometrial biopsy are rarely ideally orientated, and each individual component must be recognized and its significance evaluated if false conclusions about the variability of the endometrial appearance and maturation are to be avoided.

It is usual to find both functional and basal endometrium in curettage samples (Fig. 3.1) while, in some cases, particularly after a miscarriage or post-partum, when the tissues are soft, myometrium may be encountered (Fig. 3.2): fragments of endocervical and ectocervical tissue are also commonly present (Fig. 3.3). In biopsies that have been taken from infertile patients, simply in order to assess the quality of secretory change and exclude overt disease, it is usual to expect only functionalis, and aspiration samples are usually small and fragmented, even to the extent that epithelial and stromal fragments lie separately (Fig. 1.1).

3.1   THE ISTHMUS

Isthmic tissue may be included intentionally in the biopsy as part of a single endometrial strip taken to sample the entire endometrium from the fundus to the isthmus. In these cases,

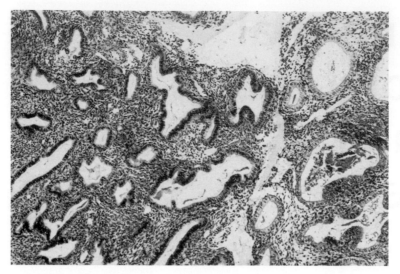

Figure 3.1 Basal and functional endometrium as they appear in a curettage sample. To the left, the basal glands are somewhat irregular, lined by a darkly staining, inactive columnar epithelium and set in a compact cellular stroma. On the right, the functional glands are in transition from early to mid-secretory phase; they are rather dilated and the stroma is less compact. Haematoxylin and eosin.

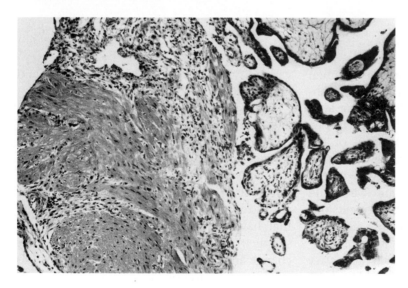

Figure 3.2 Myometrium in a curettage specimen: smooth muscle and basal endometrium lie to the left and placental villi to the right: from a patient who has suffered a miscarriage. Haematoxylin and eosin.

isthmic tissue is clearly recognizable, as the transition from endometrium to isthmus is easy to identify (Fig. 3.4). Isthmic tissue may also be intermingled with fragments from the corpus or cervix and care must be taken to recognize these lest they convey the wrong impression to the pathologist (Fig. 3.5).

Tissue from the isthmus differs from that in the corpus in so far as the stroma contains a higher proportion of fibrous tissue while glands with characteristics of both the corpus and endocervix are seen. A well-taken and well-orientated sample should present no difficulties in recognition but, in practice, irregularly orientated material is most commonly seen. It is important to remember, particularly when isthmic tissue forms the major component of the sample, that the isthmic glands and stroma do not mirror

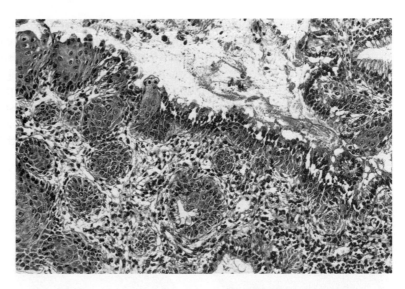

Figure 3.3 Endocervical tissue in which the surface and crypt epithelium has undergone squamous metaplasia, such fragments are common in endometrial curettings and usually come from the lower part of the endocervical canal. Care should be taken to distinguish the mucus-secreting epithelium of the cervix from the superficially similar secretory epithelium of the endometrium. Haematoxylin and eosin.

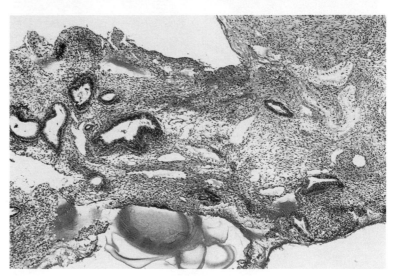

Figure 3.4 A strip of endometrium taken to include the isthmus: the upper end of the tissue, in which there are glands of endometrial type, lies to the left and endocervical crypts are seen on the right. Haematoxylin and eosin.

the hormonal-dependent changes in the uterine corpus and are thus unsuitable for determining the quality of such changes (Fig. 2.6).

3.2   BASAL ENDOMETRIUM

It is usual to see fragments of basal endometrium in curettage samples but not in the more superficial biopsies taken in the investigation of infertility or obtained by an aspiration technique. Basal tissues are easy to identify when they are orientated in their correct anatomical position in relation to the functionalis. However, difficulties are sometimes encountered when fragments of basalis are received mixed with functionalis, when basalis is cut in transverse section or when curettage has taken place shortly following an episode of bleeding, this having left basalis as the only endometrium available for sampling. In this last case, it is particularly important to recognize that the tissue is basalis or the pathologist may reach the erroneous conclusion that the endometrium is inactive.

The appearance of the basalis remains constant throughout the normal cycle. The stroma is densely cellular, the individual spindled cells having oval to elongated darkly staining nuclei, scanty cytoplasm and ill-defined cell borders. The glandular epithelium in the basalis is columnar: the cells appear tightly packed, have more scanty cytoplasm than in the functionalis and are orientated at right angles to the basement membrane of the gland, their nuclei being tall

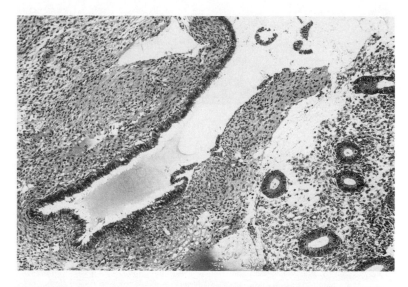

Figure 3.5 Isthmic tissue and proliferative endometrium as they appear, intermingled in a curettage sample. Haematoxylin and eosin.

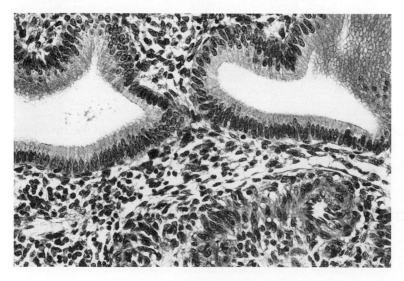

Figure 3.6 Basal endometrium. The glands are lined by a tall, columnar epithelium, which, in the reproductive years, has pale cytoplasm, parallel-sided, closely packed nuclei and low nucleo-cytoplasmic ratios. Contrast this with the cells lining the glands in the postmenopausal patient (Fig. 3.22). The thick-walled artery is typical of the basalis. Haematoxylin and eosin.

and strikingly parallel-sided (Fig. 3.6). Mitoses are not seen.

3.3 MENSTRUAL PHASE

Biopsies taken during menstruation are often difficult to interpret and provide very limited information. They are composed largely of blood in which collapsed, serrated glands, aggregates of stromal cells and small clusters of neutrophilic polymorphonuclear leucocytes are intermingled (Fig. 3.7). The normal morphology is lost after the first day of menstruation and, apart from confirming that the material came from a secretory endometrium and is thus actually menstrual and that bleeding is not the consequence of oestrogen withdrawal, the pathologist may be unable to supply any further information.

On the first day of the cycle (Fig. 3.8), in vertically orientated tissue, continuous segments of serrated, collapsed gland, including their orifices, lie in a haemorrhagic, fragmented stroma in which the stromal cells form densely cellular clusters and are admixed with neutrophil polymorphonuclear leucocytes. Aggregation of the stromal cells and interstitial haemorrhage, indicative of the onset of menstruation, is identifiable first in the spongy layer of the functionalis (Fig. 2.15), and it is at this level that the plane of cleavage will occur. The decidual appearance of the stromal cells, so characteristic of the late secretory phase, is lost as the stromal cells aggregate, although granulated lymphocytes are still apparent: spiral artery remnants also remain identifiable. The glandular epithelium is usually described as being exhausted but, in practice, even at this stage the epithelium in some glands, particularly around the margin of the sample, where fixation occurs most rapidly, remains vacuolated and of secretory appearance (Fig. 3.9). In horizontally orientated material stellate glandular remnants are seen in a fragmented stroma.

By the second to third day of the cycle, little or no stromal tissue may remain and the glands, which appear more resistant to dissolution than does the stroma, become closely packed (Fig. 3.7) and are seen in the biopsy

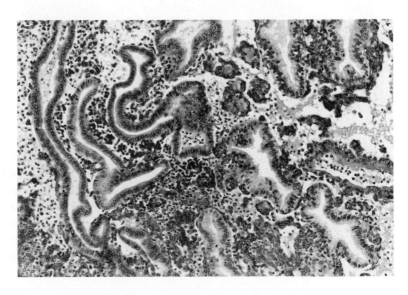

Figure 3.7 Menstrual endometrium, day 2 of the cycle. The sample often consists of no more than isolated glandular elements intermingled with stromal cell aggregates and blood clot. Secretory activity can usually still be identified in the glandular epithelium, confirming that this is in fact menstrual and not oestrogen or therapeutic hormone withdrawal bleeding (see Fig. 5.17). Haematoxylin and eosin.

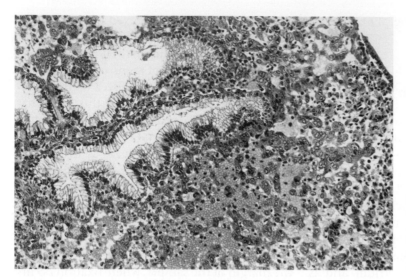

Figure 3.8 Menstrual endometrium, day 1 of the cycle. Secretory glands are set in a haemorrhagic stroma in which the cells have undergone aggregation. Haematoxylin and eosin.

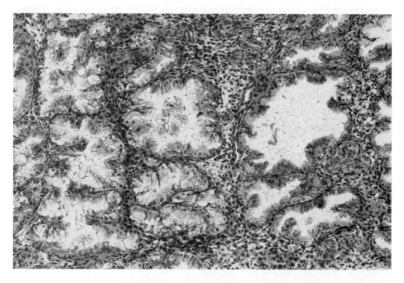

Figure 3.9 Menstrual endometrium, first day of the cycle. The cells lining the glands to the left of the tissue are large, have prominent round nuclei and more copious cytoplasm than in the glands to the right. This 'pseudo-hypersecretory' appearance is a fixation artefact. The glands showing this phenomenon lie closer to the surface of the tissue and therefore become fixed more rapidly. Haematoxylin and eosin.

in a virtually back-to-back pattern. They may therefore bear a superficial resemblance to a hyperplastic endometrium or even to an adenocarcinoma: careful attention to the cytological details should, however, clarify the position.

By the third to fourth day of the cycle, towards the end of the menstrual phase, the functionalis has been largely lost and only tiny dense basophilic cellular aggregates of indeterminate type remain (Fig. 3.10). A biopsy taken at this stage now often contains basal endometrium and the adjacent residual functionalis in which there are the remnants of secretory glands (Fig. 2.18). The surface is ragged and fragmented and there is no

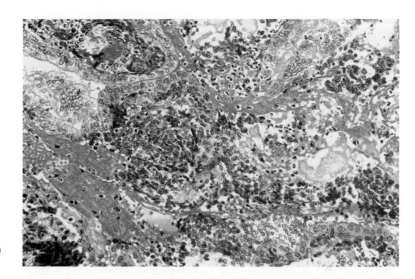

Figure 3.10 Menstrual endometrium, day 3 of the cycle. The sample consists only of blood clot containing stromal cellular aggregates, isolated epithelial fragments and blood. Haematoxylin and eosin.

epithelial covering but healing of the surface epithelium, from the glandular epithelium, is apparent by the third to fourth day (Fig. 2.7). This process appears to be independent of hormonal stimulation and therefore mitoses are often seen here, even when they are absent in the deeper parts of the glands: no abnormal mitoses occur but the epithelial cells often show a minor degree of reactive cytological atypia during healing.

3.4 PROLIFERATIVE (FOLLICULAR) PHASE

It is impossible to date precisely the endometrium in the proliferative phase but in an adequate sample some idea of the duration and adequacy of the phase can be gained from the depth of the functional layer, the degree of glandular development and tortuosity and the number of stromal and epithelial mitoses.

In the early part of the proliferative phase (days 5–7), the glands are straight, narrow (Fig. 2.1) and round in cross-section (Fig. 3.11). Their moderately basophilic epithelium is cubo-columnar with oval or rounded nuclei in which the chromatin is evenly dispersed; there is a minor degree of epithelial stratification. Occasional mitoses are seen in the glandular epithelium and are identified most easily, at this stage, in that part of the glands lying in the junctional zone between the basalis and functionalis: they may therefore be scanty in a superficial biopsy. The stromal cells show mitotic activity and are oval to elongated with scanty cytoplasm and ill-defined cell borders; the delicate, translucent appearance of the newly grown functional stroma is in sharp contrast to the darkly staining dense appearance of the underlying basalis. Scanty thin-walled blood vessels are present and the fibrous endometrial skeleton is identifiable.

Proliferative activity reaches its maximum between the 8th and 10th day of the cycle and by then the glandular epithelium is taller, stratification of the epithelium is more obvious and mitotic figures are frequently seen in both the glands and stroma (Fig. 3.12). Transient stromal oedema is common and capillaries are numerous, although arteries and arterioles are inconspicuous.

33

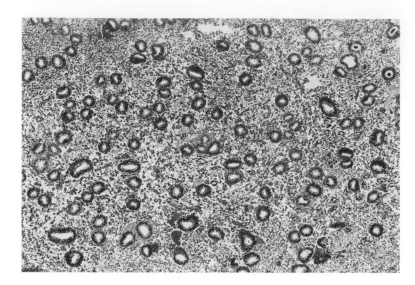

Figure 3.11 Proliferative phase endometrium. A transverse section through the narrow, tubular glands emphasizes their uniformity of shape and distribution. Haematoxylin and eosin.

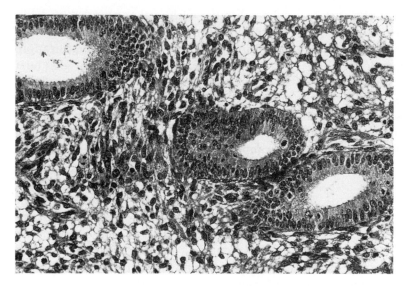

Figure 3.12 Mid-proliferative phase endometrium, 9th to 10th day of the cycle. Glandular epithelium is pseudostratified and the nuclei oval or elongated: stromal cells are immature and cell membranes and cytoplasm ill defined: mitoses are visible in both the glandular and stromal cells. Haematoxylin and eosin.

In the late proliferative phase (days 11–14), glandular growth outstrips that of the stroma and, consequently, the glands become rather tortuous. They therefore appear, in section, as more variable in size and shape (Fig. 2.8) but it is helpful to remember that their walls remain parallel no matter how oblique the plane of section. The glandular epithelium remains stratified but mitoses decline in number in both the glands and stroma.

3.5 SECRETORY PHASE

In contrast to the proliferative phase, the appearance of the endometrium in the secretory

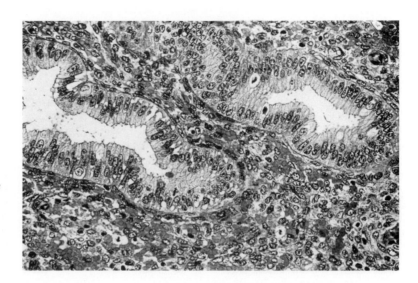

Figure 3.13 Endometrium in transition from proliferative to early secretory phase, second post-ovulatory day. The glands retain the tubular form and pseudostratified epithelium characteristic of the proliferative phase but scanty subnuclear vacuoles are present in the glandular epithelium. Haematoxylin and eosin.

phase can be related precisely to the day of the cycle and as the investigation of infertility becomes more sophisticated, with parallel sequential hormone measurements, it is useful to advise the gynaecologist of the number of days since ovulation when reporting a secretory phase endometrium.

3.5.1 Early and mid-secretory phase

Following ovulation, there may be no change in the appearance of the endometrium for between 24 h and 36 h, but at the end of that time vacuoles appear in the subnuclear cytoplasm of the glandular epithelium (Fig. 3.13). In the first 12 h these are somewhat irregularly dispersed, being most marked in the parts of the glands in the mid zone of the endometrium and least obvious in the superficial part, and occurring in some but not all the cells in a particular gland: the presence of the vacuoles appears to exaggerate the stratification of the nuclei. Not until the vacuoles are evenly distributed in at least 50 per cent of the glands can one be certain that ovulation has occurred (early secretory phase). At this stage, mitoses are still common in the glandular epithelium; in fact, they will be identified in

small numbers until day 17 (Fig. 3.14). Gland profiles remain similar to those of the proliferative phase until day 18, when subnuclear vacuoles reach their peak (Fig. 3.15) but, with the movement of the vacuolar contents from the subnuclear cytoplasm to the supranuclear cytoplasm and then into the glandular lumina, there is a progressive distension of the glands. This distension reaches a peak on days 21–22 (8th to 9th post-ovulatory day), i.e. during the mid-secretory phase, and creates the typical geometric shape of the mid-secretory gland (Fig. 3.16), which develops as secretions distend a gland tethered by the supporting stroma. As secretion of cell contents occurs, the nuclei return to a basal position in the cells and careful examination of the cell tips reveals a shaggy appearance. Secretion is usually uniform throughout the specimen but the glands tend to be a little narrower and less actively secretory in the superficial functionalis – the part that will eventually develop into the compacta of the late secretory phase (Fig. 3.17). Biopsies that include only this part of the endometrium may therefore give a false impression of poorly developed, narrow, weakly secretory glands.

35

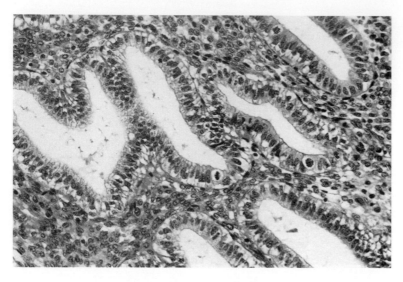

Figure 3.14 Early secretory endometrium, 3rd post-ovulatory day. Although mitoses are still present in the glandular epithelium, subnuclear vacuoles are now uniformly distributed: contrast this with Fig. 3.13. Haematoxylin and eosin.

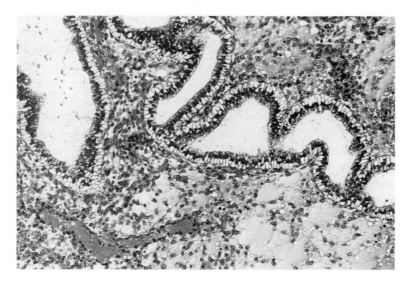

Figure 3.15 Early secretory phase endometrium, 4th post-ovulatory day. Subnuclear vacuolation of the glandular epithelium is uniform and at its peak; stromal oedema is present. Haematoxylin and eosin.

The stroma of the early secretory phase (1st to 5th post-ovulatory day), differs very little from that typical of the follicular phase but towards the end of the early secretory phase there is a progressive accumulation of oedema fluid in the stroma. This accumulation reaches a peak in the mid-secretory phase on days 22–23 of the cycle (8th to 9th post-ovulatory day) (Fig. 2.11). Stromal oedema is maximal in the spongy layer, in the mid-zone of the endometrium, and this will persist, to some extent, into the late secretory phase. The amount of oedema fluid apparent in paraffin-processed material depends upon the fixative (see Chapter 1) and it is important that one should become familiar with the normal

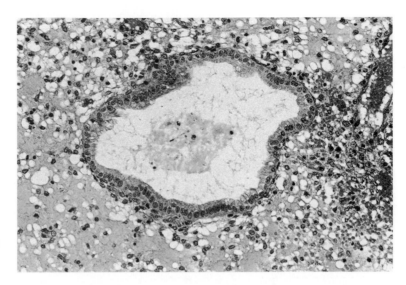

Figure 3.16 Mid-secretory endometrium, 8th post-ovulatory day. The gland is rather angular in outline, distended and contains a trace of secretion. The glandular epithelium is tall, the regular oval nuclei have returned to the base of the cells and the surrounding stroma is markedly oedematous. Haematoxylin and eosin.

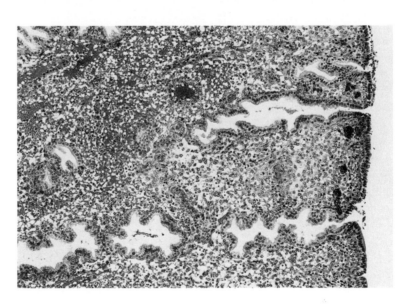

Figure 3.17 Late secretory endometrium, 12th post-ovulatory day. The superficial segments of the glands, as they pass through the compacta, are rather narrow and a biopsy in which the tissue is orientated so that the plane of section passes through these narrower segments may give a false impression that glandular development is inadequate. Haematoxylin and eosin.

appearances that occur using the different fixatives because these appearances are so variable.

3.5.2 The late secretory phase

In the late secretory phase, glandular secretion is exhausted, the glands collapse, their lumina become narrow, particularly in the most superficial part of the gland (Fig. 3.17), and their contour becomes saw-toothed (Fig. 2.15). Associated with the reduction in endometrial height, which results from the regression of stromal oedema, the glands become plicated (Fig. 3.18).

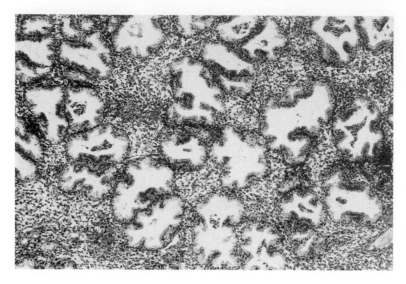

Figure 3.18 Late secretory phase endometrium, 13th post-ovulatory day. Loss of oedema in the spongy layer has resulted in close packing of the glands, which are now well past the secretory peak and have become irregular and rather serrated. Haematoxylin and eosin.

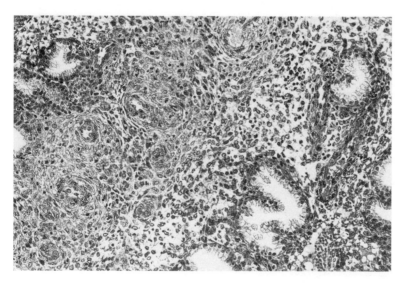

Figure 3.19 Late secretory endometrium, 13th post-ovulatory day. The spiral artery, to the left is well muscularized and surrounded by a cuff of pre-decidualized stromal cells with regular, round nuclei, copious cytoplasm and well-defined cell margins. Haematoxylin and eosin.

Spiral artery growth occurs throughout the proliferative phase but maturation of the muscular layer only becomes evident at the end of the mid-secretory phase on day 22 (8th post-ovulatory day). Stromal predecidualization occurs first in the mid-zone of the endometrium, around the spiral arteries, on day 23 (9th post-ovulatory day): it increases rapidly over the next 2 days, appearing in the infraluminal stroma on day 25. By the end of the cycle a distinct, superficial, compact layer has formed and bands of decidua traverse the spongy layer along the course of the spiral arteries (Fig. 3.19).

Mitoses reappear in the stroma by day 26 or 27 (Fig. 3.20) and are a reflection of the

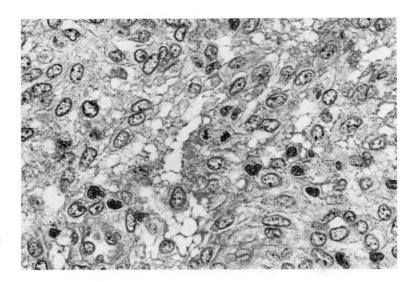

Figure 3.20 Late secretory endometrium, 13th to 14th post-ovulatory day. Within the compacta there is a sparse infiltrate of darkly staining granulated lymphocytes and a mitosis is seen in a stromal cell. Haematoxylin and eosin.

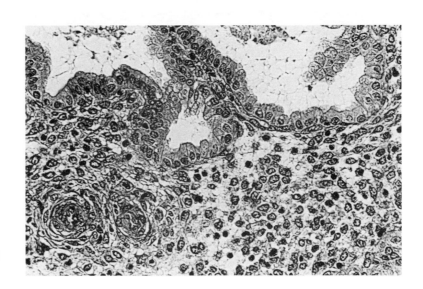

Figure 3.21 Late secretory endometrium, 13th to 14th post-ovulatory day. A scattering of granulated lymphocytes is present in the stroma and two, well-muscularized spiral arteries are seen on the left. Haematoxylin and eosin.

decrease in progestagenic activity, which marks a minor recrudescence of an oestrogenic effect. Granulated lymphocytes appear on days 27 and 28 (Fig. 3.21) and a scattering of neutrophil polymorphs infiltrates the superficial stroma in the immediate premenstrual phase.

3.6 POSTMENOPAUSAL ENDOMETRIUM

In the postmenopausal woman, the endometrium is shallow and endometrial biopsy samples are therefore often scanty, if not actually inadequate. Frequently, the material

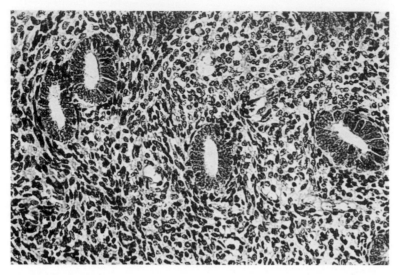

Figure 3.22 Postmenopausal endometrium; the last menstrual period had occurred 10 months previously. The stroma is composed of closely packed cells with scanty cytoplasm: the glands are narrow, tubular and lined by a single layer of cubo-columnar cells with very little cytoplasm. Contrast this with the appearance of the basal glands in the reproductive years (Fig. 3.6). Haematoxylin and eosin.

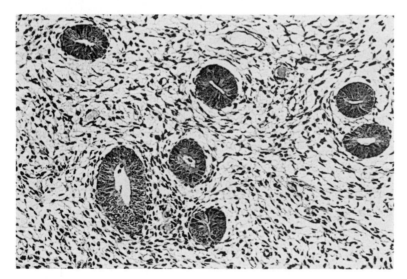

Figure 3.23 Weakly proliferative, postmenopausal endometrium. The glandular epithelium is mildly stratified and the stroma less compact than in the sample shown in Fig. 3.22. Haematoxylin and eosin.

consists only of isolated fragments of inactive, cubo-columnar epithelium of indeterminate type and fragments of fibrous stroma. In these circumstances it may be possible to tell the gynaecologist only that there is no evidence of neoplasm or proliferative activity but quite impossible to comment upon any other characteristics of the tissue.

In a more adequate sample, narrow tubular glands, lined by cuboidal epithelium showing neither secretory nor proliferative activity (Fig. 3.22), are set in a compact cellular stroma. The epithelium may remain tall and, on occasions, mildly pseudostratified (Fig. 3.23) and a shallow functionalis may persist for many years after the menopause. This is indicative of the

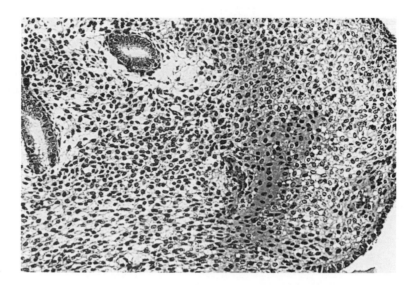

Figure 3.24 Postmenopausal endometrium in which continued, low-level oestrogen stimulation has resulted in the formation of a shallow functionalis recognized by the less compact stroma and the resemblance of the cells to those seen in the proliferative phase (Fig. 3.12). Haematoxylin and eosin.

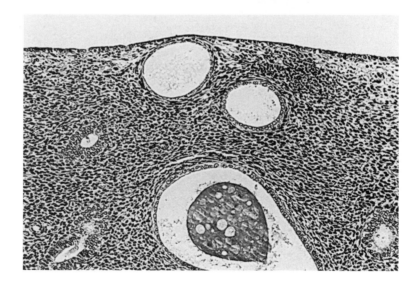

Figure 3.25 Postmenopausal endometrium, senile cystic atrophy. The cystically dilated glands are lined by a single layer of inactive, flattened cubo-columnar cells: compare this with the tall, stratified columnar epithelium lining the glands in simple hyperplasia (Figs 9.1 and 9.2). Haematoxylin and eosin.

presence of persistent very low levels of oestrogen of either endogenous or exogenous origin, e.g. from topical oestrogens used to treat vaginal atrophy (Fig. 3.24). Glandular mitoses are also sometimes encountered in patients in whom there is no proven source of oestrogenic stimulation but in whom there is a genital prolapse. More commonly, the picture of very weak proliferative activity is seen in women that have experienced postmenopausal bleeding in the years immediately following the menopause or in women in whom the menopause appears to be occurring gradually over a period of years.

Many years after the menopause, the stroma may become fibrous and this is a particularly conspicuous feature in women developing senile cystic atrophy (Fig. 3.25). The glands vary in size: some are narrow and tubular but many are dilated and cystic. The glandular epithelium is inactive and cuboidal but in the most widely dilated glands, it may be flattened and of indeterminate type. Such endometrium has a tendency to become polypoidal and this may be apparent in the biopsy.

It is also noticeable that in the post-menopausal phase there may be an increase in the number of lymphocytes and the number of lymphoid aggregates; these features appear to occur without evidence of overt infection. The development of lymphoid follicles with germinal centres, however, is normally regarded as indicating the development of infection.

4 Functional disorders of the endometrium

Those abnormalities of endometrial development and maturation which are secondary to ovarian dysfunction, are usually referred to as functional disorders. This term encompasses endometrial abnormalities caused by a paucity of oestrogen, an excess of oestrogen, an abnormality of progesterone secretion following ovulation or an abnormality in the relative proportions of oestrogen and progesterone.

4.1 ENDOMETRIAL ATROPHY AND LOW OR ABSENT OESTROGEN STATES

An atrophic endometrium and low oestrogen state is typical of the normal premenarchal child and of the postmenopausal woman (see Chapter 3) but occurs under pathological conditions in the absence of normal ovarian follicular development, following irradiation damage to the ovaries and in primary and secondary ovarian failure. Endometrial atrophy is therefore encountered in women with a wide range of abnormalities, some of which may be ovarian (e.g. 17-hydroxylase deficiency, gonadotrophin-resistant ovary syndrome and premature menopause), while others lie in the hypothalamic pituitary axis (e.g. hypopituitary states and hyperprolactinaemia).

Patients with abnormally low oestrogen levels may present with delayed puberty, delayed menarche, primary amenorrhoea, oligomenorrhoea or infertility, the clinical picture depending upon the patient's age and the severity of the abnormality. The appearance of the endometrium is, however, similar in all instances whatever the nature of the primary abnormality as it simply reflects the inadequacy of oestrogenic stimulation. A similar picture is seen in those uncommon patients whose ovulatory function is normal but in whom the endometrium is refractory to hormonal stimulation (Dallenbach-Hellweg, 1987).

The degree of endometrial atrophy varies, but in cases of the most profound oestrogen deficiency it is complete, the uterus being lined only by endometrium of basal type (Fig. 2.19): there is no functionalis and biopsy samples tend to be scanty and rather difficult to obtain. Biopsy of the endometrium reveals an inactive picture (Fig. 3.22). The stroma is composed of closely packed, spindle-shaped cells and appears densely cellular. The glands, which are usually sparse, simple and tubular, are lined by an inactive, cuboidal or cubo-columnar epithelium with scanty cytoplasm and densely staining nuclei. In women in whom oestrogen levels are lower than the physiological range but are, nevertheless, sufficient to induce a minimum of growth, there can be a minor degree of glandular epithelial stratification, occasional mitoses may be seen and a thin functionalis can form (Fig. 4.1).

In patients with inadequate, rather than absent, follicular function, a paucity of oestrogen in the follicular phase may lead to prolongation of the proliferative phase without the development of a hyperplastic endometrium. In such patients, biopsy may reveal a morphologically normal endometrium that is delayed relative to the apparent day of the cycle, or a weakly proliferative endometrium. Some patients in this category will, in due course, if oestrogen secretion is not opposed by a progestagen, develop a mild glandular architectural atypia, the so-called 'disordered proliferative endometrium' (see Chapter 5). Inadequate oestrogen secretion is also a factor in the development of luteal phase insufficiency (see below).

4.2 ANOVULATORY CYCLES AND HYPEROESTROGENIC STATES

The term 'hyperoestrogenic state' implies that the endometrium is being subjected to unopposed oestrogenic stimulation. Oestrogen levels are therefore not necessarily elevated, since normal levels of oestrogen, the action of which is not opposed or interrupted by progesterone, can produce a hyperoestrogenic state, as is the case, for example, in women having anovulatory cycles. A genuine hyperoestrogenic state with abnormally high oestrogen levels is rather uncommon but is seen, for example, in women with the polycystic ovary syndrome or with granulosa cell tumours of the ovary. It is the case that true hyperoestrogenism of this type will, by disturbing the hypothalamic feedback mechanism, also result in anovulatory cycles.

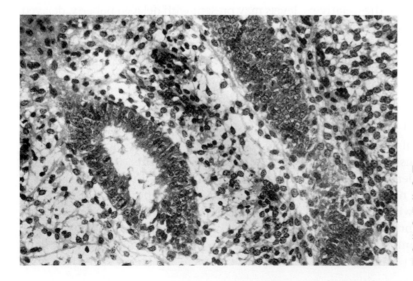

Figure 4.1 Weakly proliferative endometrium in a low oestrogen state. The glands are lined by a mildly stratified epithelium in which occasional mitoses are seen: the stroma is immature. Only scanty curettage material was received. Haematoxylin and eosin.

Clinically, the patient may have oligomenorrhoea, amenorrhoea, and infrequent heavy vaginal bleeding interspersed with episodes of scanty vaginal loss, infertility or any combination or permutations of these.

Persistent or prolonged stimulation of the endometrium by oestrogens, uninterrupted by progestagenic activity, results ultimately in the development of an endometrial hyperplasia of simple or atypical form. The appearances are similar whatever the source of the oestrogen and are fully described in Chapter 7. In some patients, however, the changes are insufficient to warrant a diagnosis of hyperplasia but are recognizable as those of a prolonged proliferative phase (Figs 4.2 and 4.3). Mitotic activity

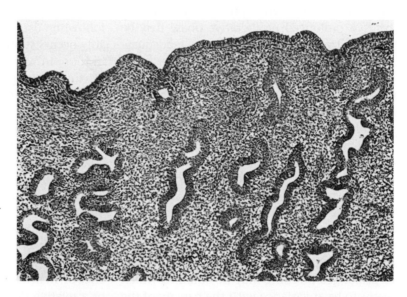

Figure 4.2 Prolonged proliferative phase endometrium. The patient menstruated only every 45–50 days: the last menstrual period had occurred 34 days previously. The endometrial glands are not dissimilar from those seen in the normal late proliferative phase but are slightly more tortuous. There is no evidence of hyperplasia. Haematoxylin and eosin.

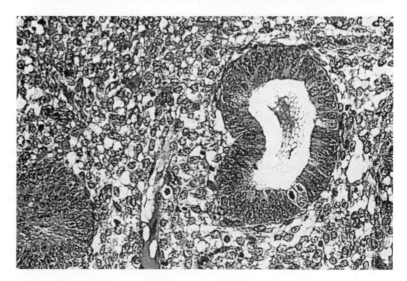

Figure 4.3 Prolonged proliferative phase endometrium. There is mild stratification of the glandular epithelium: mitoses are present in both glands and stroma. Haematoxylin and eosin.

45

continues beyond day 14 of the cycle, glandular epithelial stratification persists, a minor degree of variation in glandular size is seen, without gross cystic dilatation, a little, focal glandular crowding may be present and the stroma remains immature and cellular. These features occur in women in whom there is a failure or delay of ovulation in the current cycle, for example owing to a persistent, unruptured follicle, or in whom there has been a previous anovulatory cycle. A prolonged proliferative phase may be followed by either a normal or an inadequate luteal phase (see below).

4.2.1 Oestrogen withdrawal bleeding

Bleeding from an endometrium subjected only to oestrogenic stimulation (oestrogen withdrawal bleeding), can be recognized in endometrial biopsies. In hypo-oestrogenic states, curetting typically yields a scanty sample in which inactive glands showing no evidence of secretory activity are admixed with fragments of both crumbling and intact haemorrhagic endometrium. A history of surprisingly severe or prolonged bleeding may be obtained which seems to be at variance with the paucity of the sample. There is frequently a scanty to moderately heavy endometrial stromal infiltrate of lymphocytes, macrophages (some of which may contain haemosiderin) and plasma cells; this feature is seen particularly in women who have had repeated or prolonged bleeding.

Bleeding after, or during, a hyperoestrogenic state is characteristically irregular. The endometrium is bulky and biopsy usually yields pieces of relatively well-preserved endometrium in which areas showing focal interstitial haemorrhage and stromal disintegration are interspersed with intact proliferative or inactive endometrium showing little or no evidence of interstitial haemorrhage. A scattering of polymorphonuclear leucocytes is commonly found in the areas of stromal disintegration (Fig. 9.3).

4.3 LUTEAL PHASE INSUFFICIENCY

The terms 'luteal phase insufficiency' and 'secretory insufficiency or inadequacy' are used to describe a state characterized by a relative or absolute abnormality in progesterone secretion following ovulation. This abnormality probably occurs sporadically in normal women but in those in whom it is thought to be the cause of clinical symptoms, the diagnosis should be confirmed by repeated biopsies over several cycles.

An inadequate luteal phase can be preceded by a normal, short or inadequate follicular phase. Following ovulation, there may be a delay in progesterone secretion, a general paucity of progesterone secretion with a failure to reach physiological levels, a gradual rather than rapid rise in progesterone secretion, a premature decline in progesterone levels towards the end of the phase (short secretory phase), abnormal persistence of an active corpus luteum beyond 14 days or a relative deficiency of progesterone associated with hyperoestrogenism. The condition is most accurately expressed in terms of the hormonal abnormality but a number of morphological features may alert the histopathologist to this diagnosis.

Patients with luteal phase insufficiency may have apparently normal menstrual cycles, but many complain of premenstrual spotting, a blood-stained vaginal discharge for several days prior to the onset of menstruation, intermenstrual bleeding, irregular cycles, prolonged, though not necessarily heavy, periods or infertility. The histopathological features do not always correlate directly with either the hormone levels or the clinical abnormality, although some pictures are sufficiently specific as to suggest the nature of the underlying hormonal abnormality. Others simply allow the pathologist to suggest the possible nature of the underlying problem. The biopsies vary greatly in appearance and several patterns are recognizable.

4.3.1 Coordinated delayed endometrial transformation

In its simplest form, the endometrium is of normal morphology but shows a coordinated delay in glandular and stromal maturation relative to the day of ovulation. Such a picture may occur when progesterone secretion following ovulation is delayed, or the rise in progesterone levels is slow or inadequate. In such cases, it may be impossible to recognize the abnormality unless the gynaecologist has given the date of ovulation (Fig. 4.4). In other cases, however, if the inadequate luteal phase follows a prolonged follicular phase, the endometrium may show secretory changes superimposed upon an endometrium that exhibits features of a prolonged follicular phase (see above), an underlying simple hyperplasia or, less commonly, an atypical hyperplasia. Biopsies of this type may be seen in patients with an apparently normal menstrual cycle but the biopsy may show not only delay in maturation but frequently also premature breakdown (see below).

4.3.2 Generally inadequate secretory phase, glandular stromal asynchrony and irregular ripening

In patients with luteal phase insufficiency preceded by, or associated with, oestrogen deficiency the endometrium is poorly grown and shallow and the biopsy may be scanty and include basal endometrium or myometrium (de Brux, 1981a). The glands are sparse, straight, narrow and undistended, even 8 or 9 days after ovulation, and secretion in the glandular lumina is scanty (Fig. 4.5). The glandular cell nuclei tend to be elongated and hyperchromatic and morphometric analysis of the nuclei shows that they are different in shape from those seen at any time during the normal menstrual cycle and from basal endometrium. Nuclear expression of oestrogen and progesterone receptors in formalin-fixed and paraffin-embedded sections is also reduced. The stroma

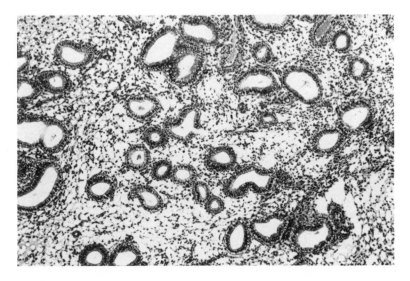

Figure 4.4 Luteal phase insufficiency, 8th post-ovulatory day. Subnuclear vacuoles are still present in the epithelium of the majority of glands and the stroma is immature, an appearance corresponding approximately to the 3rd post-ovulatory day: little glandular dilatation has occurred. Occasional less-mature glands are also seen, indicating a minor degree of irregular ripening. Haematoxylin and eosin.

47

is poorly developed; in particular, spiral arteries are few in number and inadequately developed (Thornburgh and Anderson, 1997).

When the preceding oestrogen levels have been normal, luteal insufficiency may be characterized by a generally poor, delayed glandular secretory transformation (Fig. 4.6) with narrow, straight or only mildly convoluted glands undistended by, or containing only a little, secretion or by glands showing variation in maturation. In the latter case, sometimes also called irregular ripening, glands exhibiting weak secretion, normal secretion for the stage of the cycle, inactivity and even proliferative activity may coexist (Figs 4.7 and 4.8). In a hysterectomy specimen, it is possible, in some

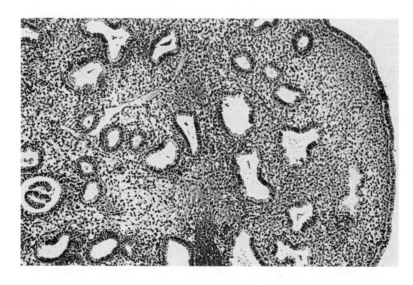

Figure 4.5 Luteal phase insufficiency. The endometrium is poorly grown, most glands are narrow and are devoid of secretion: occasional glands appear to have developed weak secretory activity: spiral artery maturation is absent. Haematoxylin and eosin.

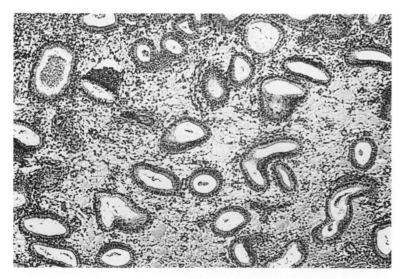

Figure 4.6 Luteal phase insufficiency, day 26 of a 28-day cycle. The endometrial glands are narrow with parallel sides similar to those seen in the proliferative phase (see Fig. 2.8). There is evidence of secretion in occasional glands but the general morphology contrasts sharply with that seen in Fig. 3.18 which was taken only 24 h later in a normal cycle. Haematoxylin and eosin.

cases, to see that the most mature glands lie in proximity to the spiral arteries, while the least well developed glands lie at the greatest distance from these vessels (Fig. 4.9). This phenomenon is, however, rarely apparent in a biopsy. The stroma may be relatively more oedematous than in the normal cycle and the stromal cells, which depend upon progesterone for their maturation to predecidual cells, may be immature (Fig. 4.10). Spiral arteries, which also depend upon progesterone for their differentiation, are few in number and poorly differentiated (Fig. 4.11).

Luteal phase insufficiency with oestrogen predominance is common. The endometrium is thick and well grown and samples therefore ample. The stroma remains cellular and rich in

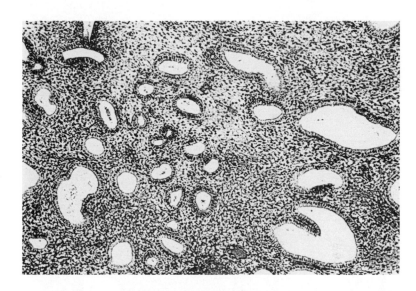

Figure 4.7 Luteal phase insufficiency, irregular ripening, day 22 to 23 of a 28-day cycle. There is a marked difference between the small, unresponsive glands in the centre of the field and the surrounding glands, which show moderate secretory activity. Haematoxylin and eosin.

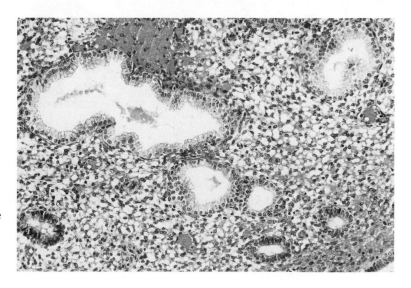

Figure 4.8 Luteal phase insufficiency, irregular ripening. This is a sample from a woman of 35 years who complained of almost continuous irregular spotting. There is a marked discrepancy between the maturation of the weakly secretory gland above and the small inactive glands below. Haematoxylin and eosin.

49

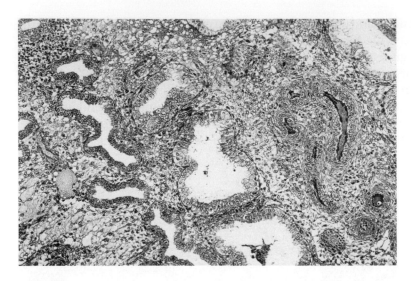

Figure 4.9 Luteal phase insufficiency, irregular ripening. The glands exhibiting the most adequate secretory transformation lie adjacent to the spiral artery. Haematoxylin and eosin.

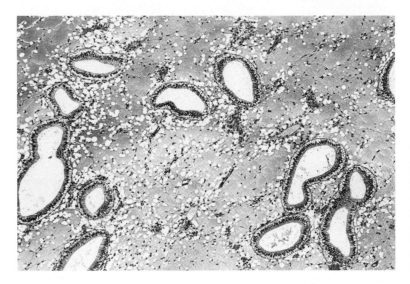

Figure 4.10 Luteal phase insufficiency, delayed secretory transformation, day 21 of a 27–28-day cycle. The glands are consistent in appearance with the 3rd post-ovulatory day and appear uniformly secretory. The stroma is immature and excessively oedematous for day 21 of the cycle. Haematoxylin and eosin.

fibroblasts, though lacking in collagen even many days after ovulation. The glands are numerous, somewhat dilated and regular or slightly convoluted. Mitoses may persist in the glandular epithelium, which may be stratified, and glycogen secretion coexists as basal and apical vacuoles. Spiral arteries are thick-walled and well differentiated (Figs 4.12 and 4.13). The picture is that of delayed endometrial glandular maturation with a discrepancy between the stromal and glandular maturation.

In those endometria in which there is a discrepancy between the maturation of the glands and stroma, glandular secretion may

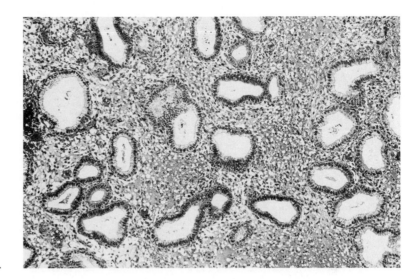

Figure 4.11 Luteal phase insufficiency, day 22 of a 28-day cycle. Glandular secretion is rather weak, spiral artery development is negligible and the stroma is immature. Haematoxylin and eosin.

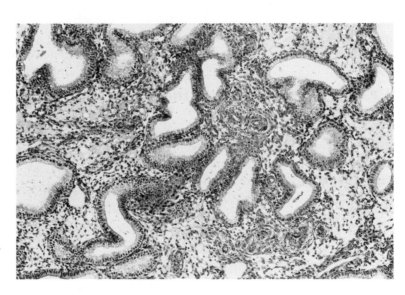

Figure 4.12 Luteal phase insufficiency, 23rd to 24th day of a 28-day cycle. Spiral arteries are well muscularized and surrounded by a cuff of decidual cells, which is consistent with the date of the cycle. In contrast, the glands are narrow and weakly secretory, approximately equivalent in activity to the 5th post-ovulatory day. Haematoxylin and eosin.

be uniformly weak, irregular or just delayed while stromal maturation, in terms of stromal decidualization and spiral artery differenti-ation, is in advance of the glandular matura-tion (Fig. 4.12). The discrepancy may vary from two to seven or more days and examination of the spiral arteries is the single most useful diagnostic clue in these cases. The reason for the usefulness of the spiral artery maturation in identifying the actual date of the cycle lies in the fact that spiral artery differentiation is exquisitely sensitive to progesterone and occurs in response to only a minute quantity of progesterone in the presence of only

51

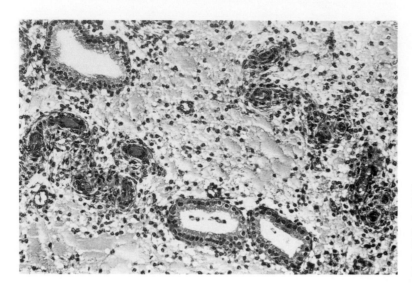

Figure 4.13 Luteal phase insufficiency, day 23 of a 28–29-day cycle. The spiral artery maturation corresponds to the day of the cycle but the glands are very narrow and only very weakly secretory. Haematoxylin and eosin.

moderate or even slight oestrogenic stimulation (de Brux, 1981b).

4.3.3 Premature failure of the corpus luteum

Premature failure of the corpus luteum leads to a short luteal phase and is sometimes encountered in patients complaining of premenstrual bleeding or spotting or of infertility. It is recognized in a biopsy by the finding of focal interstitial stromal haemorrhage and crumbling, indicative of tissue breakdown, in an endometrium that is either not fully mature or exhibits the features described above as characterizing luteal phase insufficiency. In the absence of stromal crumbling, stromal mitoses prior to the 12th post-ovulatory day, which indicate a return of oestrogen dominance, may indicate failure of the corpus luteum.

4.3.4 Delayed, prolonged or irregular shedding

In some patients, in whom there has been a premature decline in progesterone secretion,

shedding of the endometrium may not only commence early but also take longer than normal and may be associated with persistence of a functional corpus luteum. Such cases are recognized by the presence, in uterine curettings, of secretory endometrium several days after the onset of bleeding. The secretory endometrium in these cases may retain features of the luteal phase insufficiency, but if the endometrium had previously been of normal appearance this will also be apparent. In the latter case the sample most commonly consists of fragments of endometrium that have undergone regression and shrinkage rather than fragmentation and disintegration (Dallenbach-Hellweg and Bornebusch, 1970): these tend to have a rather fibrous stroma, sometimes infiltrated by a scattering of chronic inflammatory cells, and the glands have a stellate outline in transverse section (Fig. 4.14). A similar phenomenon is also encountered in patients having a spontaneous miscarriage and it is one of the common appearances observed in endometrium removed at curettage following a miscarriage (Fig. 4.15) (see Chapter 13).

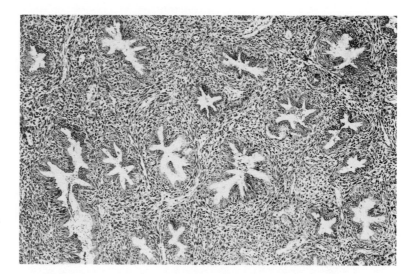

Figure 4.14 Delayed endometrial shedding. The stellate glands set in a fibrous stroma infiltrated by lymphocytes are typical of this state. This patient had been bleeding for 2 weeks at the time of the biopsy. Haematoxylin and eosin.

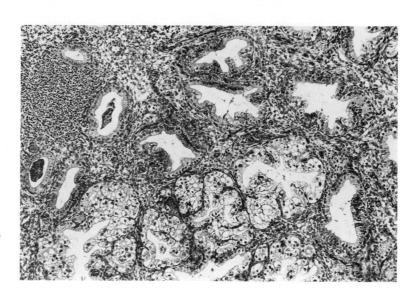

Figure 4.15 Delayed endometrial shedding. Glands exhibiting Arias-Stella change (lower part of the field) are visible in this curettage sample from a woman who had a spontaneous miscarriage 2 weeks earlier. Haematoxylin and eosin.

In certain women, in whom there is delayed or prolonged shedding, endometrial regrowth may occur before shedding is complete and, in these circumstances, curettage or biopsy material may contain a mixture of secretory endometrium showing the features of delayed shedding, menstrual type fragments and proliferative endometrium (Fig. 4.16).

4.3.5 Progesterone receptor defect

Occasionally, the endometrial appearance suggests luteal phase insufficiency yet hormonal secretion patterns are normal. It can be demonstrated that such endometria contain fewer high-affinity progesterone-binding sites in the cytosol fraction of the endometrium than

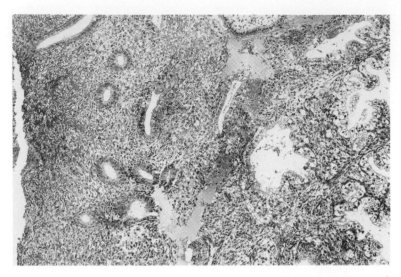

Figure 4.16 Delayed endometrial shedding. Both hypersecretory endometrium (to the right) and proliferative endometrium (to the left) are present in this curettage sample from a woman who had been bleeding for 12 days. It is likely that she had a spontaneous miscarriage. Haematoxylin and eosin.

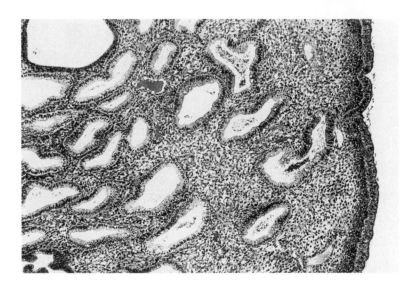

Figure 4.17 This is a biopsy from an infertile woman in whom luteal phase insufficiency had been reported in previous cycles. In view of the failure to develop an adequate secretory endometrium, norethisterone had been given in this cycle 8 days before the biopsy. Note the very poor response to the therapy. Haematoxylin and eosin.

normal (Fig. 4.17) (Cooke *et al.*, 1972; Keller *et al.*, 1979; Laatikainen *et al.*, 1983).

REFERENCES

Cooke, I.D., Morgan, C.A., Parry, T.E. (1972) Correlation of endometrial biopsy and plasma progesterone levels in infertile women. *J. Obstet. Gynaecol. Br. Cwlth.* **79**, 647–50.

de Brux, J. (1981a) Evaluation of ovarian disturbances by endometrial biopsy. In: de Brux, J., Mortel, R., Gautray, J.P. (eds), *The Endometrium. Hormonal Impacts*. New York, London: Plenum Press, 107–21.

de Brux, J. (1981b) Analysis of isolated and combined actions of ovarian steroids on the endometrium. In: de Brux, J., Mortel, R., Gautray, J.P. (eds), *The*

Endometrium. Hormonal Impacts. New York, London: Plenum Press, 31–42.

Dallenbach-Hellweg, G. (1987) Functional disturbances of the endometrium. In: Fox, H. (ed.), *Haines and Taylor: Obstetrical and Gynaecological Pathology*, 3rd edn. Churchill Livingstone, Edinburgh, 320–9.

Dallenbach-Hellweg, G. and Bornebusch, C.G. (1970) Histologische Untersuchungen über die Reaktion des Endometriums bei der verzögerten Abstossung. *Archiv Gynäkol.* **208**, 235–46.

Keller, D.W., Wiest, W.G., Askin, F.B., Johnson, L.W., Strickler, R.C. (1979) Pseudocorpus luteum insufficiency: a local defect of progesterone action on endometrial tissue. *J. Clin. Endocrinol. Metab.* **48**, 127–32.

Laatikainen, T., Andersson, B., Kärkkäinen, J., Wahlström, T. (1983) Progestin receptor levels in endometria with delayed or incomplete secretory changes. *Obstet. Gynecol.* **62**, 592–8.

Thornbugh, I., Anderson, M. C. (1997) The endometrial deficient secretory phase. *Histopathology* **30**, 11–15.

5 The effect of therapeutic and contraceptive hormones on the endometrium

Exogenous sex steroid hormones may be administered to a woman for contraceptive or therapeutic purposes, or as replacements for diminished or absent endogenous hormones. Such hormones markedly influence endometrial histology and their use, particularly for contraceptive purposes, is now so widespread that a pathologist required to interpret endometrial biopsies must insist upon receiving a history that includes details of recent exposure, and not simply current exposure, or otherwise, of the patient to exogenous steroids. In the absence of such a history the pathologist is, to a significant extent, working in the dark.

In patients receiving exogenous hormones for either replacement or therapeutic purposes, the endometrium is commonly biopsied in order to monitor the morphological changes induced in the endometrium or, in some instances, the response of the disease that is being treated. In contrast, endometrial biopsies in women using steroids for contraceptive purposes are almost invariably undertaken for purposes unrelated to hormone usage and it is under these circumstances in particular that the pathologist may, in the absence of a reliable contraceptive history, be led astray.

5.1 THE EFFECTS OF HORMONAL THERAPY

5.1.1 Oestrogens

Oestrogens are given for the relief of menopausal symptoms, as postmenopausal hormone replacement therapy, as part of the therapeutic regime for carcinoma of the breast or as a factor in the management of hypogonadal conditions, e.g. gonadal dysgenesis.

Oestrogens normally effect synchronous growth of the endometrial glands, stroma and vasculature, induce endometrial progesterone receptors and, in the normal cycle, cause the stromal oedema that characterizes the mid-secretory phase. The endometrial morphological response to exogenous hormones, however, depends not only upon the duration of administration of oestrogen, the potency of the hormonal preparation and the total dosage but also upon the endogenous hormonal status of the patient.

If oestrogens are given to a patient in the proliferative phase of the cycle, endometrial growth is prolonged and the endometrium may exhibit features of a prolonged proliferative phase (see Chapter 4), ovulation is suppressed or delayed and the secretory phase is shortened or absent (Dallenbach-Hellweg, 1981). Oestrogen administration during the secretory phase results in marked stromal oedema, incomplete secretory transformation of the glands and retarded stromal maturation (Egger and Kindermann, 1980) – a picture that resembles that of spontaneous luteal phase insufficiency.

More commonly, oestrogens are given to women with a paucity of endogenous hormone, an absence of cyclical changes and an atrophic endometrium. Under these circumstances, small doses of oestrogen induce only a weakly proliferative pattern with few visible mitoses, a poorly defined functionalis and relatively little thickening of the endometrium: there may be focal multilayering of the glandular epithelium (Fig. 5.1). If dosage at this level is given for a prolonged period, the glands may eventually show a minor degree of dilatation and architectural atypia (Figs 1.10, 5.2 and 5.3), the appearances being those of a 'disordered proliferative endometrium' (Hendrickson and Kempson, 1980). In patients given larger, physiological doses of oestrogen, either continuously or cyclically, a significant proportion will, if a progestagen is not also given, develop either a simple (cystic glandular) endometrial hyperplasia or a hyperplasia with glandular and cytological atypia (Whitehead et al., 1977; Campenhout et al., 1980; Fox and Buckley, 1982; Schiff et al., 1982) (see Chapter 9). A much smaller proportion of women on long-term oestrogen dosage will eventually develop an endometrial carcinoma (Persson et al., 1996; Cushing et al., 1998), albeit one that is usually of the well-differentiated endometrioid type. An indication that unopposed oestrogens may be implicated in the development of endometrial stromal sarcoma and carcinosarcoma has also been reported (Schwartz et al., 1996). If a

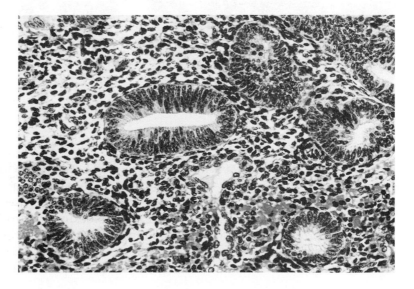

Figure 5.1 Weakly proliferative endometrium in a woman presenting with postmenopausal bleeding 6 years after the menopause. She had been treated intermittently with small doses of unopposed oestrogen. Epithelial stratification is present but the stroma remains compact. Haematoxylin and eosin.

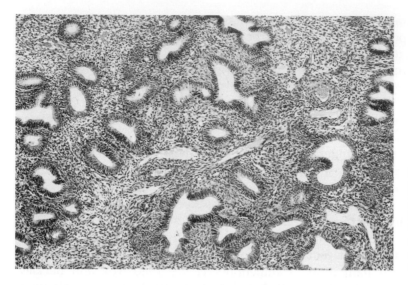

Figure 5.2 Disordered proliferation. A minor degree of glandular architectural irregularity is present in the endometrium of a woman treated with unopposed oestrogen for many years after the menopause. Haematoxylin and eosin.

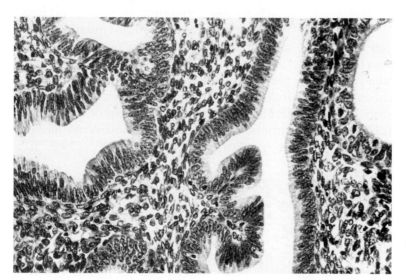

Figure 5.3 Disordered proliferation. Glandular epithelium is similar to that seen in the weakly proliferative endometrium (Fig. 5.1) and in the basalis of the reproductive years (Fig. 3.6). There is no cytological atypia and epithelial stratification is minimal: a mitosis is present in the gland to the right. Haematoxylin and eosin.

progestagen is administered with the oestrogen, either in combination or sequentially, both hyperplasia and adenocarcinoma will be prevented (Paterson *et al.*, 1980) and any hyperplastic process that has developed during unopposed oestrogenic stimulation will often be reversed.

5.1.2 Tamoxifen

Tamoxifen is a triphenylethylene compound that, as a consequence of competing for and blocking oestrogen-binding sites, has anti-oestrogenic properties. It is convenient to consider its effects here because, in a proportion of women, particularly those that are

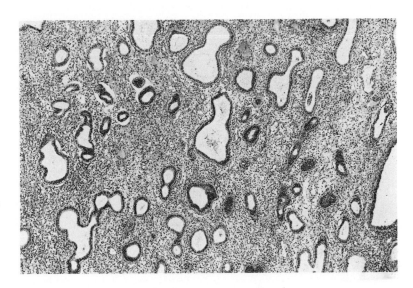

Figure 5.4 Mild simple hyperplasia in an endometrium from a patient that received tamoxifen for the treatment of breast carcinoma until 14 days before the biopsy. Haematoxylin and eosin.

postmenopausal, it induces an oestrogen-like effect. This has been described both experimentally, when the drug has been used at a level exceeding the recommended dose by over 100 times, and clinically at therapeutic levels (Legault-Poisson *et al.*, 1979).

The effects of tamoxifen on the endometrium may amount to no more than epithelial multi-layering but it can induce proliferative activity or hyperplasia in women receiving treatment for breast carcinoma (Fig. 5.4). Multiple, large, benign endometrial polyps may also develop (Ismail, 1994; Kennedy *et al.*, 1999), particularly in the postmenopausal woman and there is some evidence that these are dose-related (Cohen *et al.*, 1996a; McGonigle *et al.*, 1996); they are not necessarily prevented by the administration of progestagens (Berezowsky *et al.*, 1994). The polyps are characterized by glands aligned along the long axis of the polyps, staghorn-shaped glands, frequent areas of various epithelial metaplasia, of which mucinous metaplasia has been particularly noted (Schlesinger *et al.*, 1998), a patchy stromal cambium layer and stromal myxoid degeneration (Fig. 5.5).

Endometrial carcinoma has been reported to occur more commonly in women with breast carcinoma treated with tamoxifen than in those receiving no hormonal therapy (Fornander *et al.*, 1989; Robinson *et al.*, 1995; Mignotte *et al.*, 1998). Caution should be exercised in accepting this observation, however, as some women with breast carcinoma are also at genetic risk of developing endometrial carcinoma. In a large series, Silva *et al.* (1994) found that while endometrial carcinoma is not more common in women with breast carcinoma treated with tamoxifen, those tumours that do develop tend to be deeply penetrating at the time of presentation, high grade and more commonly serous or clear-celled. They are also more likely to be associated with polypi than in the untreated group. Tamoxifen-related severe atypical hyperplasia has also been reported following tamoxifen therapy in a patient who had previously undergone endometrial resection (Berliere *et al.*, 1999). Recent observations have suggested that a hyperoestrogenic state may be associated not only with endometrial carcinoma but also with mesenchymal or mixed epithelial mesenchymal tumours

59

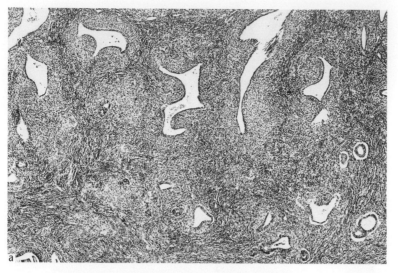

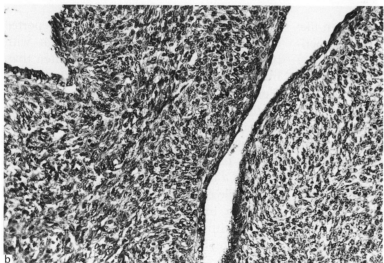

Figure 5.5 (a) A tamoxifen-associated polyp with staghorn-shaped glands and a variable cellular cambium layer around the individual glands. **(b)** The periglandular stroma is intensely cellular but note the absence of cytological atypia and mitotic activity. Haematoxylin and eosin.

(Schwartz *et al.*, 1996). A series of adenosarcomas developing in women on tamoxifen therapy (Clement *et al.*, 1996) lends support to this idea, as does the paper by McCluggage *et al.* (2000) reporting an association between long-term usage of tamoxifen and uterine carcinosarcomas. A possible association between myxoid or epithelioid features in leiomyosarcoma has also been noted (Silva *et al.*, 1994). In women

receiving tamoxifen, the administration of a progestagen results in endometrial stromal decidualization, indicating that progesterone receptors have been induced (Cohen *et al.*, 1996b).

Tamoxifen has also been used to suppress ovulation temporarily in the treatment of infertility, with the intention of causing 'rebound' ovulation when the drug is withdrawn. The

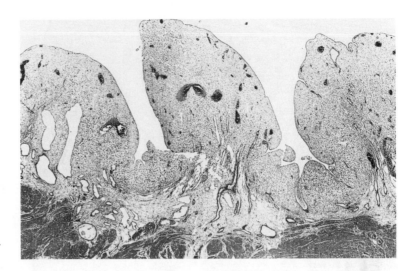

Figure 5.6 Progestagen therapy. The polypoidal appearance of the endometrium develops following treatment by norethisterone. Note the marked pseudodecidualization of the superficial part of the stroma, the paucity of glands and the congested thin-walled blood vessels. Haematoxylin and eosin.

endometrium from such patients may, both prior to treatment and following therapy, exhibit a wide variety of appearances.

5.1.3 Progestagens

Progestagens are used in the management of dysfunctional uterine bleeding, endometriosis, endometrial hyperplasia and some cases of endometrial adenocarcinoma. They act only on an endometrium in which progesterone receptors have been induced by prior exposure to oestrogen. Progestagens exert an anti-oestrogenic effect, with inhibition of endometrial growth, and induce differentiation or maturation of the glands and stroma.

When exogenous progestagens are given in therapeutic doses to a patient, the appearance of her endometrium will depend upon the extent to which the endometrium has been primed by oestrogen and upon the biochemical characteristics of the particular hormone. If progestagens are given early in the proliferative phase, little stromal decidualization occurs and there may be only a minor degree of abortive secretory activity in glands that remain narrow and tubular: spiral artery differentiation is not

seen. The administration of a progestagen to a patient late in the proliferative phase will induce marked pseudodecidualization of the functionalis (Figs 5.6 and 5.7) and transitory glandular secretory activity, this reflecting the widespread prior induction of progesterone receptors. The glands rapidly exhaust their secretory activity and become small and inactive, though occasional glands may retain a secretory or even hypersecretory appearance. Granulated lymphocytes are scattered throughout the decidualized stroma and these may form small aggregates (Fig. 5.8): it is important to distinguish these from polymorphonuclear leucocytes, which they may, at first sight, resemble (Fig. 5.9). This pattern can be confused with that of early pregnancy in which, however, the glands are, at least focally, hypersecretory and there is good growth of the spiral arteries (Figs 13.1 and 13.2).

Prolonged progestagen therapy results in an atrophic endometrium with sparse glands set in a shallow, compact stroma; the glands are inactive, though their epithelium may remain columnar rather than cuboidal (Fig. 5.10). It is usual for the large granulated lymphocyte

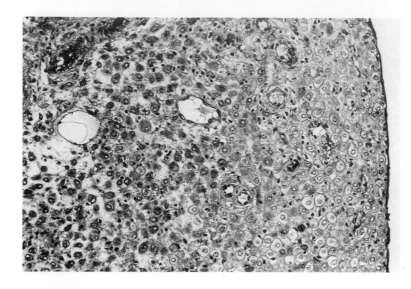

Figure 5.7 Progestagen therapy. The florid pseudodecidualization of the endometrial stroma that follows treatment with norethisterone: stromal cells are enlarged and have well-demarcated cell borders. Haematoxylin and eosin.

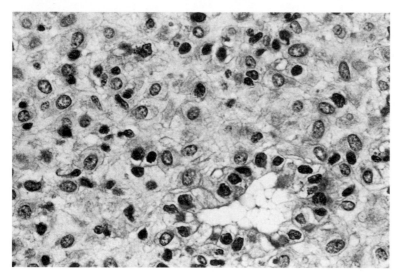

Figure 5.8 Progestagen therapy. The stroma is pseudodecidualized and the gland, to the right is narrow and lined by inactive, cuboidal clear cells. Granulated lymphocytes are scattered throughout the stroma. Haematoxylin and eosin.

infiltrate to persist while thin-walled vascular channels of indeterminate type are a conspicuous feature (Fig. 5.11), these possibly being the source of the intermittent breakthrough bleeding experienced by these patients; spiral artery growth is absent. Endometrial atrophy of this type, which results from the anti-oestrogenic effect of the progestagens, will persist as long as the progestagen therapy is continued but

usually recovers rapidly after withdrawal of the exogenous hormone: permanent atrophy with stromal hyalinization has been described (Dallenbach-Hellweg, 1980) but is very rarely encountered.

The appearances described above are seen most markedly in patients receiving 19-nor-testosterone-derived progestagens: in women given the weakly progestagenic synthetic

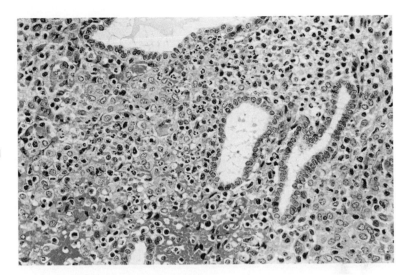

Figure 5.9 Progestagen withdrawal bleeding. The stroma in the centre of the field is undergoing necrosis and there is focal haemorrhage: an infiltrate of polymorphonuclear leucocytes contrasts with the granulated lymphocytes seen in Fig. 5.8. Note the inactivity of the glands. Haematoxylin and eosin.

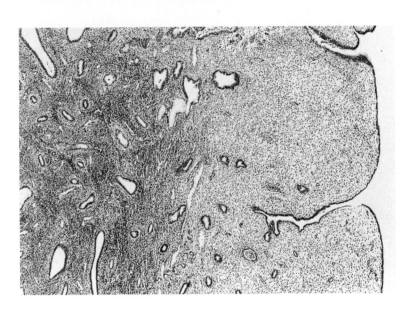

Figure 5.10 Prolonged progestagen therapy: moderate atrophy. Endometrial depth is much reduced; the marked polypoidal appearance associated with the recent commencement of progestagen is not seen. There is a shallow functionalis with pseudodecidualized stroma, almost devoid of glands and most glands are inactive. Spiral arteries are not differentiated. Haematoxylin and eosin.

anti-gonadotrophic androgen Danol (danazol), used particularly in the treatment of endometriosis, a moderately atrophic endometrium lacking stromal decidualization and glandular secretory activity develops rapidly *ab initio* (Fig. 5.12).

In women treated with progestagens for dysfunctional uterine bleeding, the typical changes described above are commonly seen. However, in many cases of dysfunctional uterine bleeding there is an underlying endometrial hyperplasia, upon which secretory changes may be superimposed (Figs 5.13 and 5.14); this appearance is sometimes known as 'secretory hyperplasia'. With continued therapy simple hyperplasia may regress completely but atypical

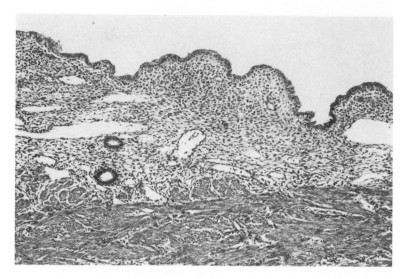

Figure 5.11 Prolonged progestagen therapy with profound atrophy. The uterus is lined only by a shallow, inactive endometrium containing narrow tubular glands and thin-walled vascular channels: vascular and stromal differentiation is absent. There is no functionalis. Haematoxylin and eosin.

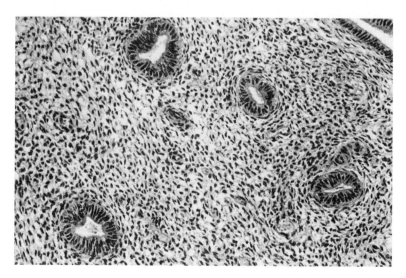

Figure 5.12 Danazol therapy. The endometrial glands are narrow, tubular and inactive and the stroma is immature and spindle-celled. The appearance is similar to that seen following prolonged treatment with norethisterone (Fig. 5.11). Haematoxylin and eosin.

hyperplasia may regress only partly, leaving islands of architecturally atypical glands set in an endometrium that is otherwise relatively normal in appearance, pseudodecidualized or possibly atrophic (Fig. 5.15). In rare cases, when endometrial hyperplasia is treated with progestagens, squamous metaplasia may develop despite its absence in the pretreatment hyperplasia (Miranda and Mazur, 1995).

Hormonally responsive endometrial adenocarcinomas, which are usually well differentiated (Grade 1) tumours, may also show secretory changes within 10–14 days of commencing progestagen therapy (Fig. 10.12), while the stromal cells of the neoplasm can show pseudodecidualization (Ferenczy, 1980). Tumour growth may be suppressed and focal areas of regression or degeneration may be apparent

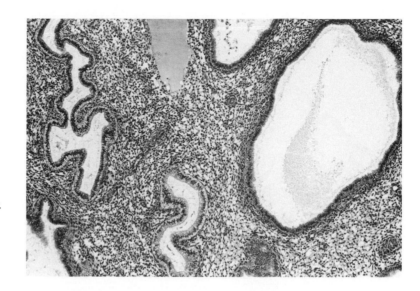

Figure 5.13 Progestagen therapy. Patchy, weak secretory activity superimposed on a simple hyperplasia: the patient had been treated with norethisterone. Haematoxylin and eosin.

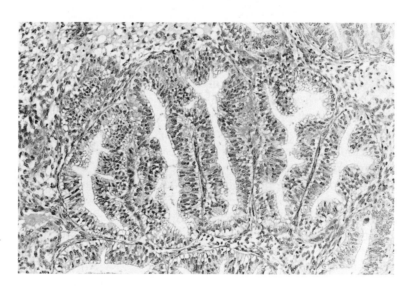

Figure 5.14 Progestagen therapy. Secretory transformation superimposed on an endometrium with the features of complex hyperplasia: uniform subnuclear vacuoles are present in the glandular epithelial cells. Haematoxylin and eosin.

(Anderson, 1972; Rosier and Underwood, 1974; Dallenbach-Hellweg, 1980; Ferenczy, 1980).

5.1.4 Antiprogestagens

Antiprogestagens such as mifepristone and onapristone, when given as a single dose after the luteinizing hormone (LH) surge, delay the onset of secretory changes but do not prolong the length of the cycle. When given daily, they also have an antiproliferative effect (Cameron *et al.*, 1996a, b). A possible use as a post-ovulatory contraceptive has been suggested. Murphy *et al.* (1995) reported that the endometrial morphology was abnormal in all patients treated with low doses. The glands varied in shape and size and were lined by a combination of epithelial

65

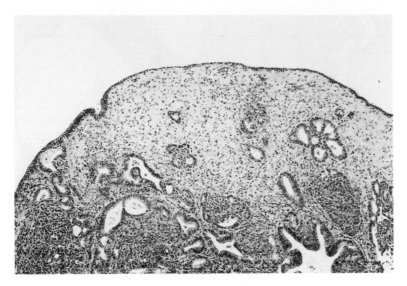

Figure 5.15 Progestagen therapy, persistent atypical hyperplasia. The stroma is pseudodecidualized and the glands in the superficial part of the tissue are narrow and tubular, those in the deeper part remain architecturally and cytologically atypical and many contain foci of squamous metaplasia. Haematoxylin and eosin.

types, some of which were secretory; the stroma was dense and cellular.

5.1.5 Gonadotrophin-releasing hormone agonists

Endometrial cell proliferation is suppressed by gonadotrophin-releasing hormone agonists, thus resulting in an inactive, or even atrophic endometrium. Even in women with endometrial hyperplasia, the hormone can induce atrophy, although when the therapy is stopped the hyperplastic state may recur if the underlying cause is not treated (Agorastos *et al.*, 1997).

5.2 THE EFFECTS OF CONTRACEPTIVE HORMONES

Steroid contraceptives fall into two main groups, those in which an oestrogen and progestagen are given in combination and those containing only a progestagen.

Most women follow a regimen in which between 20 and 50 µg of oestrogen, usually ethinyloestradiol, combined with a progestagen

is taken for 21 days out of every 28. The proportion of hormone in the preparation may be identical throughout the 21 days or there may be a phased formulation in which the hormone content of the pill is increased in the middle of the cycle. It is usual to commence therapy on the first day of the cycle, as it has been shown that by postponing the commencement to day 5, as was previously recommended, ovulation may not be inhibited in the first cycle. On the seven hormone-free days, either a placebo is taken or there are seven pill-free days.

Some women, particularly those over the age of 35 years, heavy smokers and those in whom oestrogens induce severe side-effects, may use a progestagen-only contraceptive. The progestagen, which is taken every day, may be administered in several ways, the effects upon the endometrium being independent of the mode of administration.

5.2.1 Combined steroid contraceptives

In the first few months in which a combined steroid contraceptive is used, the pattern of

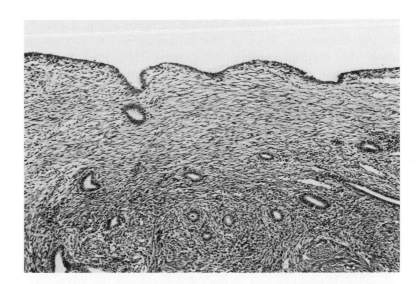

Figure 5.16 Long-term combined steroid contraceptive, monophasic pattern. The endometrium is moderately atrophic and resembles that seen in progestagen users (Fig. 5.10). The patient had used a combination of 30 μg of ethinyloestradiol with 150 μg levonorgestrel. Haematoxylin and eosin.

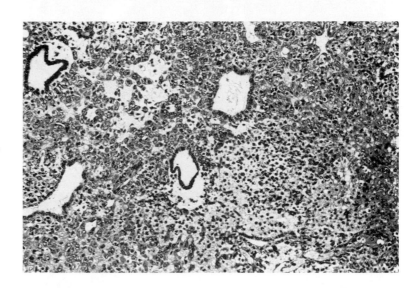

Figure 5.17 Combined steroid contraceptive, monophasic pattern. Hormone withdrawal bleeding on the second day of the cycle: the glands are small and inactive, there is no evidence of secretory change and the stroma is crumbling and haemorrhagic. Contrast this with the appearance of menstrual endometrium (Fig. 3.8). Haematoxylin and eosin.

endometrial changes may be cyclical but after prolonged usage the regenerative capacity of the endometrium may be diminished, because of progestagen predominance, and an atrophic picture ensues (Fig. 5.16). The morphological effects of combined steroid contraceptives, while being generally similar whatever the precise hormone combination and dosage, show sufficient variation for the relative importance of the oestrogen and progestagen in the combination to be recognized and for this to be associated in some patients with particular problems.

Following hormonal withdrawal bleeding at the end of each cycle of hormone usage (Fig. 5.17) the endometrium regenerates and there is a proliferative phase, which is curtailed by the inhibitory effect of the progestagen upon the oestrogen-stimulated growth; the endometrium therefore remains shallow. The glands, which are narrow, sometimes extremely so, lack the tortuosity of the normal proliferative phase and may appear sparse. They are lined by a single layer of cubo-columnar cells in which a small number of mitoses are seen (Fig. 5.18). The stromal cells, in which only occasional mitoses appear, remain spindled and have the so-called 'naked-nucleus' appearance.

Between days 8 and 10 of the cycle, the progestagen effect becomes apparent and subnuclear vacuoles appear in the glandular epithelial cells (Fig. 5.19) but, because of the brief, inadequate oestrogenic priming, progestagen

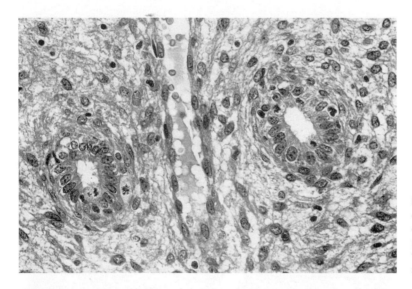

Figure 5.18 Combined steroid contraceptive, monophasic pattern, day 8 of the cycle, the proliferative phase: mitoses are present in both the glandular epithelium and in the stroma. Haematoxylin and eosin.

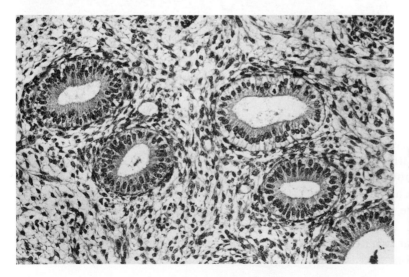

Figure 5.19 Combined steroid contraceptive, day 8 of the cycle in a phased contraceptive user. Subnuclear vacuoles are present in all the glands and there is a resemblance to the early secretory phase of the physiological cycle. Gland size, however, remains small. Haematoxylin and eosin.

receptors are few in number and the secretory changes are weak and poorly developed. By day 10, the subnuclear secretory vacuoles move into the supranuclear cytoplasm and there is a short, premature secretory phase lasting until day 14 or 15. The glands remain narrow, or only minimally dilated, and straight or only gently convoluted: the cytoplasm of the glandular epithelium, which is columnar, appears faintly eosinophilic, the apices of the cells remain, for the most part, intact and there is only a trace of secretion within the lumina (Fig. 5.20). There is, in some patients, a little stromal oedema. In the latter half of the cycle there is regression of secretory change and the endometrium becomes inactive (Fig. 5.21).

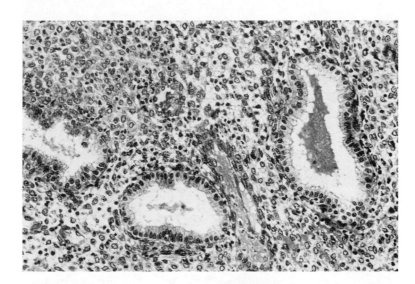

Figure 5.20 Combined steroid contraceptive, monophasic pattern. A weak secretory transformation with poor vascular differentiation: a sprinkling of granulated lymphocytes is present. Haematoxylin and eosin.

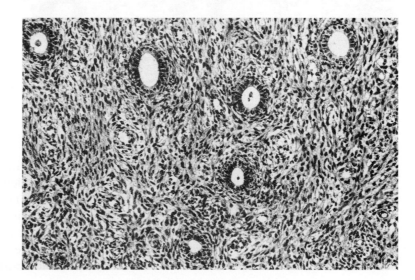

Figure 5.21 Combined steroid contraceptive, monophasic pattern, day 24 of the cycle. The glands are extremely narrow and inactive and the stroma densely cellular with a pseudodecidualized appearance. Haematoxylin and eosin.

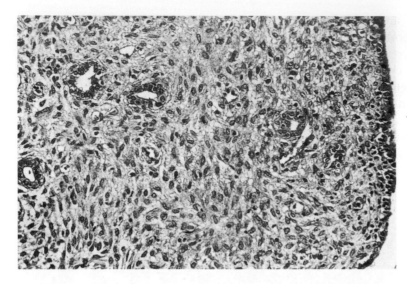

Figure 5.22 Combined steroid contraceptive, monophasic pattern, 50 μg ethinyloestradiol, 250 μg levonorgestrel, day 26 of the cycle. The glands are extremely narrow and inactive, the stroma is markedly pseudodecidualized, forming a compacta, and there is a granulated lymphocyte infiltrate. Haematoxylin and eosin.

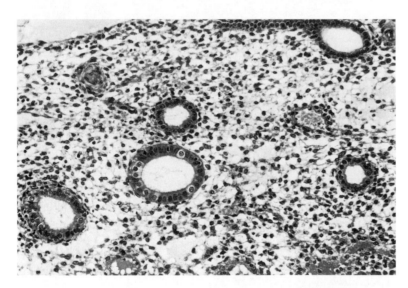

Figure 5.23 Combined steroid contraceptive, monophasic pattern, 30 μg ethinyloestradiol, 250 μg levonorgestrel, 3 weeks since hormone withdrawal bleeding. Compared with Fig. 5.22, the glands are less atrophic and the stroma is immature; there is no decidualization. Haematoxylin and eosin.

The degree of spiral artery differentiation and growth, the quality of the pseudodecidualization and the extent of the glandular secretory transformation vary according to the relative potency of the oestrogen and progestagen in the combination (Buckley, 1995) and the duration of use (Figs 5.22–5.25).

The alternating nodules of stromal hyperplasia and oedema described by Dallenbach-Hellweg (1981) and the bizarre stromal pseudosarcomatous changes reported by Dockerty *et al.* (1959) are not, in our experience, encountered in users of modern, low-dose, steroid contraceptives.

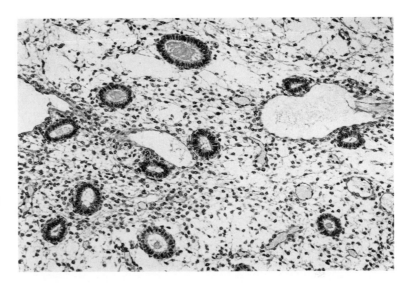

Figure 5.24 Combined steroid contraceptive, monophasic pattern, 35 μg ethinyloestradiol, 1 mg norethisterone. The glands are small and inactive, the stroma is immature and there is no spiral artery differentiation; thin-walled vascular channels are present. The appearance is similar to that seen in Fig. 5.23. Haematoxylin and eosin.

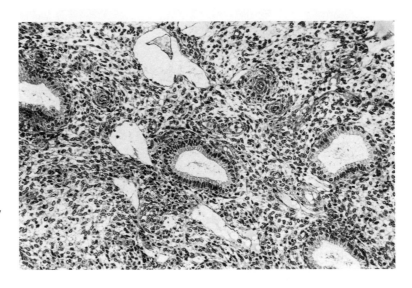

Figure 5.25 Combined steroid contraceptive, monophasic pattern, 30 μg ethinyloestradiol, 150 μg levonorgestrel, 3 weeks since hormone withdrawal bleeding. In contrast to the three preceding figures, the glands are moderately well grown, exhibit secretory activity and spiral artery differentiation has occurred: a granulated lymphocyte infiltrate is present. Haematoxylin and eosin.

The appearance observed after the 15th day of the cycle is more variable in users of the phased contraceptives. In some patients, a picture indistinguishable from that seen in conventional combined steroid contraceptive users is observed (Fig. 5.26). In others, there is less glandular regression, a persistence of weak secretory activity to the time of hormone withdrawal and, in those preparations with increased mid-cycle oestrogen (and hence more adequate progestagen receptor induction) better growth and muscularization of the spiral arteries (Fig. 5.27).

An unexpected, asymptomatic, chronic, non-specific endometritis has been identified in a

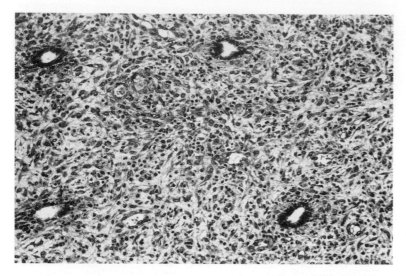

Figure 5.26 Phased steroid contraceptive. The glands are small, narrow, tubular and devoid of secretion: the stroma is pseudodecidualized and infiltrated by granulated lymphocytes. The degree of glandular regression is similar to that seen in Fig. 5.22. Haematoxylin and eosin.

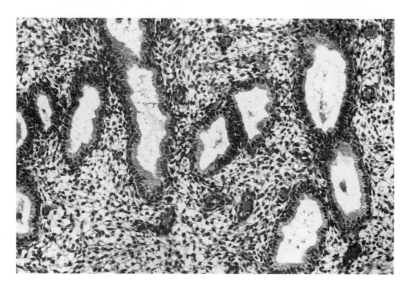

Figure 5.27 Phased steroid contraceptive. This biopsy was from a patient receiving a hormone combination identical to that given to the woman whose biopsy appears in Fig. 5.26. In striking contrast, glandular growth and secretion are much better developed, there is a minor degree of spiral artery differentiation and granulated lymphocyte infiltration is absent. Haematoxylin and eosin.

small proportion of women that use steroid contraceptives but have no symptoms of pelvic inflammatory disease (Ness *et al.*, 1997). In such cases, the possibility of chlamydial infection should be considered.

We do not in the UK currently encounter women using sequential steroid contraceptives in which a period of oestrogen therapy is followed by a short phase of progestagen–oestrogen combination.

In contrast to patients receiving oestrogen therapy, women using combined steroid contraceptives are protected against the risk of developing endometrial carcinoma: they have

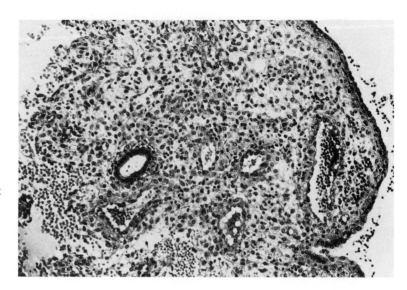

Figure 5.28 Progestagen contraceptive. A fragment of endometrium which is typical of that obtained from a woman using a depot progestagen for contraceptive purposes. A single inactive gland and several abnormal, dilated vascular channels are present. Haematoxylin and eosin.

only half the risk compared with 'never-users' (Huggins and Giuntoli, 1979; Kaufman *et al.*, 1980; Weiss and Sayvetz, 1980; Hulka *et al.*, 1982; WHO, 1982). This beneficial effect persists after the menopause provided that the woman is not given unopposed oestrogen replacement therapy. Maximum protection is afforded to those who are nulliparous and have used the pill for more than 1 year.

5.2.2 Progestagen-only contraceptives

A very variable endometrial picture is encountered in women using a progestagen-only contraceptive. The dose is small and its contraceptive effect depends not upon suppression of ovulation but upon alterations in tubal transport and in the quality of the cervical mucus. Ovulation is suppressed in only about 50 per cent of cycles and, consequently, the underlying, endogenous hormone pattern may vary from cycle to cycle and from patient to patient. In addition, it is usual to give the same dose of progestagen every day, or administer it systemically by depot injection, rather than in a cyclical pattern and amenorrhoea or breakthrough bleeding with intermittent healing therefore occurs.

The most commonly encountered pattern is one in which glands of rather variable size and secretory activity are set in a spindle-celled stroma containing thin-walled vascular channels and showing little or no evidence of decidualization (Figs 5.28 and 5.29): the appearance is reminiscent of that sometimes encountered in luteal phase insufficiency. If bleeding has occurred recently, mitoses may be seen in both glandular epithelium and stromal cells and if ovulation has occurred there may be sufficient proliferative activity both to increase the general thickness of the endometrium and to permit spiral artery growth and muscularization. Their appearances do not resemble those seen in patients receiving high doses of progestagen for therapeutic purposes (see above).

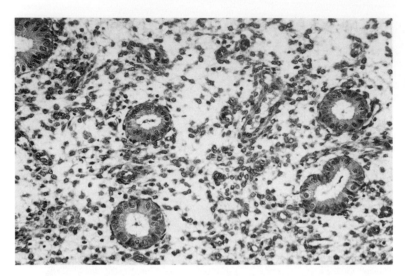

Figure 5.29 Progestagen contraceptive, daily dose of 0.35 mg of norethisterone. The appearance of the endometrium in progestagen-only contraceptive users is very variable. In this case it resembles that seen in Figs 5.23 or 5.24, in which combinations with relatively high doses of progestagen have been taken: spiral artery differentiation has not occurred, the glands are small and inactive and the stroma is immature. Haematoxylin and eosin.

5.3 HORMONE REPLACEMENT THERAPY

It is now considered unwise to use oestrogens alone for replacement therapy when the uterus is *in situ* because of the risk that endometrial carcinoma may develop: nonetheless, we occasionally encounter patients in whom this has occurred (Figs 1.10, 5.2 and 5.3). More commonly, oestrogen is given for between 10 and 15 days, on average, and then a progestagen is added to the regime for the next 5–10 days: this eliminates the risk of inducing endometrial carcinoma (Whitehead *et al.*, 1982). Some women also use a regimen in which progestagen is given only four to six times per year to elicit hormone withdrawal bleeding. The appearance of the endometrium in such cases will, therefore, depend very much on the time in this prolonged cycle at which the endometrium is sampled. Increasingly nowadays, a combined oestrogen plus progestagen preparation is given continuously and, in these women, the endometrium is generally shallow, inactive or mildly atrophic and the glands narrow and inactive (Fig. 5.30). The stroma is usually spindle-celled but a pseudodecidual change sometimes occurs (Piegsa *et al.*, 1997). Such prolonged, balanced hormone replacement therapy appears to have no adverse, long-term consequences upon the endometrium (Sturdee, 1996). Other less commonly used combinations include combining an oestrogen with testosterone. We have not, however, had the opportunity of examining the endometria of women using this regimen.

Following the administration of oestrogen, the endometrium proliferates and grows normally for the first part of the cycle and after introduction of the progestagen there is a brief, poorly developed, delayed secretory phase, which may not appear until shortly before hormone withdrawal bleeding. There is little or no stromal decidualization, though stromal oedema may be marked as a reflection of oestrogenic activity (Fig. 5.31), and granulated lymphocytes are sparse or absent. In a proportion of women, oestrogen is administered by means of a skin patch and progestagen given either as an intramuscular depot injection or by mouth. In such cases, endometrial appearance is variable, depending upon the dose and

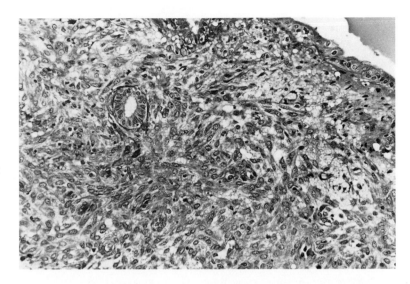

Figure 5.30 Hormone replacement therapy, continuous combined pattern. The endometrial gland is narrow and inactive and the stroma cellular and compact in a woman taking 2 mg oestradiol combined with 1 mg norethisterone acetate daily.

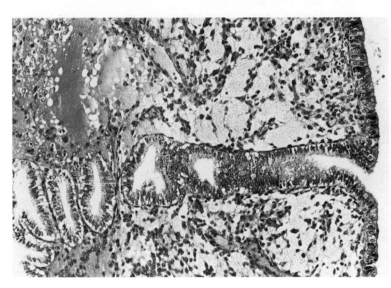

Figure 5.31 Hormonal replacement therapy, sequential pattern. The sample was taken on the 23rd day of an artificial 28-day cycle. The endometrium is well-grown and there is subnuclear vacuolation of the glandular epithelium: stromal oedema is marked and spiral artery differentiation has not yet occurred. Haematoxylin and eosin.

interval between administration of the two hormones and the biopsy. In many women, endometrial morphology approximates to the normal, particularly in those in whom there has been premature ovarian failure (Fig. 5.32). Polyps may be found in a small number of women who experience irregular bleeding while using hormone replacement therapy (Maia *et al.*, 1996).

5.3.1 Tibolone

Tibolone combines oestrogenic and progestagenic activity with a weak androgenic effect. It is used as a form of hormone replacement therapy and may produce a weakly proliferative endometrium. When bleeding occurs in postmenopausal women using this preparation, there is a likelihood that a pathological process will be identified in the endometrium.

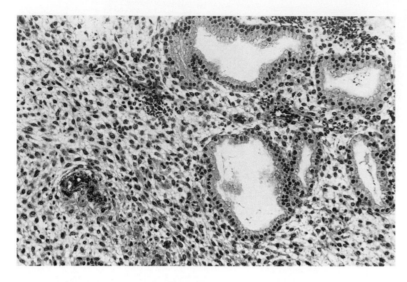

Figure 5.32 Hormone replacement therapy. Glands are well-grown, secretory activity is present, spiral artery differentiation has occurred and mild stromal pseudodecidualization has developed. Haematoxylin and eosin.

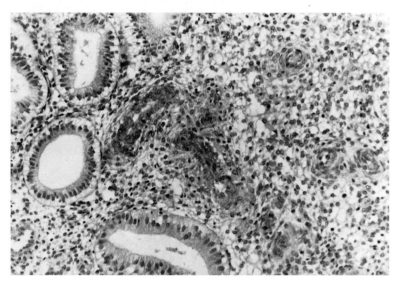

Figure 5.33 Assisted reproduction: premature spiral artery development consistent in appearance with the 9th to 10th post-ovulatory day contrasts with the subnuclear secretory vacuoles in the glands, which are characteristic of the early secretory phase. Haematoxylin and eosin.

This is most commonly a polyp but simple hyperplasia and atypical hyperplasia have also been reported (Ginsburg and Prelevic, 1996).

5.4 ASSISTED REPRODUCTION

The chance of collecting large numbers of ova from women undergoing assisted reproduction is improved by prior downregulation by gonadotrophin-releasing hormone analogues followed by the administration of human chorionic gonadotrophin (hCG). Biopsy of the endometrium on the fourth day after administration of hCG will reveal glandular/stromal asynchrony (Fig. 5.33). It differs, however, from spontaneously developing luteal phase defect because, in these cases, the stromal maturation,

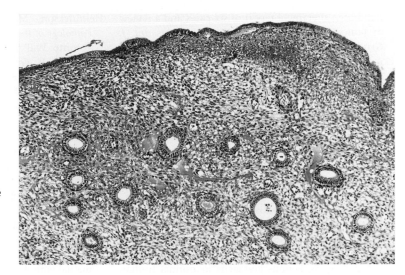

Figure 5.34 Hormone therapy. The narrow glands and cellular stroma seen in a woman taking 35 µg ethinyloestradiol in combination with 2 mg cyproterone for 21 days out of 28. Haematoxylin and eosin.

specifically the spiral artery development, is precocious and the glandular maturation is appropriate for the day of the cycle. In spontaneously occurring luteal phase defect, the stromal maturation is consistent with the correct day of the cycle while glandular maturation is usually retarded (Seif *et al.*, 1992; Noci *et al.*, 1997).

5.5 OTHER HORMONE PREPARATIONS

It should be noted that oestrogen-containing preparations may be used in combination with cyproterone in the treatment of acne or hirsutism and this produces an endometrium in which the glands are narrow, or minimally dilated and inactive, and the stroma is compact and cellular (Fig. 5.34).

REFERENCES

Agorastos, T., Bontis, J., Vakiani, A., Vavilis, D., Constantinidis, T. (1997) Treatment of endometrial hyperplasias with gonadotropin-releasing hormone agonists: pathological, clinical, morphometric, and DNA-cytometric data. *Gynecol. Oncol.* **65**, 102–14.

Anderson, D.G. (1972) The possible mechanisms of action of progestins on endometrial adenocarcinoma. *Am. J. Obstet. Gynecol.* **113**, 195–211.

Berliere, M., Galant, C., Donnez, J. (1999) The potential oncogenic effect of tamoxifen on the endometrium. *Hum. Reprod.* **14**, 1381–3.

Berezowsky, J., Chalvardjian, A., Murray, D. (1994) Iatrogenic endometrial megapolyps in women with breast carcinoma. *Obstet. Gynecol.* **84**, 727–30.

Buckley, C.H. (1995) Pathology of contraception and of hormonal therapy. In Fox, H. (ed.), *Haines and Taylor Obstetrical and Gynaecological Pathology*, 4th edn. Edinburgh: Churchill Livingstone, 1137–82.

Cameron, S.T., Critchley, H.O.D., Buckley, C.H., Chard, T., Kelly, R.W., Baird, D.T. (1996a) The effects of post-ovulatory onapristone on the development of a secretory endometrium. *Hum. Reprod.* **11**, 40–9.

Cameron, S.T., Critchley, H.O.D., Thong, K.J., Buckley, C.H., Williams, A.R., Baird, D.T. (1996b) Effects of daily low dose mifepristone on endometrial maturation and proliferation. *Hum. Reprod.* **11**, 2518–26.

Campenhout, J., van, Choquette, P., Vauclair, R. (1980) Endometrial pattern in patients with primary hypo-estrogenic amenorrhoea receiving estrogen replacement therapy. *Obstet. Gynecol.* **56**, 349–55.

Clement, P.B., Oliva, E., Young, R.H. (1996) Müllerian adenosarcoma of the uterine corpus associated with tamoxifen therapy: a report of six cases and a review of tamoxifen-associated endometrial lesions. *Int. J. Gynecol. Pathol.* **15**, 222–9.

Cohen, I., Altaras, M.M., Shapira, J. *et al.* (1996a) Time-dependent effect of tamoxifen therapy on endometrial pathology in asymptomatic postmenopausal breast cancer patients. *Int. J. Gynecol. Pathol.* **15**, 152–7.

Cohen, I., Figer, A., Altaras, M.M. *et al.* (1996b) Common endometrial decidual reaction in postmenopausal breast cancer patients treated with tamoxifen and progestogens. *Int. J. Gynecol. Pathol.* **15**, 17–22.

Cushing, K.L., Weiss, N.S., Voigt, L.F., McKnight, B., Beresford, S.A. (1998) Risk of endometrial cancer in relation to use of low-dose, unopposed estrogens. *Obstet. Gynecol.* **91**, 35–9.

Dallenbach-Hellweg, G. (1980) Morphological changes induced by exogenous gestagens in normal human endometrium. In: Dallenbach-Hellweg, G. (ed.), *Functional Morphologic Changes in Female Sex Organs Induced by Exogenous Hormones*. Berlin, Heidelberg, New York: Springer-Verlag, 95–100.

Dallenbach-Hellweg, G. (1981) *Histopathology of the Endometrium*, 3rd Edn. Berlin, Heidelberg, New York: Springer-Verlag, 126–256.

Dockerty, M.B., Smith, R.A., Symmonds, R.E. (1959) Pseudomalignant endometrial changes induced by the administration of new synthetic progestins. *Proc. Mayo Clinic* **34**, 321–8.

Egger, H., Kinderman, G. (1980) Effects of high oestrogen doses on the endometrium. In: Dallenbach-Hellweg, G. (ed.), *Functional Morphologic Changes in Female Sex Organs Induced by Exogenous Hormones*. Berlin, Heidelberg, New York: Springer-Verlag, 51–3.

Ferenczy, A. (1980) Morphological effects of exogenous gestagens on abnormal human endometrium. In: Dallenbach-Hellweg, G. (ed.), *Functional Morphologic Changes in Female Sex Organs Induced by Exogenous Hormones*. Berlin, Heidelberg, New York: Springer-Verlag, 101–10.

Fornander, T., Rutqvist, L.E., Cedermark, B. *et al.* (1989) Adjuvant Tamoxifen in early breast cancer: occurrence of new primary cancers. *Lancet* **i**, 117–20.

Fox, H., Buckley, C.H. (1982) The endometrial hyperplasias and their relationship to neoplasia. *Histopathology* **6**, 493–510.

Ginsburg, J., Prelevic, G.M. (1996) Cause of vaginal bleeding in postmenopausal women taking tibolone. *Maturitas* **24**, 107–10.

Hendrickson, M.R., Kempson, R.L. (1980) *Surgical Pathology of the Uterine Corpus*. Philadelphia, London, Toronto: W.B. Saunders.

Huggins, G.R., Giuntoli, R.L. (1979) Oral contraceptives and neoplasia. *Fertil. Steril.* **32**, 1–23.

Hulka, B.S., Chambless, L.E., Kaufman, D.G., Fowler, W.C., Greenberg, B.G. (1982) Protection against endometrial carcinoma by combination-product oral contraceptives. *J. Am. Med. Assoc.* **247**, 475–7.

Ismail, S.M. (1994) Pathology of endometrium treated with tamoxifen. *J. Clin. Pathol.* **47**, 827–33.

Kaufman, D.W., Shapiro, S., Slone, D. *et al.* (1980) Decreased risk of endometrial cancer among oral contraceptive users. *New Engl. J. Med.* **303**, 1045–7.

Kennedy, M.M., Baigrie, C.F., Manek, S. (1999) Tamoxifen and the endometrium: review of 102 cases and comparison with HRT-related and non-HRT-related endometrial pathology. *Int. J. Gynecol. Pathol.* **18**, 130–7.

Legault-Poisson, S., Jolivet, J., Poisson, R., Beretta-Piccoli, M., Band, R.R. (1979) Tamoxifen induced tumour stimulation and withdrawal response. *Cancer Treat. Rep.* **63**, 1839–41.

McCluggage, W.G., Abdulkader, M., Price, J.H. *et al.* (2000) Uterine carcinosarcoma in patients receiving tamoxifen. A report of 19 cases. *Int. J. Gynecol. Cancer* **10**, 280–4.

McGonigle, K.F., Lantry, S.A., Odom-Maryon, T.L., Chai, A., Vasilev, S.A., Simpson, J.F. (1996) Histopathologic effects of tamoxifen on the uterine epithelium of breast cancer patients: analysis by menopausal status. *Cancer. Lett.* **101**, 59–66.

Maia Jr, H., Barbosa, I.C., Marques, D., Calmon, L.C., Ladipo, O.A., Coutinho, E.M. (1996) Hysteroscopy and transvaginal sonography in menopausal women receiving hormone replacement therapy. *J. Am. Assoc. Gynecol. Laparosc.* **4**, 13–18.

Mignotte, H., Lasset, C., Bonadona, V. *et al.* (1998) Iatrogenic risks of endometrial carcinoma after treatment for breast cancer in a large French case-control study. Federation Nationale des Centres de Lutte Contre le Cancer (FNCLCC). *Int. J. Cancer* **76**, 325–30.

Miranda, M.C., Mazur, M.T. (1995) Endometrial squamous metaplasia. An unusual response to progestin therapy of hyperplasia. *Arch. Pathol. Lab. Med.* **119**, 458–60.

Murphy, A.A., Kettel, L.M., Morales, A.J., Roberts, V., Parmley, T., Yen, S.S. (1995) Endometrial effects of long-term low-dose administration of RU486. *Fertil. Steril.* **63**, 761–6.

Ness, R.B., Keder, L.M., Soper, D.E. *et al.* (1997) Oral contraception and the recognition of endometritis. *Am. J. Obstet. Gynecol.* **176**, 580–5.

Noci, I., Borri, P., Coccia, M.E. *et al.* (1997) Hormonal patterns, steroid receptors and morphological pictures of endometrium in hyperstimulated IVF cycles. *Eur. J. Obstet. Gynecol. Reprod. Biol.* **75**, 215–20.

Paterson, M.E.L., Wade-Evans, T., Sturdee, D.W., Thom, M.H., Studd, J.W.W. (1980) Endometrial disease after treatment with oestrogens and progestogens in the climacteric. *BMJ* 1, 822–4.

Persson, I., Yuen, J., Bergkvist, L., Schairer, C. (1996) Cancer incidence and mortality in women receiving estrogen and estrogen–progestin replacement therapy – long-term follow-up of a Swedish cohort. *Int. J. Cancer* **67**, 327–32.

Piegsa, K., Calder, A., Davis, J.A., McKay-Hart, D., Wells, M., Bryden, F. (1997) Endometrial status in post-menopausal women on long-term continuous combined hormone replacement therapy (Kliofem). A comparative study of endometrial biopsy, outpatient hysteroscopy and transvaginal ultrasound. *Eur. J. Obstet. Gynecol. Reprod. Biol.* **72**, 175–80.

Robinson, D.C., Bloss, J.D., Schiano, M.A. (1995) A retrospective study of tamoxifen and endometrial cancer in breast cancer patients. *Gynecol. Oncol.* **59**, 186–90.

Rosier, J.G., Underwood, P.B. (1974) Use of progestational agents in endometrial adenocarcinoma. *Obstet. Gynecol.* **44**, 60–4.

Schiff, I., Sela, H.Km., Cramer, D., Tulchinsky, D., Ryan, K.J. (1982) Endometrial hyperplasia in women on cyclic or continuous estrogen regimens. *Fertil. Steril.* **37**, 79–82.

Schlesinger, C., Kamoi, S., Ascher, S.M., Kendell, M., Lage, J.M., Silverberg, S.G. (1998) Endometrial polyps: a comparison study of patients receiving tamoxifen with two control groups. *Int. J. Gynecol. Pathol.* **17**, 302–11.

Schwartz, S.M., Weiss, N.S., Daling, J.R. *et al.* (1996) Exogenous sex hormone use, correlates of endogenous hormone levels, and the incidence of histologic types of sarcoma of the uterus. *Cancer* **77**, 717–24.

Seif, M.W., Pearson, J.M., Ibrahim, Z.H.Z. *et al.* (1992) Endometrium in *in-vitro* fertilization cycles: morphological and functional differentiation in the implantation phase. *Hum. Reprod.* **7**, 6–11.

Silva, E.G., Tornos, C.S., Follen-Mitchell, M. (1994) Malignant neoplasms of the uterine corpus in patients treated for breast carcinoma: the effects of Tamoxifen. *Int. J. Gynecol. Pathol.* **13**, 248–58.

Sturdee, D.W. (1996) Endometrial morphology and bleeding patterns as a function of progestogen supplementation. *Int. J. Fertil. Menopausal. Stud.* **41**, 22–8.

Weiss, M.I., Sayvetz, T.A. (1980) Incidence of endometrial cancer in relation to the use of oral contraceptives. *N. Engl. J. Med.* **302**, 551–4.

Whitehead, M.I., McQueen, J., Beard, R.J., Minardi, J., Campbell, S. (1977) The effects of cyclical oestrogen therapy and sequential oestrogen/progestagen therapy on the endometrium of post-menopausal women. *Acta Obstet. Gynecol. Scand.* **65**(Suppl.), 91–101.

Whitehead, M.I., Townsend, P.T., Pryse-Davies, J. *et al.* (1982) Effect of various types and dosages of progestogens on the postmenopausal endometrium. *J. Reprod. Med.* **27**, 539–48.

World Health Organisation (1982) Non-communicable disease surveillance: oral contraceptives and cancer risk. *WHO Weekly Epidemiol. Rec.* **57**, 281–8.

6   Endometrial changes associated with intrauterine contraceptive devices

Three basic types of intrauterine contraceptive device (IUCD) are currently encountered: the inert plastic device, which is now rarely used but may still be found in women who have been wearing a device for many years; copper-coated plastic devices, which are in current vogue; and, less commonly, progestagen-impregnated devices. About 50 per cent of women wearing an IUCD have no symptoms attributable to the presence of the device but others may have symptoms of intermenstrual spotting, menorrhagia, uterine colic or dysmenorrhoea, which tend to diminish when the device has been in place some time (Tindall, 1987). A small proportion of women using a device complain of symptoms, such as irregular bleeding associated with pelvic pain and vaginal discharge, which suggest a complicating uterine infection. Endometrial biopsy in IUCD wearers may, therefore, be undertaken for the investigation of symptoms secondary to IUCD usage, to confirm or refute the presence of an endometritis or for reasons not directly related to the IUCD, and to which the presence of the device is incidental.

In endometrial biopsies from women wearing an IUCD, the principal problem posed to the pathologist is that of distinguishing between inflammatory changes due solely to the mechanical and irritative effects of the IUCD and those caused by a superimposed endometrial infection. The local, non-infective, morphological changes induced by an IUCD are largely confined to the superficial layer of the functionalis and are, indeed, localized to the areas of contact between the superficial endometrium and the device. In contrast, changes caused by infection are more widespread and extend more deeply into the tissues. If therefore, an endometrial biopsy sample contains only tissue from the superficial part of the endometrium, it may be possible to assess the direct local effects of the device but impossible to give a histological opinion as to whether or not there is a complicating endometrial infection (Buckley, 1995).

6.1 LOCAL, MECHANICAL AND IRRITATIVE CHANGES

Local changes are limited to the contact site of the device and it is, to some extent, a matter of chance whether this site is included in the biopsy: in the absence of tissue from the contact site a biopsy may show no histological evidence of the presence of an IUCD. It should be noted also that the changes at the contact site are least easily assessed during the late secretory and premenstrual phases of the cycle, when they may be masked by the normal physiological changes in the endometrium.

The local pressure of an inert device produces a smooth-contoured depression (Fig. 6.1), while the copper wire on the stem of a copper-covered device may leave an accurate imprint on the endometrial surface (Fig. 6.2) with the formation of a fine papillary pattern, the papillae lying between the coils of the copper wire. The endometrium lying between the device

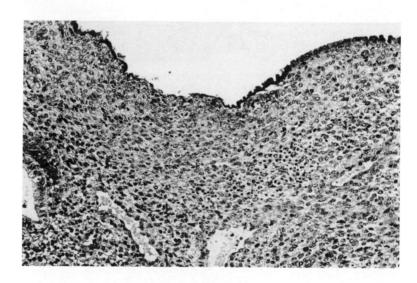

Figure 6.1 Inert intrauterine contraceptive device contact site. The surface of the endometrium is depressed, the epithelium flattened and the underlying stroma pseudodecidualized and infiltrated by a round cell population. Haematoxylin and eosin.

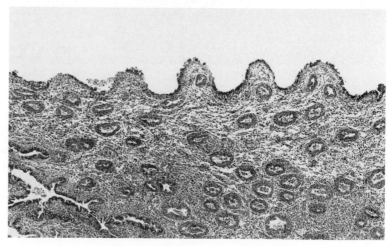

Figure 6.2 Copper-covered intrauterine contraceptive device contact site. The regular indentations created by the copper wire on the shaft of the device are clearly seen. Note that in this case there is little or no underlying inflammation. Haematoxylin and eosin.

81

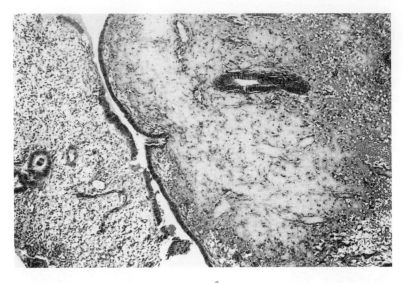

Figure 6.3 The marked oedema which sometimes develops in the stroma between the contact sites of an intrauterine contraceptive device is seen in the fragment of endometrium to the right; the endometrium to the left is of more normal appearance. Haematoxylin and eosin.

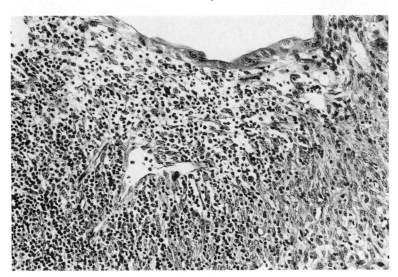

Figure 6.4 Intrauterine contraceptive device contact site. A flattened surface epithelium lies over a stroma that is devoid of glands, infiltrated by chronic inflammatory cells and partly replaced by maturing non-specific granulation tissue. Haematoxylin and eosin.

coils or arms may be normal but it is sometimes thrown into oedematous folds, particularly during the early secretory phase (Fig. 6.3). In some endometria, these folds form polypoidal projections with focally congested and inflamed tips. The surface epithelium at the contact site may be flattened but is sometimes absent, having been stripped away by the removal of the device prior to the taking of the biopsy. Beneath

some devices there can, however, be true ulceration with the formation of non-specific granulation tissue (Fig. 6.4). The epithelium at the margins of an ulcerated contact site may show evidence of regrowth, with mitotic activity and non-specific reactive changes such as nuclear enlargement, nuclear pleomorphism and an increased nucleocytoplasmic ratio (Fig. 6.5). Infrequently, when the device has been worn

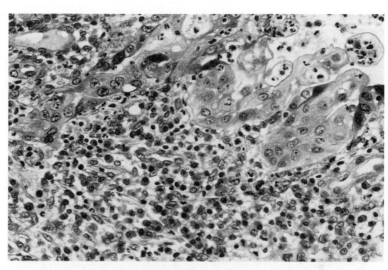

Figure 6.5 Intrauterine contraceptive device contact site: reactive epithelial changes. The surface epithelium, to the upper right, is formed by cells that vary in shape and size, have lost their polarity and are moderately pleomorphic: the underlying stroma is heavily infiltrated by plasma cells and lymphocytes and the epithelium contains polymorphonuclear leucocytes. Haematoxylin and eosin.

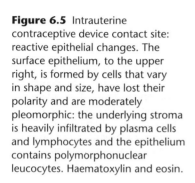

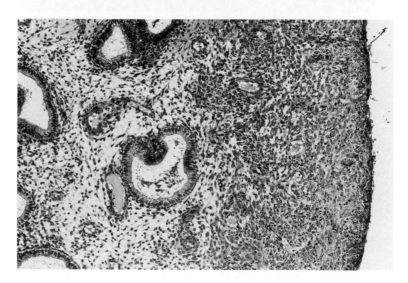

Figure 6.6 Pseudodecidualization of the superficial part of the endometrial stroma (to the right) beneath the contact site of an intrauterine contraceptive device: a focal inflammatory infiltrate is also present. Haematoxylin and eosin.

for many years there can be focal squamous metaplasia at the contact site.

The endometrium immediately below the device is sometimes extremely atrophic and represented by only a thin wisp of stroma, occasionally fibrotic, and lacking any glands (Fig. 6.4). More commonly, the subjacent stroma shows foci of superficial or, less commonly, deep pseudodecidualization (Fig. 6.6). Such foci may, in an otherwise unremarkable endometrium, be a clue to the presence of an IUCD. On occasions the endometrial glands immediately deep to the contact site show a pattern of maturation that differs slightly from that in the adjacent areas; the glands may, for example, show delayed maturation, premature secretory maturation or can, rarely, be inactive. A greater secretory phase glandular epithelial height has also been reported in IUCD wearers (Wang *et al.*, 1995).

83

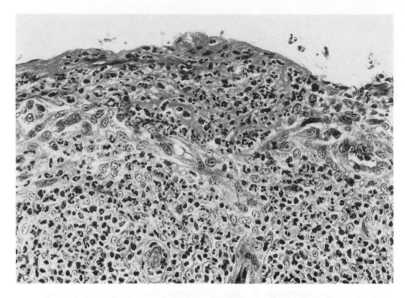

Figure 6.7 Acute inflammation at the contact site of an intrauterine contraceptive device. The surface epithelium is intact but shows marked reactive changes and is covered by a layer of acute fibrinous exudate containing numerous polymorphonuclear leucocytes: the underlying stroma is also inflamed. Haematoxylin and eosin.

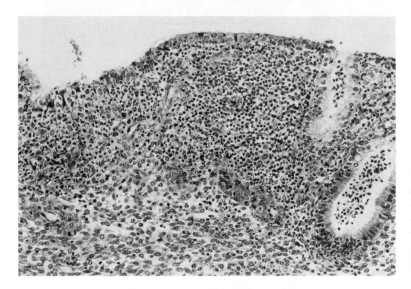

Figure 6.8 A well-demarcated, discrete inflammatory focus at the contact site of an intrauterine contraceptive device. In this example, the inflammatory infiltrate is composed predominantly of lymphocytes and plasma cells. Haematoxylin and eosin.

At the contact site, it is usual to find a few polymorphonuclear leucocytes in the surface epithelium (Fig. 6.7), together with a focal, mild, non-specific chronic inflammatory cell infiltrate in the subjacent stroma. This infiltrate occasionally forms a sharply defined focus (Fig. 6.8) within which the glands may contain occasional polymorphonuclear leucocytes together with nuclear debris. This appearance cannot always be distinguished from early tuberculosis (see Chapter 7) but the presence of the other features of a contact site should serve to negate this diagnosis. A foreign-body response to an IUCD is distinctly unusual. However, occasionally, intraglandular macrophage giant cells are seen (Fox and Buckley, 1983), while foreign-body

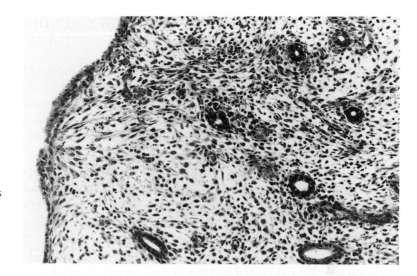

Figure 6.9 Narrow inactive glands set in a pseudodecidualized stroma in the endometrium of a progestagen-impregnated intrauterine contraceptive device user. Haematoxylin and eosin.

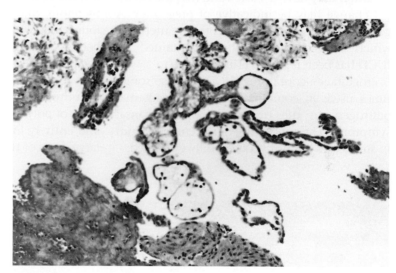

Figure 6.10 Micropapillae, which have formed on the surface of the endometrium in a progestagen-impregnated intrauterine contraceptive device user. Haematoxylin and eosin.

granulomas may form around fragments of debris that have become detached from the surface of the device: these are small, associated with minimal local damage and can be in either the deep or superficial layers of the endometrium.

In women wearing a progestagen-impregnated device there are, in addition to the local irritative effects described above, changes attributable to the progestagen. The appearances are similar regardless of the phase of the menstrual cycle, the duration of IUCD use or the type of progestagen-containing device (Silverberg *et al.*, 1986; Critchley *et al.*, 1998). Stromal pseudodecidualization, which is usually most marked in the first months after insertion, and glandular atrophy are typical (Fig. 6.9); surface micropapillae may also develop (Fig. 6.10). Stromal calcification, small polyps, and thick-walled fibrotic blood vessels, similar to those seen in endometrial polyps, may develop after several years of use. Rarely, cells with slight nuclear atypia, resembling those in the Arias-Stella phenomenon, are seen in glands lined by otherwise inactive cells. The appearance of the stroma close to the device and distant from the IUCD may differ. The decidual cells adjacent to the device tend to be well rounded and of normal decidual appearance, while the stromal cells remote from the device tend to be more spindle-shaped and of artificial appearance (Critchley *et al.*, 1998).

It should always be borne in mind, when interpreting decidual changes in the endometria of IUCD wearers, that an intrauterine or ectopic gestation may have occurred and that the decidual change may be indicative of pregnancy. A gestation in one horn of a bicornuate uterus in which the contralateral horn contained an IUCD has been reported (Tindall, 1987).

Progestagen-containing IUCDs are also sometimes used, in combination with transdermal oestrogen, in the treatment of menopausal symptoms. The appearance of the endometrium in such cases has not yet been fully evaluated.

6.2 ENDOMETRIAL INFECTION IN IUCD WEARERS

Some women wearing an IUCD develop a true infective endometritis, probably due to an ascending infection, although this has become less common with the change from inert plastic devices to those covered with copper. Infection results in a diffuse endometrial inflammation superimposed on the local inflammatory response evoked by the device acting as an irritative foreign body. Recognition of a complicating endometrial infection depends, therefore, upon the finding of an inflammatory cell infiltrate that extends beyond the contact sites. To establish this diagnosis in a biopsy specimen requires, therefore, that endometrial fragments must be found that, while inflamed, show no evidence of being part of the contact site – a task that is not always easy and sometimes impossible.

In relatively mild cases of endometrial infection the salient feature is the presence of aggregates of polymorphonuclear leucocytes within, and entirely limited to, glandular lumina over large areas of the endometrium (Fig. 6.11). It is

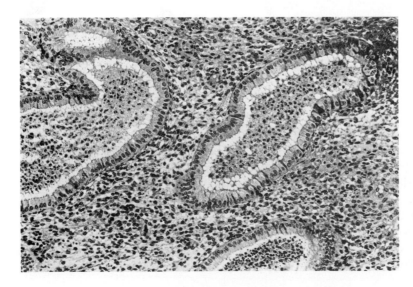

Figure 6.11 Infection of the uterine cavity in a intrauterine contraceptive device user. The glands, which are in the mid-secretory phase, are filled by a polymorphonuclear leucocyte exudate. Haematoxylin and eosin.

unusual for every gland to be affected and, indeed, it is more common to find some variation both in the number of glands affected in a given area and in the degree of involvement. There is usually little or no disturbance of endometrial cyclical maturation with inflammation of this severity and the appearance may suggest a diagnosis of early tuberculosis (Chapter 7).

Distinction from tuberculosis is usually possible if all the other IUCD-related changes in the endometrial biopsy are taken into account, but in occasional cases of real doubt it may prove necessary to suggest bacteriological cultures.

With more severe infections, the intraglandular polymorphonuclear leucocyte exudate in areas away from the contact site is associated with a diffuse lymphoplasmacytic infiltrate of the stroma (Fig. 6.12), the plasma cell component of which is sometimes concentrated around the glands. Infections of this severity tend to inhibit hormone receptor synthesis and hence normal cyclical endometrial maturation is usually disturbed (Fig. 6.13). Marked reactive cytological atypia is also a feature commonly found in severe infections (Fig. 7.3),

while biopsies from these patients may also include fragments of heavily inflamed myometrium. Severe infections are most commonly encountered in women wearing an inert plastic device and are thus, in our experience, becoming less frequent as inert devices are progressively replaced by less infection-prone copper-coated varieties.

Most endometrial infections complicating IUCD usage are polymicrobial in nature and the inflammatory changes evoked are entirely non-specific. In rare instances, however, an actinomycotic infection occurs, a condition associated with a significant risk of pelvic infection and portal pyaemia (Schiffer *et al.*, 1975; Lomax *et al.*, 1976; Witwer *et al.*, 1977; Schmidt *et al.*, 1980). Actinomycotic pyometra has also been described in a woman 13 years after the menopause (Kriplani *et al.*, 1994). The organisms may be identified in the superficial layers of the endometrium and are accompanied by a polymorphonuclear leucocyte infiltrate. The colonies (sulphur granules) form stellate basophilic structures in haematoxylin and eosin stained sections.

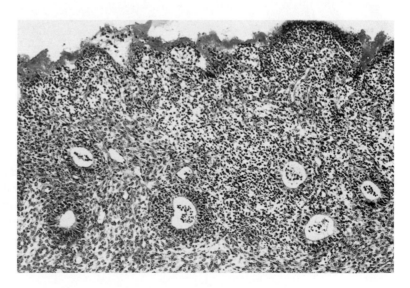

Figure 6.12 Severe, non-specific, chronic inflammation in the endometrium of an intrauterine contraceptive device user. A predominantly round cell population infiltrates the stroma and the epithelium of the glands. Haematoxylin and eosin.

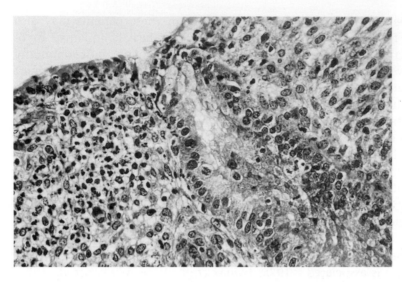

Figure 6.13 Severe, non-specific, chronic inflammation in the endometrium of an intrauterine contraceptive device wearer, 24th day of the cycle in a woman with a regular 28-day cycle. Secretory changes are absent and mitotic activity is present in the glandular epithelium. Haematoxylin and eosin.

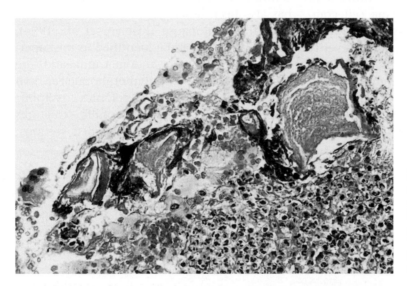

Figure 6.14 The debris from the surface of an intrauterine contraceptive device as it appears in an endometrial curetting: the so-called 'pseudo-sulphur' granules. These may bear a resemblance to bacterial colonies. Haematoxylin and eosin.

With Gram stain, the peripheral margins of the colony are Gram negative while the colony is Gram positive.

Correct identification of *Actinomyces* in an endometrial biopsy is important and can present difficulties for the typical appearances may be mimicked by other intrauterine organisms and by debris (Luff *et al.*, 1978; Jones *et al.*, 1979; Duguid *et al.*, 1980). It is only possible to make an accurate diagnosis of *Actinomyces* if culture or immunohistochemical techniques are employed (Spence *et al.*, 1978; Fry *et al.*, 1980). However, even if the presence of *Actinomyces* is proven, a diagnosis of actinomycotic endometritis is not justified unless there is a definite tissue response to the organism, which can be present as only a commensal. A further factor complicating the diagnosis of actinomycosis in IUCD users is the presence of 'pseudo-sulphur granules' (O'Brien *et al.*, 1981). These are fragments of debris from the surface of the device which form amorphous eosinophilic or basophilic aggregates that bear some resemblance to the sulphur granules found in actinomycotic abscesses (Fig. 6.14). Careful histological examination and the employment of a Gram stain usually reveal the true nature of this material, which is composed of a mixture of calcium carbonate and apatite in an organic matrix (Patai *et al.*, 1998).

6.3 IUCD USE AND MALIGNANT CHANGE IN THE ENDOMETRIUM

An endometrial carcinoma may, by chance, be identified in an endometrial biopsy from an IUCD-wearer but there is some evidence that IUCD use protects against the development of endometrial carcinoma (Hill *et al.*, 1997). The reason for this protective effect is uncertain, particularly as it applies to inert and copper-containing device users and is independent of duration of use.

REFERENCES

Buckley, C.H. (1995) Pathology of contraception and of hormonal therapy. In: Fox, H. (ed.), *Haines and Taylor Obstetrical and Gynaecological Pathology,* 4th edn. Edinburgh: Churchill Livingstone, 1137–82.

Critchley, H.O.D., Wang, H., Jones, R.L. *et al.* (1998) Morphological and functional features of endometrial decidualization following long-term intrauterine levonorgestrel delivery. *Hum. Reprod.* **13**, 1218–24.

Duguid, H.L., Parratt, D., Traynor, R. (1980) Actinomyces-like organisms in cervical smears from women using intrauterine contraceptive devices. *BMJ* **281**, 534–7.

Fox, H., Buckley, C.H. (1983) *Atlas of Gynaecological Pathology.* Lancaster: M.T.P. Press, 159–62.

Fry, R., Linder, A.M., Bull, M.M. (1980) Actinomyces-like organisms in cervicovaginal smears. *S. Afr. Med. J.* **57**, 1041–3.

Hill, D.A., Weiss, N.S., Voigt, L.F., Beresford, S.A. (1997) Endometrial cancer in relation to intra-uterine device use. *Int. J. Cancer* **70**, 278–81.

Jones, M.C., Buschmann, B.O., Dowling, E.A., Pollock, H.M. (1979) The prevalence of actinomycetes-like organisms found in cervico-vaginal smears of 300 IUD wearers. *Acta Cytol.* **23**, 282–6.

Kriplani, A., Buckshee, K., Relan, S., Kapila, K. (1994) 'Forgotten' intrauterine device leading to actinomycotic pyometra – 13 years after menopause. *Eur. J. Obstet. Gynecol. Reprod. Biol.* **15**, 215–16.

Lomax, C.W., Harbert Jr, E.M., Thornton Jr, W.N. (1976) Actinomycosis of the female genital tract. *Obstet. Gynecol.* **48**, 341–6.

Luff, R.D., Gupta, P.K., Spence, M.R., Frost, J.K. (1978) Pelvic actinomycosis and the intra-uterine contraceptive device: a cyto-histomorphologic study. *Am. J. Clin. Path.* **69**, 581–6.

O'Brien, P.K., Roth-Moyo, L.A., Davis, B.A. (1981) Pseudo-sulfur granules associated with intrauterine contraceptive devices. *Am. J. Clin. Path.* **75**, 822–5.

Patai, K., Berenyi, M., Sipos, M., Noszal, B. (1998) Characterization of calcified deposits on contraceptive intrauterine devices. *Contraception* **58**, 305–8.

Schiffer, M.A., Elguezabal, A., Sultana, M., Allen, A.C. (1975) Actinomycosis infections associated with intrauterine contraceptive devices. *Obstet. Gynecol.* **45**, 67–72.

Schmidt, W.A., Bedrossian, C.W.M., Ali, V., Webb, J.A., Bastian, F.O. (1980) Actinomycosis and intrauterine contraceptive devices: the clinicopathologic entity. *Diagn. Gynecol. Obstet.* **2**, 165–77.

Silverberg, S.G., Haukkamaa, M., Arko, H., Nilsson, C.G., Luukkainen, T. (1986) Endometrial morphology during long-term use of Levonorgestrel-releasing intrauterine devices. *Int. J. Gynecol. Pathol.* **5**, 235–41.

Spence, M.R., Gupta, P.K., Frost, J.K., King, T.M. (1978) Cytologic detection and clinical significance of *Actinomyces israelii* in women using intrauterine contraceptive devices. *Am. J. Obstet. Gynecol.* **131**, 295–8.

Tindall, V.R. (1987) *Jeffcoate's Principles of Gynaecology.* London: Butterworths, 608.

Wang, I.Y., Russell, P., Fraser, I.S. (1995) Endometrial morphometry in users of intrauterine contraceptive devices and women with ovulatory dysfunctional uterine bleeding: a comparison with normal endometrium. *Contraception* **51**, 243–8.

Witwer, M.W., Farmer, M.F., Wand, J.S., Solomon, L.S. (1977) Extensive actinomycosis associated with an intrauterine contraceptive device. *Am. J. Obstet. Gynecol.* **128**, 913–14.

7 Inflammation of the endometrium

Endometrial inflammation may be of infective or non-infective origin and is recognized, histologically, by the identification of an abnormal pattern of inflammatory cell infiltrate and by disturbances in the normal processes of endometrial growth and maturation. The diagnosis of endometritis depends entirely upon such histopathological criteria because the clinical correlates of endometrial inflammation are both variable and inconsistent.

The diagnosis of an endometritis is complicated by the fact that many of the features that, in other tissues, indicate the presence of an inflammatory process are found in the normal endometrium. Thus, for example, a polymorphonuclear leucocytic infiltrate, interstitial haemorrhage and tissue necrosis accompany menstruation or hormone withdrawal bleeding, while tissue regeneration occurs not only following inflammation but also in the immediate post-menstrual phase. Furthermore, lymphocytes, lymphoid aggregates and lymphoid follicles with germinal centres, which, in association with macrophages, are regarded elsewhere in the body as indicators of chronic inflammation all occur in the normal endometrium (Payan et al., 1964; Sen and Fox, 1967). Other, more precise, criteria are therefore needed for the diagnosis of inflammation in the endometrium and paramount among these are the finding of plasma cells and eosinophils, both of which are absent from the normal endometrium (Hendrickson and Kempson, 1980). It is important to distinguish an inflammatory cell infiltrate alone, from foci of haemopoiesis, which, although rare, may develop in the endometrium in the presence of inflammation (Sirgi et al., 1994).

The reported incidence of chronic endometritis ranges from 2.8 per cent (Vasudeva et al., 1972) to 19.2 per cent (Farooki, 1967) in series that included biopsy, curettage and hysterectomy specimens and samples from non-pregnant, post-miscarriage and postpartum patients.

Excluding post-miscarriage and postpartum material, the incidence in our practice of active, chronic endometritis is 3.08 per cent in biopsy material, which is much lower than the 10.86 per cent recorded for hysterectomy specimens in the same hospital. This suggests that there may be a sampling error when only small biopsies are examined or, alternatively, that superficial specimens fail to detect inflammation in the deeper parts of the functionalis or in the basalis (Kitching, 1984).

Cases of endometrial inflammation are usually classified into those in which the pathological features are non-specific and those in which the findings are sufficiently typical as to suggest a specific aetiological factor.

7.1 NON-SPECIFIC ENDOMETRITIS

The term 'non-specific endometritis' refers to the presence within the endometrium of a range of inflammatory changes that offer little or no clue to their cause. However, it is customary to distinguish pathologically between the acute and chronic phases of the disorder and between infective and non-infective causes, although the clinical correlates are rarely so clearly defined and, in the absence of microbiological studies, it is impossible to distinguish infective from non-infective endometritis. Further, many conditions in which the cause may initially be non-infective, such as the inflammation which accompanies tissue breakdown, may, if they persist, predispose to the establishment of non-specific infection. The distinction between the acute and chronic phases may also become blurred as the two often have a common origin and similar clinico-pathological correlates (Buckley, 1995).

7.1.1 The aetiology and clinical correlates of non-specific endometritis

Non-specific endometrial inflammation occurs under a variety of conditions, many of which have in common one or more of the following factors: disruption of the cervical mucous barrier, intrauterine stasis or necrosis, interruption of regular endometrial shedding and hindrance to natural drainage. Disruption of the cervical mucous barrier occurs when an organism has the capacity to penetrate the mucus, when there is cervical infection or surgery (Rotterdam, 1978; Greenwood and Moran, 1981), when the tail of an IUCD protrudes through the external os (see Chapter 6) and, during menstruation (Korn *et al.*, 1998). Non-specific endometritis has also been reported in steroid contraceptive users (Ness *et al.*, 1997) and in patients with immunological impairment, such as that which occurs in patients with HIV infection, where it is a predominantly plasma cell endometritis (Kerr-Layton *et al.*, 1998). A plasma cell endometritis is also encountered in women who have bacterial vaginosis (Korn *et al.*, 1995).

Intrauterine necrosis may occur under a wide variety of circumstances, for example, on the tip of a polyp or submucous leiomyoma, during a spontaneous miscarriage, around an IUCD, after miscarriage or in the postpartum state, or in patients with an intrauterine neoplasm (where it may also be part of an immunological response) or dysfunctional uterine haemorrhage. Intrauterine stasis may also occur in many of the preceding circumstances but more typically results from stenosis of the cervix or distortion of the cavity by a space-occupying lesion.

Pregnancy may be associated with an acute or chronic inflammatory cell infiltrate (see below) and low birth weight is more common in women that subsequently develop puerperal infection (Bergstrom and Libombo, 1995), possibly owing to a subclinical antenatal intrauterine infection, predisposing to both adverse fetal and maternal outcomes of pregnancy.

Following radiotherapy to the genital tract a non-specific or, less commonly, a granulomatous

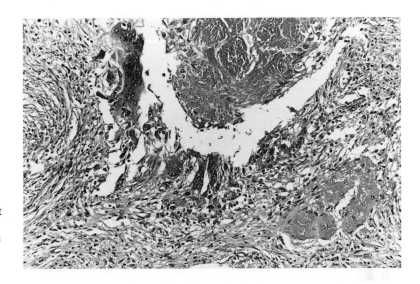

Figure 7.1 A granulomatous response seen at the site of a recent endometrial resection. A layer of foreign-body type giant cells lines a cavity in which there is coagulated tissue. Haematoxylin and eosin.

inflammation may occur and granulomas, which may be of foreign body type, may occur in response to the presence of necrotic myometrium (Silvernagel *et al.*, 1997; Colgan *et al.*, 1999) following endometrial ablation (Fig. 7.1). On rare occasions, there may be a systemic cause for a granulomatous lesion (see below).

In patients with acute endometritis, there is commonly an immediately recognizable predisposing factor such as pregnancy, miscarriage, parturition or a recent surgical procedure in the cervix or corpus uteri. In patients with chronic inflammation of the endometrium, there are, in contrast, rarely any identifiable causes and the patient can be asymptomatic or may present with abnormal uterine bleeding, abdominal pain, infertility or vaginal discharge.

Recurrent endometrial infections associated with postmenopausal bleeding may also be a feature of the postmenopausal state, as secretory immunoglobulin A may be reduced in postmenopausal women because of oestrogen deficiency (Barrington *et al.*, 1994).

7.1.2 The diagnosis of non-specific endometritis

The morphological response of the endometrium to inflammatory agents is of limited range and, strictly speaking, a diagnosis of infection should be made only when both an infecting organism and a morphological response can be identified. However, in practice, microbiological studies are not always performed and the finding of an inflammatory process in the endometrium should always raise the suspicion that it may be of an infective origin.

Mild acute inflammation (Fig. 7.2) is often limited to the superficial layers of the endometrium and is recognized by the presence of a polymorphonuclear leucocytic infiltrate within the glands and in the endometrial stroma. There may be a minor degree of stromal necrosis, together with epithelial disruption on the endometrial surface and in the superficial parts of the glands. Inflammation of this degree can occur at any stage of the endometrial cycle and in the non-cycling endometrium and may be diffuse and widespread or focal and local: it

93

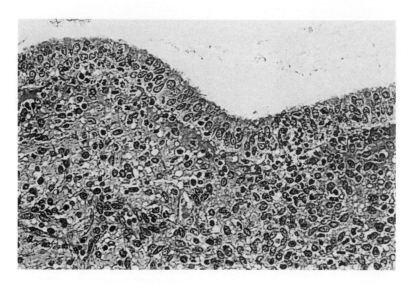

Figure 7.2 Mild acute, non-specific endometritis. The surface epithelium and underlying stroma contains a scanty infiltrate of polymorphonuclear leucocytes. The aetiology in this case was unknown. Haematoxylin and eosin.

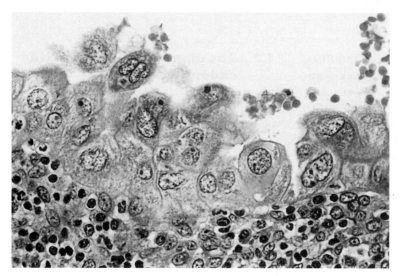

Figure 7.3 Pyometra. The surface epithelium of the endometrium in a 72-year-old woman who had a pyometra with utero-colonic fistula associated with diverticular disease of the large bowel. The epithelial cells are enlarged, the nuclei are pleomorphic and have lost their polarity: one nucleus contains a nucleolus, one cell is binucleate and nuclear chromatin is coarse. Haematoxylin and eosin.

must be distinguished from the physiological infiltrate of normal menstruation and the scanty, multifocal aggregates of polymorphonuclear leucocytes, which are a normal concomitant of decidual remodelling in early pregnancy.

When the inflammatory process is severe, the infiltrate extends through the full thickness of the endometrium to involve the basalis. There is almost invariably a non-specific reactive change in the endometrial epithelium, characterized by variation in cell size, nuclear enlargement and pleomorphism, formation of nucleoli and mitotic activity (Fig. 7.3). The more severe the inflammation, the more likely it is to disturb the normal process of endometrial maturation, although this is a more common feature of the chronically inflamed endometrium (see below).

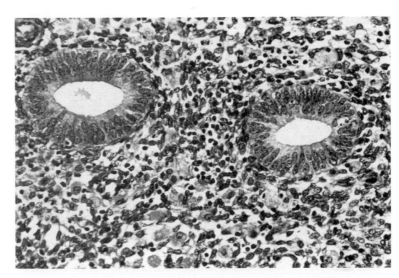

Figure 7.4 Non-specific chronic endometritis. The basalis of a patient who presented with secondary infertility. The stroma is heavily infiltrated by histiocytes and lymphocytes. A similar appearance is sometimes seen in women with polymenorrhoea. Haematoxylin and eosin.

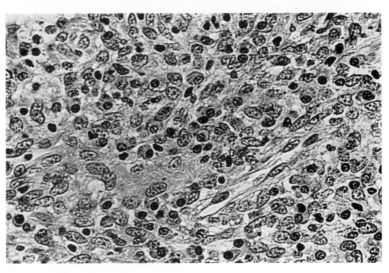

Figure 7.5 Non-specific active chronic endometritis, 3 months postpartum, in a patient with irregular and excessive bleeding. The stroma is heavily infiltrated by plasma cells and occasional lymphocytes. An inflammatory infiltrate so long after delivery is abnormal. Haematoxylin and eosin.

Chronic non-granulomatous inflammation of the endometrium (Fig. 7.4) is recognized by those features that in other tissues also constitute the hallmarks of chronic inflammation, these being the presence of a cellular infiltrate containing plasma cells, lymphocytes, macrophages (which may contain haemosiderin), occasional polymorphonuclear leucocytes and eosinophils. In the active chronic phase (Fig. 7.5), it is usual to identify polymorphonuclear leucocytes and plasma cells and, in some instances, the pattern may be characterized by an accumulation of polymorphonuclear leucocytes in the glands and a plasma cell infiltrate that is concentrated in the periglandular stroma (Fig. 7.6). Sometimes, there is a conspicuous infiltrate in the superficial layers of the functionalis (Fig. 7.7). More commonly, however, even in moderately severe, active chronic inflammation, plasma

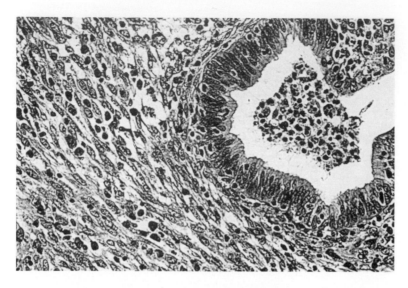

Figure 7.6 Non-specific endometritis. The inflammatory infiltrate is characterized by stromal plasma cells and lymphocytes, intraglandular polymorphonuclear leucocytes and histiocytes. Haematoxylin and eosin.

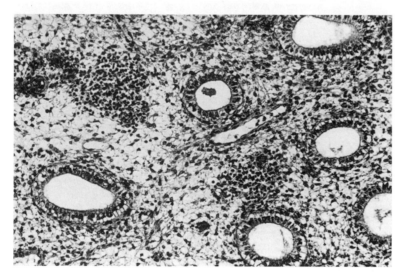

Figure 7.7 Non-specific active chronic endometritis. Aggregates of lymphocytes and plasma cells in the functionalis of an endometrium from a patient whose intrauterine contraceptive device had been removed 17 days previously because of pelvic pain and vaginal discharge. Haematoxylin and eosin.

cells are relatively few in number and are most easily identified in the endometrium at the junction of the basalis and functionalis; they may therefore be overlooked in a superficial biopsy. In the puerperium, a similar infiltrate of plasma cells, lymphocytes and macrophages can be regarded as physiological (Hendrickson and Kempson, 1980), although its persistence beyond the fourth week of the puerperium is abnormal and usually associated with persistent bleeding, retained products of conception or infection. The endometrium of a woman with perimenopausal bleeding also often contains a non-specific inflammatory cell infiltrate and in such cases, the inflammation may be the consequence of the repeated or persistent breakdown of tissue rather than its cause.

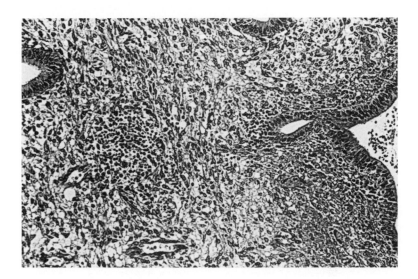

Figure 7.8 Chronic non-specific endometritis. Lymphocytic aggregates in the functionalis in an asymptomatic patient. The biopsy was taken routinely prior to sterilization. Haematoxylin and eosin.

In a less active chronic endometritis, the inflammatory cell infiltrate may be almost entirely lymphocytic (Fig. 7.8) and it is this form that is most difficult both to identify and to differentiate from the normal lymphocytic complement. Indeed, many regard the presence of eosinophils or plasma cells as a prerequisite for the diagnosis of chronic endometritis (Brudenell, 1955; Cadena *et al.*, 1973) and will not entertain this diagnosis in their absence. In this respect, the use of immunohistochemical techniques (Crum *et al.*, 1983) for the identification of immunoglobulins may prove helpful in the recognition of small numbers of plasma cells, particularly if the tissues are first trypsinized. Others have found Unna–Pappenheim stained sections useful for the same purpose (Horton and Wilkes, 1976). Certainly, a diagnosis based upon the recognition of an increased number of lymphocytes and the occurrence of more than the usual number of lymphoid aggregates or lymphoid follicles is often more subjective than objective, and genuine cases of chronic inflammation are undoubtedly overlooked in the anxiety not to succumb to overdiagnosis. We would regard as suspicious those

cases in which the lymphoid aggregates or follicles occur in the functional layers of the endometrium, or when patchy lymphocytic infiltrates are present (Fig. 7.9).

A dense chronic inflammation must be distinguished from the monotonous infiltrate of a leukaemia, or lymphoma and from an endometrial stromal sarcoma (see Chapters 11 and 12).

Fibrosis and the formation of non-specific granulation tissue are distinctly uncommon in the endometrium, even in long established disease (Hendrickson and Kempson, 1980). However, these may sometimes be found when an IUCD is present (Fig. 6.4) or when there has been a particularly destructive inflammation, such as that which can complicate pregnancy or a miscarriage, or occur in a polypoidal leiomyoma or endometrial polyp that has undergone torsion or prolonged ischaemia. The possibility that non-specific granulation tissue in an endometrial biopsy may have come from the cervix should always be considered.

In both severe acute and chronic inflammation the endometrium is often poorly developed. It is shallow, the glands are tubular and inactive,

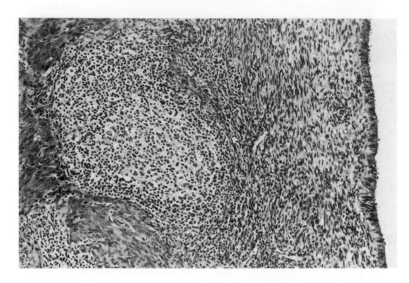

Figure 7.9 Chronic non-specific endometritis. Lymphoid follicles are seen in the basalis and superficial myometrium in a hysterectomy specimen. There was cervical stenosis and the patient had had a pyometra that had been treated by antibiotics for several weeks prior to surgery. Haematoxylin and eosin.

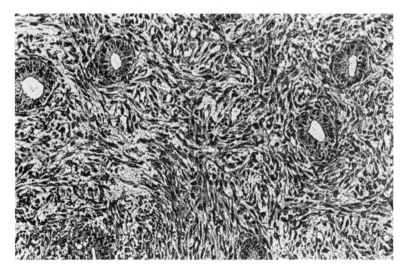

Figure 7.10 Non-specific chronic endometritis. This endometrium, from a patient who had worn an inert intrauterine contraceptive device, has a rather fibrous stroma in which there is a scanty lymphocytic infiltrate: the glands are poorly responsive. Haematoxylin and eosin.

or only weakly proliferative and their lining epithelium may show severe, non-specific reactive changes. The cells become stratified, tend to have an increased nucleocytoplasmic ratio and can show some loss of nuclear polarity with nuclear pleomorphism and the formation of nucleoli: cytoplasmic vacuolation may be prominent. Indeed, the atypia of these cells can be so marked as to mimic a neoplastic process. The stroma may be unusually compact (Fig. 7.10) and have a rather fibrotic appearance, while the stromal cells often palisade around the glands to create a 'pinwheel' effect (Kurman, 1982). The poor or negligible response to hormonal stimulation that occurs in the severely inflamed endometrium (van Bogaert *et al.*, 1978) is the consequence of a failure of hormone receptor formation. It is difficult or impossible, therefore, in these samples to assess the patient's hormonal status.

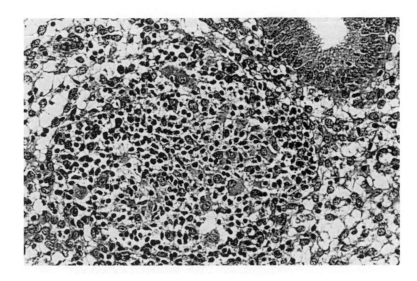

Figure 7.11 Non-tuberculous granulomatous endometritis. The centre of the field is occupied by a well-formed foreign-body type granuloma. Microbiological studies were negative and no foreign material was identified. The cause remains unknown. Haematoxylin and eosin.

We have only rarely encountered non-specific granulomatous endometritis, usually in the presence of an IUCD, following radiotherapy for carcinoma of the cervix, following endometrial resection (Fig. 7.1) or in response to keratin from metaplastic foci or carcinoma. The granulomas tend to be very poorly formed and consist of no more than an aggregate of macrophages or foreign body giant cells (Fig. 7.11).

7.1.2 Morphologically distinct forms of non-specific chronic endometritis

7.1.2.1 Histiocytic endometritis
The end stage of a pyometra or haematometra may be recognized by the presence of a histiocytic endometritis (Buckley and Fox, 1980), a lesion also known as xanthogranulomatous endometritis. The endometrium is replaced or heavily infiltrated by foamy, lipid-containing histiocytes intermingled with macrophage giant cells, in which there may be cholesterol clefts, plasma cells, lymphocytes and occasional polymorphonuclear leucocytes (Fig. 7.12). The histiocytes stain positively with Sudan Black and Oil Red-O and are periodic acid–Schiff reagent (PAS), diastase resistant positive. The haemosiderin content in the histiocytes is variable and dependent upon the degree of preceding haemorrhage. The absence of Michaelis–Gutmann bodies distinguishes the condition from malakoplakia. A similar, though less intense histiocytic infiltrate is seen in a wide variety of other conditions such as the post-miscarriage or post-delivery endometrium (Fig. 7.13) or in association with chronic cervical stenosis, endometrial hyperplasia or carcinoma (Fig. 10.4).

7.1.2.2 Malakoplakia
Malakoplakia is a histological expression of an abnormal immunological response to bacteria. The histological appearance of endometrial malakoplakia is similar to that of histiocytic endometritis. The stroma of the endometrium is heavily infiltrated, and may be entirely replaced, over large areas, by sheets of foamy histiocytes (von Hansemann's histiocytes) that differ in appearance from those seen in histiocytic endometritis only by the presence of Michaelis–Gutmann bodies (Fig. 7.14).

99

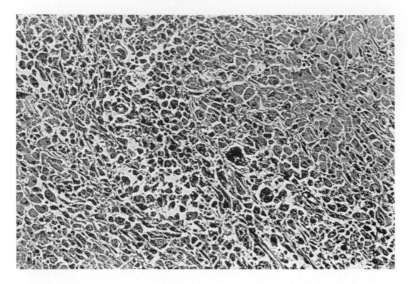

Figure 7.12 Histiocytic (xanthogranulomatous) endometritis. The endometrium is almost entirely replaced by sheets of histiocytes, many of which contain haemosiderin: a lymphocytic infiltrate is also present. In this case, the condition represents the end stage of a haematometra. Haematoxylin and eosin.

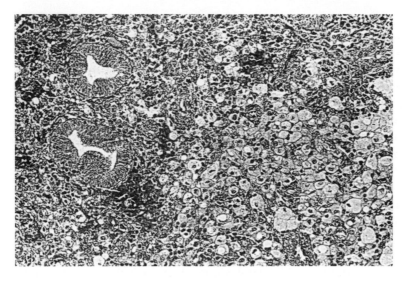

Figure 7.13 Chronic endometritis characterized by histiocytic infiltration. The specimen was taken 6 weeks postpartum from a woman who complained of continued bleeding: note that the glands (to the left) show no evidence of cyclical changes. Haematoxylin and eosin.

These are small, round, laminated calcispherites, which are found not only in the cytoplasm of the histiocytes but also extracellularly. They contain calcium, which can be identified using von Kossa's stain: they are also PAS positive and contain lysozyme (Molnar and Poliak, 1983). A mixed inflammatory infiltrate of plasma cells, polymorphonuclear leucocytes and lymphocytes is usually mixed with the histiocytes.

Admixed bacteria, most commonly *Escherichia coli*, which are retained within the phagolysosomes of the macrophages are not digested and can be identified, by light and electron microscopy, in the cytoplasm of the histiocytes in extracellular sites.

Clinically, malakoplakia is a rare cause of postmenopausal bleeding (Thomas *et al.*, 1978; Molnar and Poliak, 1983; Chadha *et al.*, 1985).

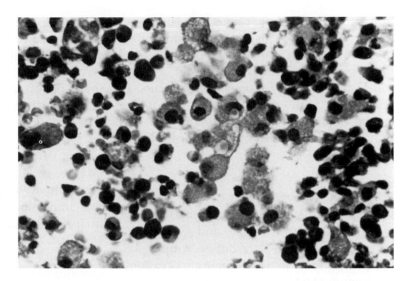

Figure 7.14 Malakoplakia. The specimen consists almost entirely of histiocytes, lymphocytes and plasma cells. In the centre of the field, there are several histiocytes in which spherical intracytoplasmic inclusions, Michaelis–Gutmann bodies, can be seen. Haematoxylin and eosin.

7.1.2.3 *Focal necrotizing endometritis*

In a small group of premenopausal women with irregular vaginal bleeding, there may be patchy, focal inflammation characterized by the presence of lymphocytes, with a variable number of neutrophil polymorphonucleocytes, centred on individual endometrial glands (Bennett *et al.*, 1999). The lesions are usually scanty and can be easily overlooked. Plasma cells are not seen. There may be mild reactive changes in the gland epithelium and the affected stroma may contain spindle cells. In addition, in some cases, there are lymphoid aggregates, some of which contain macrophages and polymorphs, adjacent to the spiral arteries or beneath the surface epithelium. Some of these women will have received exogenous hormone therapy, most commonly Provera, but no consistent aetiological factor has been identified. One explanation may be that it is a response to the bleeding rather than its cause. The possibility of progression is suggested by a case in which, in a subsequent hysterectomy, the lesions were more widespread, the inflammatory infiltrate more severe and the glands dilated; the glandular lumina contained inflammatory cells and cellular debris.

7.2 SPECIFIC FORMS OF ENDOMETRITIS

7.2.1 **Viral infections**

7.2.1.1 *Herpes virus hominis*

Herpetic endometritis is characterized by the presence of enlarged epithelial nuclei of ground-glass appearance, beading of the nuclear membranes and epithelial multinucleation. Eosinophilic intranuclear viral inclusions with clear haloes can be seen in both stromal and epithelial cells in haematoxylin and eosin stained sections (Abraham, 1978; Schneider *et al.*, 1982); their presence is confirmed by either electron microscopy or immunohistochemical techniques. There may also be endometrial necrosis and a lymphocytic infiltrate. In the absence of virological investigations, difficulties have been reported in distinguishing intranuclear pseudoinclusions in a patient with

101

Arias-Stella change from those caused by herpes (Dardi *et al.*, 1982). This is an important distinction as herpetic endometritis has been described in the postpartum period (Hollier *et al.*, 1997).

Infection of the endometrium occurs in association with herpetic infection of the cervix, vagina and vulva (Goldman, 1970) and immunosuppression may predispose to its development.

7.2.1.2 *Cytomegalovirus*

Cytomegalovirus infection of the endometrium is rare (Weller, 1971; Dehner and Askin, 1975) and is characterized by a diffuse lymphoplasmacytic infiltrate in which there are occasional eosinophils (McCracken *et al.*, 1974) and lymphoid follicles with poorly formed germinal centres (Wenkebach and Curry, 1976). In the nuclei of both stromal and glandular epithelial cells, there are large amphophilic to basophilic inclusions measuring $20–25\,\mu m$ in diameter; these are separated from the nuclear membrane by a clear space traversed by fine chromatin strands. The same cells also contain small, basophilic, PAS-positive cytoplasmic inclusions.

An Arias-Stella reaction with marked nuclear enlargement may be confused histologically with cytomegalovirus infection (Kurman, 1982), but the recognition of pregnancy-type hypersecretory endometrium throughout the biopsy specimen should make it possible to avoid this diagnostic error.

7.2.2 **Chlamydial infections**

The intensity of the inflammatory infiltrate in chlamydial endometritis is variable. In the acute phase there may be a non-specific, polymorphonuclear leucocyte infiltrate of such severity that it suggests a pyogenic infection, while in the chronic phase the infiltrate is predominantly plasmalymphocytic (Schachter, 1978a–c; Paukku *et al.*, 1999) and may include

lymphoid aggregates and follicles. Stromal necrosis is a common finding and this may be so severe that it mimics menstrual breakdown (Winkler *et al.*, 1984). As with other severe inflammatory processes, reactive atypia of the endometrial epithelium is commonly seen.

Typical *Chlamydia trachomatis* inclusion bodies have been demonstrated in the epithelial cells of patients with chlamydial endometritis (Mårdh *et al.*, 1981; Ingerslev *et al.*, 1982; Weström, 1982) but these are difficult, if not impossible, to detect with confidence in haematoxylin and eosin stained sections. However, they can be seen a little more easily in Giemsa stained material and identified specifically using immunohistochemical techniques (Winkler *et al.*, 1984). Using a specific antibody and an immunoperoxidase technique, staining is focal and localized to the epithelial cells, where it appears as dark-brown stippling within well circumscribed rounded, supranuclear, intracytoplasmic vacuoles. These positive areas correspond in haematoxylin and eosin stained sections to intracytoplasmic vacuoles filled with pale staining, faintly basophilic, particles. Positive granules are also seen in mucus, within polymorphonuclear leucocytes and on the surface epithelium.

Chlamydial infection has been implicated not only as a cause of acute and chronic endometritis but also as a possible aetiological factor in otherwise unexplained infertility (Gump *et al.*, 1981; Mårdh *et al.*, 1981; Ingerslev *et al.*, 1982; Wølner-Hanssen *et al.*, 1982). It is a recognized cause of menometrorrhagia, intermenstrual bleeding, pelvic pain and yellow–white vaginal discharge (Gump *et al.*, 1981; Mårdh *et al.*, 1981; Winkler *et al.*, 1984).

7.2.3 **Bacterial infections**
7.2.3.1 *Tuberculosis*

This endometrial disease is now rather uncommon in most Western countries but still occurs with considerable frequency in many countries of the developing world. Tuberculosis of the endometrium is generally most common in the reproductive years, reaching a peak in the third and fourth decades (Schaefer *et al.*, 1972) and there appears to be a trend in recent years for the disease to affect a slightly older age group (Hutchins, 1977), with a mean of 42 years. During the reproductive years it is diagnosed most commonly during the investigation of infertility and presents less commonly as amenorrhoea, pelvic pain or heavy and irregular menses (Sutherland, 1949; Schaefer, 1970; Bazaz-Malik *et al.*, 1983). On very rare occasions, normal intrauterine pregnancy and tuberculous endometritis have been found to coexist (Yip *et al.*, 1999). After the menopause, tuberculous endometritis is most likely to present as abnormal uterine bleeding in a parous patient (Schaefer *et al.*, 1972).

Infection of the endometrium usually occurs by direct transluminal spread from the Fallopian tube to the superficial layers of the functionalis and, unless ovulation and hence menstruation ceases, the infected endometrium will be shed monthly, thus allowing only

22–23 days for the establishment of infection. It is therefore uncommon, in endometrial biopsies, to see well-established tuberculoid granulomas, which typically take a minimum of 15 days to form (Rotterdam, 1978). Biopsies taken in the premenstrual phase have the greatest chance of providing a positive morphological diagnosis as the granulomas have had the longest time to develop (Fig. 7.15). However, despite regular shedding of the endometrium, infection is known to affect the basalis in up to 40 per cent of cases (Nogales-Ortiz *et al.*, 1979) and tuberculosis of the endometrium can develop, probably from this source but possibly from haematogenous spread, even after removal of the Fallopian tubes.

The most typical findings in tuberculosis occur in the regularly menstruating woman. Small, isolated, frequently sparse, ill-formed granulomas are scattered throughout the functionalis. They consist of an aggregate of epithelioid macrophages surrounded by a cuff of lymphocytes (Govan, 1962) and do not often contain giant cells (Fig. 7.16). Caseation is rarely observed in these granulomas (Haines and Stallworthy, 1952) except after the

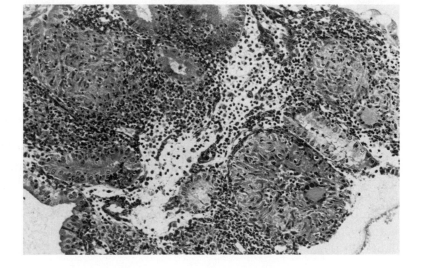

Figure 7.15 Tuberculous endometritis. A curettage sample containing particularly well-developed tuberculous granulomas: Langerhans giant cells are prominent and there is a marked lymphocytic infiltrate. Haematoxylin and eosin.

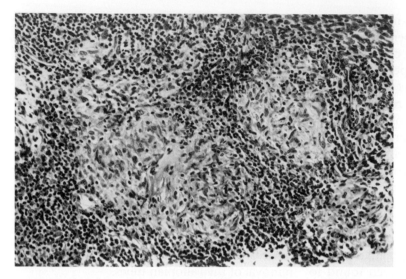

Figure 7.16 Tuberculous endometritis. The ill-formed granulomas that are more typical of tuberculosis in the endometrium: epithelioid macrophages form aggregates and have a cuff of lymphocytes but there is no caseation or giant cell formation. Haematoxylin and eosin.

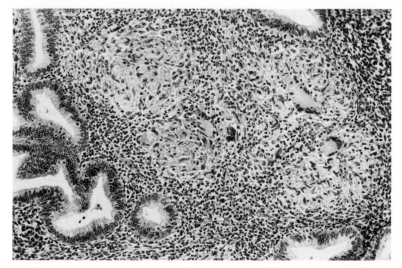

Figure 7.17 Tuberculous endometritis. There are well-formed granulomas in the basalis of this sample. Their presence suggests that shedding of the infected tissue was incomplete in the previous cycle and demonstrates that even in the reproductive years infection is not limited to the functionalis. Haematoxylin and eosin.

menopause, or in the unusual event that the severity of the systemic disease impairs ovulation. Sometimes, however, granulomas in different stages of development coexist, suggesting that complete shedding of the functionalis has not occurred and that some granulomas have persisted from the previous cycle. These are identified by their morphological maturity and by the more frequent presence of giant cells (Fig. 7.17).

Granulomas often lie adjacent to, and bulge into glands and lymphocytes from their peripheral cuff may infiltrate into the glandular epithelium (Fig. 7.18): these individual glands frequently show a lack of secretory response (Nogales-Ortiz *et al.*, 1979). Less commonly, there may be a generalized 'poor secretory' pattern (Govan, 1962) in which the endometrium is oedematous and the stromal cells spindle-shaped and lacking in decidual

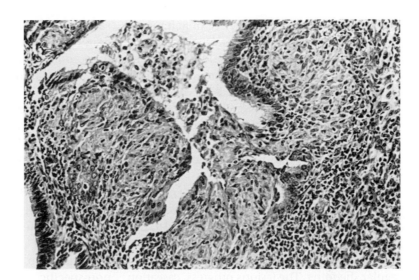

Figure 7.18 Tuberculous endometritis. Granulomas often form on the margins of glands and protrude into their lumens: glandular epithelium may be disrupted by their presence, as in this case. Haematoxylin and eosin.

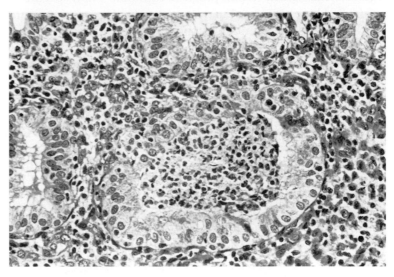

Figure 7.19 Tuberculous endometritis, non-specific appearance. In this area, in the endometrium of a patient with positive cultures for *Mycobacterium tuberculosis*, there is no evidence of granuloma formation but the gland contains polymorphonuclear leucocytes and the surrounding stroma contains lymphocytes. Haematoxylin and eosin.

change. The glandular epithelium is cuboidal and has glassy, translucent cytoplasm with well-defined cell borders. Many glands are empty but in some, there may be a trace of PAS positive material.

Biopsies taken in the early part of the menstrual cycle may fail to show evidence of granulomatous inflammation and reveal only a non-specific picture of intrastromal plasma cells and lymphocytes or intraglandular polymorphonuclear leucocytes, seen particularly in dilated glands in the deeper part of the functionalis (Govan, 1962) (Fig. 7.19). The presence of plasma cells in the endometrium of a woman with tuberculosis may indicate that there is a secondary infection (Govan, 1962). This is clinically important as the patient may develop acute symptoms following curettage.

In some cases, tuberculous granulomas of the endometrium closely resemble those seen in sarcoidosis, even to the presence of Schauman bodies (see below). As a general working rule, however, all granulomas should initially be regarded as tuberculous in nature until proved otherwise. Since acid-/alcohol-fast bacilli are seldom found in Ziehl–Neelsen stained sections of the endometrium, confirmatory cultures should be carried out in all cases in which histological examination raises the possibility of tuberculosis.

After the menopause, tuberculous endometritis is rare – a fact attributed to the diminished vascularity of the tissue (Schaefer *et al.*, 1972) – but when it does occur the infection may become well established because of the lack of regular shedding. The lesions progress, caseation occurs and biopsy material may consist only of confluent caseating granulomas; there may also be calcification. Residual endometrial glands may show non-specific, reactive changes of the type described in active, non-specific, chronic inflammation (see above).

The differential diagnosis of tuberculosis of the endometrium should include infections due to fungi, schistosomiasis (see Section 7.2.6.2), pinworm infestations, *Mycoplasma* infection,

sarcoidosis (see Section 7.2.7), foreign-body granulomas, post-irradiation granulomas and granulomas associated with giant cell vasculitis (see Section 8.6).

7.2.3.2   Gonorrhoea

Neisseria gonorrhoea is one of the relatively few organisms that have the ability to penetrate the cervical mucous barrier (Moyer, 1975) and can induce an acute, though transient, endometritis.

The superficial layers of the endometrium become heavily infiltrated by polymorphonuclear leucocytes and there is a variable degree of superficial necrosis (Fig. 7.20). This organism has also been implicated in chronic, non-specific endometritis. It has been our experience that the endometrial damage is limited to the superficial layers and that this finding was quite unexpected in patients who were asymptomatic but in whom, nevertheless, microbiological studies demonstrated the presence of *N. gonorrhoea*.

7.2.3.3   Neisseria meningitidis

Neisseria meningitidis has been isolated from a patient with endometritis-salpingitis-peritonitis

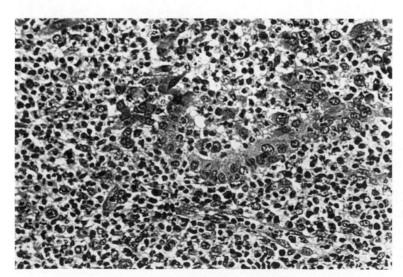

Figure 7.20 Gonococcal endometritis. A severe, necrotizing endometritis from a patient with positive cultures for *Neisseria gonorrhoea*: the gland in the centre of the field contains polymorphonuclear leucocytes and its wall is partly destroyed: the surrounding stroma contains a mixture of plasma cells and lymphocytes. Haematoxylin and eosin.

(Monif, 1981), although no details were given of the histopathological features of the endometrial infection. In practice, the organism is hard to identify and Gram-negative, oxidase-positive diplococci are usually assumed to be gonococci.

7.2.3.4 Actinomyces israelii
Actinomycosis of the endometrium is rare but has been reported in patients wearing an IUCD (see Chapter 6).

7.2.3.5 Treponema pallidum
Syphilitic infection of the endometrium is rare but in a woman with a spontaneous, incomplete first trimester miscarriage, histological examination of the evacuated decidua revealed a plasmalymphocytic infiltrate, tissue necrosis and numerous spirochaetes (Lee *et al.*, 1994).

7.2.4 *Mycoplasma hominis*
Patients in whom cultures for *Mycoplasma hominis* are positive have a subtle endometritis with minute, focal collections of lymphocytes, macrophages, occasional polymorphonuclear leucocytes and rare plasma cells (Horne *et al.*, 1973). The infiltrate tends to lie immediately below the endometrial surface epithelium, adjacent to glands or around spiral arteries.

This organism has been implicated, not always convincingly, as an aetiological factor in infertility, pelvic inflammatory disease (Møller, 1983), post-partum endometritis (Gibbs *et al.*, 1983) and non-specific plasma cell endometritis (Paavonen *et al.*, 1983).

7.2.5 Mycoses
Fungal endometritis is distinctly rare. *Blastomyces dermatitidis* (Hamblen *et al.*, 1935; Farber *et al.*, 1968), *Coccidioides immitus* (Saw *et al.*, 1975; Hart *et al.*, 1976) and *Cryptococcus glabratus* (Plaut, 1950) all elicit a granulomatous inflammatory response with epithelioid

tubercles, which must be distinguished from tuberculosis by using silver stains to demonstrate the fungi. Each organism has distinctive morphological characteristics. *Blastomyces* has a single budding yeast form, *Coccidioides* forms a large spherule in which endospores can be seen and *Cryptococcus* grows as a round or oval budding intracellular or extracellular organism with a thick, mucicarmine-positive gelatinous capsule. Sometimes *Cryptococcus* elicits not a granulomatous but a neutrophil polymorphonuclear leucocytic exudative reaction. *Candida* (Rodriguez *et al.*, 1972) tends to grow over the surface of the endometrium and is associated with a plasmalymphocytic infiltrate in the adjacent stroma. It has an oval yeast-like form and produces pseudohyphae, which can be demonstrated in histological preparations using a PAS stain or a silver technique such as Gomori methenamine silver.

7.2.6 Protozoan infections
7.2.6.1 Toxoplasma gondii
The inflammatory response to *Toxoplasma gondii* is entirely non-specific. The predominantly extracellular organisms are scattered throughout the endometrial stroma and are difficult to detect with light microscopy. The parasites have been identified in the endometrium and menstrual blood of women with habitual miscarriage (Stray-Pedersen and Lorentzen-Styr, 1977).

7.2.6.2 Schistosomiasis
The presence, in the endometrium, of the ova of *Schistosoma haematobium* or, less commonly, *Schistosoma mansoni* (Billy Brissac *et al.*, 1994) elicits a granulomatous inflammation. The ova are surrounded by multinucleated macrophage giant cells, epithelioid cells, eosinophils, lymphocytes and plasma cells, with fibroblasts forming a peripheral zone. Frequently, by the

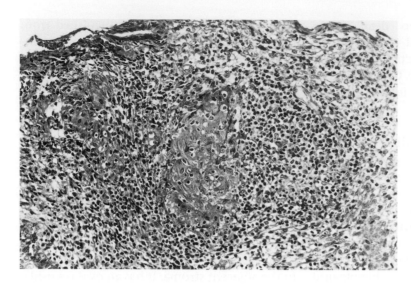

Figure 7.21 Sarcoid. Granulomas were identified in curettings 4 months before the patient developed the typical pulmonary and dermatological lesions of sarcoidosis. Haematoxylin and eosin.

time of diagnosis the ova have calcified and the inflammatory response may be mild (Berry, 1966; Williams, 1967) or occasionally so severe that the consequent fibrosis may result in amenorrhoea (Moukthar, 1966).

7.2.6 Miscellaneous parasitic infestations

Other parasitic infections of the endometrium are exceptionally rare. Pinworms (*Enterobius vermicularis*) produces a granulomatous endometritis characterized by the presence of the female worm in the basalis surrounded by successive zones of coagulative necrosis, eosinophils, epithelioid cells, lymphocytes and fibrous tissue (Schenken and Tamisiea, 1956).

7.2.7 Sarcoidosis

Sarcoidosis has been reported only rarely in the endometrium (Ho, 1979; Pearce and Nolan, 1996; Sherman *et al.*, 1997) and, until recently, it was thought to occur only in women with widespread systemic disease. This is not, however, always the case and it may, rarely, present as postmenopausal bleeding, and be limited to the endometrium (Pearce and Nolan, 1996),

or it may be the presenting sign in women who have, or who subsequently develop sarcoidosis (Elstein *et al.*, 1994) (Fig. 7.21).

REFERENCES

Abraham, A.A. (1978) Herpes virus hominis endometritis in a young woman wearing an intrauterine contraceptive device. *Am. J. Obstet. Gynecol.* **131**, 340–2.

Bazaz-Malik, G., Maheshwari, B., Lal, N. (1983) Tuberculous endometritis: a clinico-pathological study of 1000 cases. *Br. J. Obstet. Gynaecol.* **90**, 84–6.

Barrington, J.W., Papagiannis, A., Roberts, A. (1994) Immunoglobulin deficiency and recurrent postmenopausal endometritis. *Am. J. Obstet. Gynecol.* **171**, 1389–90.

Bennett, A.E., Rathore, S., Rhatigan, R.M. (1999) Focal necrotizing endometritis: a clinicopathologic study of 15 cases. *Int. J. Gynecol. Pathol.* **18**, 220–5.

Bergstrom, S., Libombo, A. (1995) Low birthweight and post partum endometritis–myometritis. *Acta Obstet. Gynecol. Scand.* **74**, 611–13.

Berry, A. (1966) A cytopathological and histopathological study of bilharziasis of the female genital tract. *J. Pathol. Bacteriol.* **91**, 325–38.

Billy Brissac, R., Foucan, L., Gallais, A., Wan Ajouhu, G., Roudier, M. (1994) Genital *Schistosoma mansoni* bilharziasis in women: apropos of 2 cases in Guadeloupe. (Bilharziose genitale de la femme a Schistosoma mansoni: a propos de deux cas en Guadeloupe). *Med. Trop. Mars.* **54**, 345–8.

Brudenell, J.M. (1955) Chronic endometritis and plasma cell infiltration of the endometrium. *J. Obstet. Gynaecol. Br. Emp.* **62**, 269–74.

Buckley, C.H. (1995) Endometrial inflammation. In: Fox, H. (ed.), *Haines and Taylor Obstetrical and Gynaecological Pathology,* 4th edn. Edinburgh: Churchill Livingstone, 405–20.

Buckley, C.H., Fox, H. (1980) Histiocytic endometritis. *Histopathology* **4**, 105–10.

Cadena, D., Cavanzo, F.J., Leone, C.L., Taylor, H.B. (1973) Chronic endometritis: A comparative clinico-pathologic study. *Obstet. Gynecol.* **41**, 733–8.

Chadha, S., Vurevski, S.D., Ten Kate, F.J.W. (1985) Malakoplakia of the endometrium: a rare cause of postmenopausal bleeding. *Eur. J. Obstet. Gynecol. Rep. Biol.* **20**, 181–9.

Colgan, T.J., Shah, R., Leyland, N. (1999) Post-hysteroscopic ablation reaction: a histopathologic study of the effects of electrosurgical ablation. *Int. J. Gynecol. Pathol.* **18**, 325–31.

Crum, C.P., Egawa, K., Fenoglio, C.M., Richart, R.M. (1983) Chronic endometritis: the role of immunohistochemistry in the detection of plasma cells. *Am. J. Obstet. Gynecol.* **147**, 812–15.

Dardi, L.E., Ariano, L., Ariano, M.C., Gould, V.E. (1982) Arias-Stella reaction with prominent nuclear pseudoinclusions simulating herpetic endometritis. *Diag. Gynecol. Obstet.* **4**, 127–32.

Dehner, L.P., Askin, F.B. (1975) Cytomegalovirus endometritis. Report of a case associated with spontaneous abortion. *J. Obstet. Gynecol.* **45**, 211–14.

Elstein, M., Woodcock, A., Buckley, C.H. (1994) An unusual case of sarcoidosis. *Br. J. Obstet. Gynaecol.* **101**, 452–3.

Farber, E.R., Leahy, M.S., Meadows, T.R. (1968) Endometrial blastomycosis acquired by sexual contact. *Obst. Gynecol.* **32**, 195–9.

Farooki, M.A. (1967) Epidemiology and pathology of chronic endometritis. *Int. Surg.* **48**, 566–73.

Gibbs, R.S., O'Dell, T.N., MacGregor, R.R., Schwarz, R.H., Morton, H. (1975) Puerperal endometritis: a prospective microbiologic study. *Am. J. Obstet Gynecol.* **121**, 919–25.

Gibbs, R.S., Blanco, J.D., St Clair, P.J., Castaneda, Y.S. (1983) *Mycoplasma hominis* and intrauterine infection in late pregnancy. *Sex. Trans. Dis.* **10**(Suppl. 4), 303–6.

Goldman, R.L. (1970) Herpetic inclusions in the endometrium. *Obstet. Gynecol.* **36**, 603–5.

Govan, A.D.T. (1962) Tuberculous endometritis. *J. Path. Bact.* **83**, 363–72.

Greenwood, S.M., Moran, J.J. (1981) Chronic endometritis: morphologic and clinical observations. *Obstet. Gynecol.* **58**, 176–84.

Gump, D.W., Dickstein, S., Gibson, M. (1981) Endometritis related to *Chlamydia trachomatis* infection. *Ann. Intern. Med.* **95**, 61–3.

Haines, M., Stallworthy, J.A. (1952) Genital tuberculosis in the female. *J. Obstet. Gynaecol. Br. Emp.* **59**, 721–47.

Hamblen, E.C., Baker, R.D., Martin, D.S. (1935) Blastomycosis of the female genital tract with report of case. *Am. J. Obstet. Gynecol.* **30**, 345.

Hart, W.R., Prins, R.P., Tsai, J.C. (1976) Isolated coccidioidomycosis of the uterus. *Hum. Pathol.* **7**, 235–9.

Hendrickson, M.R., Kempson, R.L. (1980) *Surgical Pathology of the Uterine Corpus.* Philadelphia, London, Toronto: W.B. Saunders.

Ho, K.-L. (1979) Sarcoidosis of the uterus. *Hum. Pathol.* **10**, 219–22.

Hollier, L.M., Scott, L.L., Murphree, S.S., Wendel Jr, G.D. (1997) Postpartum endometritis caused by herpes simplex virus. *Obstet. Gynecol.* **89**, 836–8.

Horne, H.W., Hertig, A.T., Kundsin, R.B. (1973) Subclinical endometrial inflammation and *T. mycoplasma*: a possible cause of human reproductive failure. *Int. J. Fertil.* **18**, 226–31.

Horton, L., Wilkes, J. (1976) Chronic non-specific endometritis. *Lancet* **ii**, 366.

Hutchins, C.J. (1977) Tuberculosis of the female genital tract. A changing picture. *Br. J. Obstet. Gynaecol.* **84**, 534–8.

Ingerslev, H.J., Møller, B.R., Mårdh, P.-A. (1982) Chlamydia trachomatis in acute and chronic endometritis. *Scand. J. Inf. Dis.* **32**(Suppl.), 59–63.

Kerr-Layton, J.A., Stamm, C.A., Peterson, L.S., McGregor, J.A. (1998) Chronic plasma cell endometritis in hysterectomy specimens of HIV-infected women: a retrospective analysis. *Infect. Dis. Obstet. Gynecol.* **6**(4), 186–90.

Kitching, A.J. (1984) Endometritis: a clinicopathological and immunohistochemical study. BSc Hons Thesis, Victoria University of Manchester, UK.

Korn, A.P., Bolan, G., Padian, N., Ohm-Smith, M., Schachter, J., Landers, D.V. (1995) Plasma cell

109

endometritis in women with symptomatic bacterial vaginosis. *Obstet. Gynecol.* **85**, 387–90.

Korn, A.P., Hessol, N.A., Padian, N.S. *et al.* (1998) Risk factors for plasma cell endometritis among women with cervical *Neisseria gonorrhoeae*, cervical *Chlamydia trachomatis*, or bacterial vaginosis. *Am. J. Obstet. Gynecol.* **178**, 987–90.

Kurman, R.J. (1982) Benign diseases of the endometrium. In: Blaustein, A. (ed.), *Pathology of the Female Genital Tract*, 2nd Edn. New York: Springer-Verlag, 279–310.

Lee, W.K., Schwartz, D.A., Rice, R.J., Larsen, S.A. (1994) Syphilitic endometritis causing first trimester abortion: a potential infectious cause of fetal morbidity in early gestation. *South. Med. J.* **87**, 1259–61.

Mårdh, P.-A., Møller, B.R., Ingerslev, H.J., Nüssler, E., Weström, L., Wøllner-Hanssen, P. (1981) Endometritis caused by *Chlamydia trachomatis*. *Br. J. Vener. Dis.* **57**, 191–5.

McCracken, A.W., D'Agostino, A.N., Brucks, A.B., Kingsley, W.B. (1974) Acquired cytomegalovirus infection presenting as a viral endometritis. *Am. J. Clin. Pathol.* **61**, 556–60.

Møller, B.R. (1983) The role of mycoplasma in the upper genital tract of women. *Sex. Trans. Dis.* **10**(Suppl. 4), 281–4.

Molnar, J.J., Poliak, A. (1983) Recurrent endometrial malakoplakia. *Am. J. Clin. Pathol.* **80**, 762–4.

Monif, G.R.G. (1981) Recovery of *Neisseria meningitidis* from the cul-de-sac of a woman with endometritis-salpingitis-peritonitis. *Am. J. Obstet. Gynecol.* **139**, 108–9.

Mouktar, M. (1966) Functional disorders due to bilharzial infection of the female genital tract. *J. Obstet. Gynaecol. Br. Commonw.* **73**, 307–10.

Moyer, D.L. (1975) Endometrial diseases in infertility. In: Behrman, S.J., Kistner, R.W. (eds), *Progress in Infertility*, 2nd Edn. Boston: Little Brown, 91–115.

Ness, R.B., Keder, L.M., Soper, D.E. *et al.* (1997) Oral contraception and the recognition of endometritis. *Am. J. Obstet. Gynecol.* **176**, 580–5.

Nogales-Ortiz, F., Taracon, I., Nogales, F.F. (1979) The pathology of female genital tract tuberculosis. A 31-year study of 1436 cases. *Obstet. Gynecol.* **53**, 422–8.

Paavonen, J., Miettinen, A., Stevens, C.E., *et al.* (1983) *Mycoplasma hominis* in cervicitis and endometritis. *Sex. Trans. Dis.* **10**(Suppl. 4), 276–80.

Paukku, M., Puolakkainen, M., Paavonen, T., Paavonen, J. (1999) Plasma cell endometritis is associated with *Chlamydia trachomatis* infection. *Am. J. Clin. Pathol.* **112**, 211–15.

Payan, H., Daino, J., Kish, M. (1964) Lymphoid follicles in endometrium. *Obstet. Gynecol.* **23**, 570–3.

Pearce, K.F., Nolan, T.E. (1996) Endometrial sarcoidosis as a cause of postmenopausal bleeding. A case report. *J. Reprod. Med.* **41**, 878–80.

Plaut, A. (1950) Human infection with *Cryptococcus glabratus*. Report of case involving uterus and fallopian tube. *Am. J. Clin. Pathol.* **20**, 377–80.

Rodriguez, M., Okagaki, T., Richart, R.M. (1972) Mycotic endometritis due to *Candida*, a case report. *Obstet. Gynecol.* **39**, 292–4.

Rotterdam, H. (1978) Chronic endometritis: a clinicopathologic study. *Pathology Annu.* **13**, 209–31.

Saw, E.C., Smale, L.E., Einstein, F.H., Huntington, R.W. (1975) Female genital tract Coccidioidomycosis. *Obstet. Gynecol.* **45**, 199–202.

Schachter, J. (1978a) Chlamydial infection. I. *N. Engl. J. Med.* **298**, 428–35.

Schachter, J. (1978b) Chlamydial infection. II. *N. Engl. J. Med.* **298**, 490–5.

Schachter, J. (1978c) Chlamydial infection. III. *N. Engl. J. Med.* **298**, 540–9.

Schaefer, G. (1970) Tuberculosis of the female genital tract. *Clin. Obstet. Gynecol.* **13**, 965–98.

Schaefer, G., Marcus, R.S., Kramer, E.E. (1972) Postmenopausal endometrial tuberculosis. *Am. J. Obstet. Gynecol.* **112**, 681–7.

Schenken, J.R., Tamisiea, J. (1956) *Enterobius vermicularis* (pinworm) infection of the endometrium. *Am. J. Obstet. Gynecol.* **72**, 913–14.

Schneider, V., Behm, F.G., Mumaw, V.R. (1982) Ascending herpetic endometritis. *Obstet. Gynecol.* **59**, 259–62.

Sen, D.K., Fox, H. (1967) The lymphoid tissue of the endometrium. *Gynaecologia* **163**, 371–8.

Sherman, M.D., Pince, K.J., Farahmand, S.M. (1997) Sarcoidosis manifesting as uveitis and menometrorrhagia. *Am. J. Ophthalmol.* **123**, 703–5.

Silvernagel, S.W., Harshbarger, K.E., Shevlin, D.W. (1997) Postoperative granulomas of the endometrium: histological features after endometrial ablation. *Ann. Diagn. Pathol.* **1**, 82–90.

Sirgi, K.E., Swanson, P.E., Gersell, D.J. (1994) Extramedullary hematopoiesis in the endometrium. Report of four cases and review of the literature. *Am. J. Clin. Pathol.* **101**, 643–6.

Stray-Pedersen, B., Lorentzen-Styr, A.M. (1977) Uterine toxoplasma infections and repeated abortions. *Am. J. Obstet. Gynecol.* **128**, 716–21.

Sutherland, A.M. (1949) The histology of the endometrium in 'functional uterine haemorrhage': analysis of 1000 cases and review of the literature. *Glasgow Med. J.* **30**, 1–28.

Thomas Jr, W.R., Sadeghieh, B., Fresco, R., Rubenstone, A.I., Stepto, R.C., Carasso, B. (1978) Malakoplakia of the endometrium, a probable cause of post-menopausal bleeding. *Am. J. Clin. Pathol.* **69**, 637–41.

van Bogaert, L.-J. (1983) A clinicopathological study of IUCD users with special reference to endometrial patterns and endometritis. *Gynecol. Obstet. Invest.* **16**, 129–35.

Vasudeva, K., Thrasher, T.V., Richart, R.M. (1972) Chronic endometritis: a clinical and electron microscopic study. *Am. J. Obstet. Gynecol.* **112**, 749–58.

Weller, T.H. (1971) The cytomegaloviruses: ubiquitous agents with protean clinical manifestations I. *N. Engl. J. Med.* **285**, 203–14.

Wenkebach, G.F.C., Curry, B. (1976) Cytomegalovirus infection of the female genital tract. Histologic findings in three cases and review of the literature. *Arch. Pathol. Lab. Med.* **100**, 609–12.

Weström, L. (1982) Gynecological chlamydial infections. *Infection* **10**(Suppl.), S40–5.

Williams, A.O. (1967) Pathology of Schistosomiasis of the uterine cervix due to *S. haematobium*. *Am. J. Obstet. Gynecol.* **98**, 784–91.

Winkler, B., Reumann, W., Mitao, M., Gallo, L., Richart, R.M., Crum, C.P. (1984) Chlamydial endometritis. A histological and immunohistochemical analysis. *Am. J. Surg. Pathol.* **8**, 771–8.

Wølner-Hanssen, P., Mårdh, P.-A., Møller, B., Weström, L. (1982) Endometrial infection in women with Chlamydial salpingitis. *Sex. Trans. Dis.* **9**, 84–8.

Yip, S.K., Wong, S.P., Fung, T.Y., Haines, C.J. (1999) Unassisted conception with a normal pregnancy outcome in a woman with active *Mycobacterium tuberculosis* infection of the endometrium. A case report. *J. Reprod. Med.* **44**, 974–6.

8   Miscellaneous benign conditions of the endometrium

The lesions discussed in this chapter have three characteristics in common: they are all benign, all occur in the endometrium and all fall outside the major categories of pathological processes.

8.1   ENDOMETRIAL CHANGES IN UTERINE PROLAPSE

In most patients with a uterine prolapse, the appearances of the endometrium are precisely those that would be expected for the woman's age and hormonal status. In some postmenopausal women, however, the endometrium is less atrophic than would be anticipated and shows an appearance suggestive of persistent low-grade oestrogenic stimulation, the glands being lined by a pseudostratified columnar epithelium and sometimes showing weak proliferative activity. These appearances occur in the absence of high levels of oestrogen and it is assumed that they are a reactive response to congestion. Whatever their pathogenesis these changes are entirely banal, and when encountered in biopsies from patients with a prolapse they can safely be ignored, provided that a distinction has been drawn between these minor abnormalities and a true endometrial hyperplasia.

8.2   ENDOMETRIAL ABNORMALITIES ASSOCIATED WITH SUBMUCOUS LEIOMYOMAS

The endometrium overlying a small submucous leiomyoma does not differ histologically from that in other areas of the uterine cavity but when the myometrial tumour is large, the overlying endometrium may be thinned and represented only by a layer of columnar epithelium with a wisp of subjacent stroma (Fig. 1.6). In less extreme cases the overlying endometrium is shallow but contains short, sparse glands or is of moderate thickness and contains glands in which maturation is delayed relative to the endometrium elsewhere in the uterine cavity. Hence, in biopsy specimens the admixture of endometrium overlying a large submucous leiomyoma with endometrium from elsewhere in the uterine cavity may produce a confusing picture that can lead to an erroneous diagnosis of luteal inadequacy. Not uncommonly, however, fragments of the underlying leiomyoma are included in such biopsy specimens and these may yield a clue to the true diagnosis.

8.3   ENDOMETRIAL METAPLASIA

Metaplastic changes occur with some frequency in the endometrium (Table 8.1), particularly in its epithelial component (Hendrickson and Kempson, 1980); these are of no clinical importance but may give rise to diagnostic confusion when encountered in biopsies.

The high incidence of metaplasia in the endometrium is, to a considerable extent, an eloquent tribute to the plasticity of Müllerian ductal derivatives (undifferentiated cells in such tissues having a potential to differentiate along any of the various Müllerian pathways). Thus, undifferentiated stem cells in endometrial epithelium can differentiate along endometrial lines but can also pursue alternative tubal or endocervical pathways with resulting tubal (ciliated cell) or mucinous metaplasia. Müllerian tissues also have a marked capacity for squamous metaplasia and can undergo intestinal metaplasia. This does, however, raise the question of terminology. If these 'metaplastic' tissues develop from undifferentiated cells should they not be classed as types of 'differentiation' rather than as 'metaplasias'. Thus we have the anomalous situation that the occurrence of squamous tissue in a benign epithelium is called 'squamous metaplasia' while the appearance of similar epithelium in a malignant endometrial lesion is classed as 'squamous differentiation' (see Chapter 10). All endometrial metaplasia should probably be classed as aberrant forms of differentiation but the use of the word 'metaplasia' is so firmly embedded both in the pathological literature and in the minds of pathologists that it will be used in this chapter despite our misgivings about its correctness.

Some alterations in endometrial cell morphology, such as eosinophilic or surface syncytial-like change, have sometimes been included within the general concept of endometrial metaplasias but appear (to us) to fall outside the definition of a metaplastic change; these are therefore considered separately in a later portion of this chapter.

Metaplastic changes may be encountered in normally cycling, atrophic, hyperplastic or neoplastic endometria and their presence, although sometimes confusing, does not alter or modify the primary histological diagnosis of the state of the endometrium. It is notable that epithelial metaplasias (of all types) are found with unusual frequency (up to 78 per cent) in

---

Table 8.1 Classification of endometrial metaplasias

Epithelial metaplasias
  Squamous metaplasia and morule
    formation
  Ciliated cell metaplasia
  Mucinous metaplasia
  Hob-nail metaplasia
  Clear cell metaplasia
  Gastrointestinal metaplasia

Stromal metaplasias
  Myomatous metaplasia
  Osseous metaplasia
  Chrondroid metaplasia

association with well-differentiated endometrioid adenocarcinomas, particularly those arising from a background of atypical hyperplasia (Andersen *et al.*, 1987; Kaku *et al.*, 1992, 1993). Since endometrial neoplasms of this type are thought to be oestrogen-induced, this acts as good circumstantial evidence that oestrogens may also play a role in the pathogenesis of endometrial epithelial metaplasias. It should be stressed that although endometrial epithelial metaplasias are often found in association with an adenocarcinoma there is no evidence that they are in any way premalignant conditions.

8.3.1 Epithelial metaplasias

8.3.1.1 *Squamous metaplasia and morule formation*

Squamous metaplasia is extremely common in the endometrium (Baggish and Woodruff, 1967) and areas of such metaplasia may show overt evidence of squamous differentiation (Fig. 8.1), such as keratinization or intercellular bridge formation, or can take the form of morules (Dutra, 1959) (Fig. 8.2). Morules are rounded or ovoid aggregates of cells that have indistinct margins, a modest amount of

eosinophilic cytoplasm and rounded, ovoid or spindly nuclei. Central necrosis is sometimes seen in large morules but the cells in a morule are always cytologically bland and usually devoid of mitotic activity. Morules can show focal squamous differentiation and it is generally believed that they represent a form of immature squamous metaplasia.

Both squamous metaplasia and morules usually occur within the endometrial glands, the metaplastic cells blending with the glandular epithelial cells and tending to fill, partially or completely, the glandular lumina. Foci of both squamous metaplasia and morules, particularly the latter, can, however, expand to an extent that they obliterate both the lumina and the lining epithelium of the glands in which they have arisen. Subsequent fusion of squamous or morular masses then results in the formation of sheets of metaplastic cells. Uncommonly, metaplastic squamous tissue can be seen on the outer aspect of the glandular epithelium, forming a focus that bulges into the stroma.

Although squamous metaplasia occurs most frequently within the endometrial glands, it is also seen in, and is sometimes confined to,

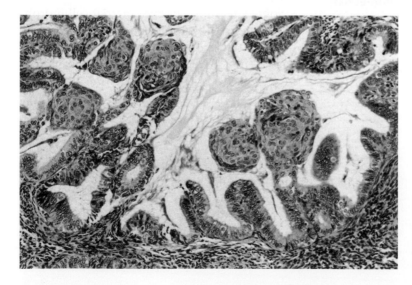

Figure 8.1 Squamous metaplasia. Foci of mature metaplastic squamous epithelium are present in the columnar epithelium of this hyperplastic endometrium. Haematoxylin and eosin.

the surface epithelium. Occasionally, the entire surface epithelium is replaced by metaplastic squamous epithelium (Fig. 8.3); this condition (ichthyosis uteri) is seen most commonly in, but is not confined to, elderly women with pyometra.

Intraglandular squamous metaplasia, cytologically bland and devoid of mitotic activity, usually presents few diagnostic difficulties in biopsies. However, morules pose a wider range of diagnostic possibilities. When growing in sheets, and especially if showing central necrosis, they may resemble poorly differentiated solid adenocarcinoma but consideration to the bland nature of the morular cells and their lack of mitotic activity should lead to avoidance of a diagnostic error. Morules can, perhaps somewhat surprisingly, bear a resemblance to epithelioid granulomas but the type of cell involved and

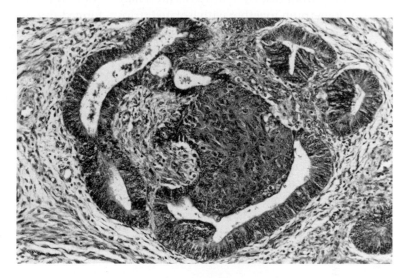

Figure 8.2 Squamous metaplasia. A gland in an endometrial polyp, exhibiting mild complex hyperplasia, contains a squamous morule. Haematoxylin and eosin.

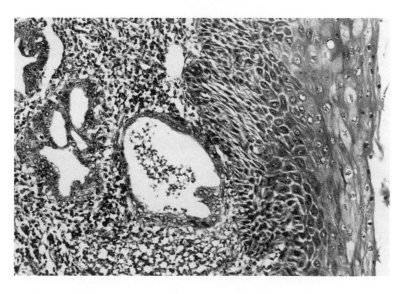

Figure 8.3 Squamous metaplasia. The surface epithelium of the endometrium, to the right, is replaced by a mature, stratified squamous epithelium. The underlying endometrium is inactive and the stroma infiltrated by chronic inflammatory cells. Haematoxylin and eosin.

115

the absence of any rim of surrounding chronic inflammatory cells should make the distinction between these two conditions a relatively easy task. Morules with spindly nuclei can mimic a focus of smooth muscle metaplasia or a stromal nodule from which they differ, however, in their lack of individual cell reticulin envelopment, their positive staining for keratins and their negative reaction for vimentin.

Curettings from cases of ichthyosis uteri may yield endometrium together with isolated strips of mature squamous epithelium. It is natural in such circumstances to conclude, despite any protestations from the gynaecologist, that the squamous tissue is derived from the cervix rather than from the uterine cavity, and in most biopsies showing this pattern that conclusion will indeed be correct. The possibility of ichthyosis uteri, should, however, always be borne in mind, particularly in elderly women, and mentioned in the report. If curettings contain benign squamous epithelium that clearly overlies subjacent endometrial glands, the diagnosis of ichthyosis uteri will present no difficulties.

8.3.1.2 Ciliated cell (tubal) metaplasia

Strictly speaking, the term 'metaplasia' should not be used to describe the presence of ciliated cells in endometrial glandular epithelium because such cells are normal constituents of this epithelium, particularly during the proliferative phase of the menstrual cycle (Fruin and Tighe, 1967). Ciliated cell metaplasia, however, describes the situation encountered most commonly in endometria subjected to prolonged unopposed oestrogenic stimulation, in which pyramidal ciliated cells predominate in the epithelial lining of an endometrial gland (Fig. 8.4) or group of glands (Hendrickson and Kempson, 1980). These ciliated cells have eosinophilic, often vacuolated cytoplasm and central round or ovoid nuclei. A perinuclear clearing of the cytoplasm (perinuclear halo) is commonly seen. There is a tendency for these ciliated cells to stratify and they may form intraglandular tufts or papillae. Any confusion with a neoplastic process should be dispelled by the bland nature of the cells and their lack of mitotic figures.

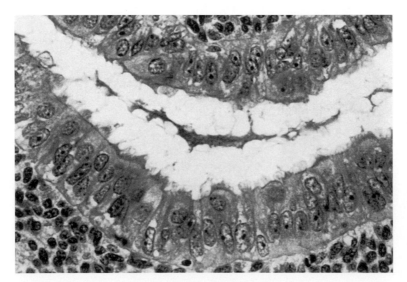

Figure 8.4 Ciliated cell metaplasia in an endometrium showing simple hyperplasia. The gland is lined by an almost pure population of ciliated cells. Note that despite the mild pseudostratification of the epithelium there is no evidence of cytological atypia: perinuclear cytoplasmic clearing is quite prominent. Haematoxylin and eosin.

8.3.1.3 *Mucinous metaplasia*

The lining of a single endometrial gland, or a group of endometrial glands or, occasionally, of the entire endometrial glandular population may be replaced by an epithelium which is histologically identical to that of the endocervix (Hendrickson and Kempson, 1980; Desmopoulos and Greco, 1983). Such an epithelium is formed by columnar cells with central

or basal, regular nuclei and abundant clear cytoplasm which stains positively for mucin (Fig. 8.5). The mucinous epithelium is usually non-stratified but can show pseudostratification, budding and papillary projections. Occasionally, the surface, rather than the glandular epithelium undergoes mucinous metaplasia (Fig. 8.6). There is no development of a microglandular pattern and no cytological

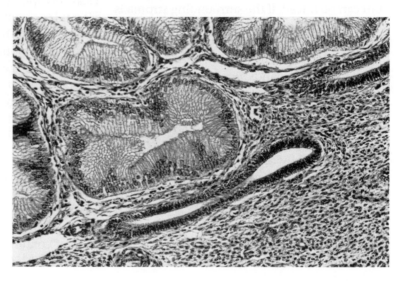

Figure 8.5 Mucinous metaplasia. The glands, in the lower part of the field, are lined by cubo-columnar cells with scanty cytoplasm which show neither secretory nor proliferative activity. The glands in the upper part of the field are lined by tall, mucus-secreting columnar cells of the type found in the endocervix. There is no cytological atypia. Haematoxylin and eosin.

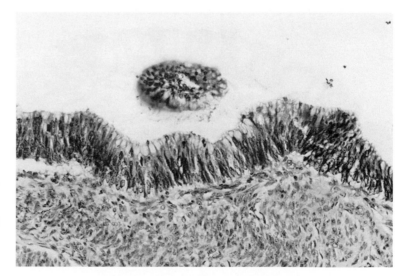

Figure 8.6 Mucinous metaplasia. In this hysterectomy specimen the uterine body was lined by a stratified mucinous epithelium, which replaced the endometrium. Haematoxylin and eosin.

117

atypia – these distinguishing a simple metaplasia from other mucinous lesions of the endometrium (Nucci *et al.*, 1999).

Mucinous metaplasia occurs predominantly in postmenopausal women and can, when extensive, be associated with a mucometra. When seen in curettings mucinous metaplasia must be distinguished from endocervical glandular epithelium. This is only possible if a direct transition from endometrial to mucinous epithelium can be traced, if the surrounding stroma is of endometrial rather than endocervical type or if there is an admixture within a single tissue fragment, in a specimen that is not from the isthmic area, of glands lined by endometrial and mucinous type epithelium.

8.3.1.4   Hob-nail metaplasia

This very rare endometrial metaplastic change is characterized by the presence of cells having a typical 'hob-nail' appearance which replace, to a variable degree, the normal, glandular epithelium (Fechner, 1968). These cells have a teardrop appearance, with their narrow point towards the basal lamina; the cells are cytologically bland with dense regular nuclei and clear or eosinophilic cytoplasm. The lack of any cytological atypia and of mitotic activity serves to distinguish these metaplastic cells from those seen in a clear cell adenocarcinoma of the endometrium.

8.3.1.5   Clear cell metaplasia

In this extremely uncommon form of endometrial metaplasia, cuboidal cells with strikingly clear cytoplasm focally replace endometrial glandular epithelium (Hendrickson and Kempson, 1980). These cells contain glycogen and small amounts of mucin. The lack of any cytological atypia allows for distinction from a clear cell adenocarcinoma while the absence of decidual change and of hypersecretory epithelium, typical of pregnancy, excludes a diagnosis of Arias-Stella change.

8.3.1.6   Intestinal metaplasia

Very occasionally, intestinal metaplasia is encountered in the endometrium (Fig. 8.7). The metaplastic epithelium is formed principally of columnar cells with ovoid nuclei and a prominent brush border. Interspersed with these

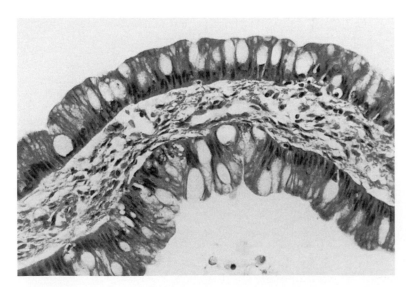

Figure 8.7 Enteric metaplasia. The epithelium in this endometrium was replaced focally by an enteric epithelium containing goblet cells. Mucin stains showed a specific intestinal pattern. Haematoxylin and eosin.

are enteric-type goblet cells, while argyrophil cells may also be present. The goblet cells give a strongly positive reaction with the periodate borohydrate/potassium hydroxide/PAS stain, thus indicating that they contain *o*-acetylated sialomucins of enteric type (Wells and Tiltman, 1989).

8.3.2 Stromal metaplasias

8.3.2.1 Cartilaginous metaplasia

Foci of mature cartilage are occasionally found in the endometrial stroma (Roth and Taylor, 1966). It is often possible to trace a peripheral transition between the surrounding stromal cells and the metaplastic cartilaginous cells.

Metaplastic cartilage must be differentiated from fetal remnants; the observation of a transition from stromal to cartilaginous, cells at the margin of the focus, the absence of any other tissue elements and the lack of a recent history of pregnancy or miscarriage would all favour a diagnosis of metaplasia rather than fetal implantation. Metaplastic cartilage also has to be distinguished from that found as a heterologous element in some mixed Müllerian tumours.

The absence of any other tissues and of any evidence of a neoplastic process makes this distinction easy.

8.3.2.2 Osseous metaplasia

Metaplastic bone formation is sometimes seen in the endometrial stroma (Ganem *et al.*, 1962; Courpas *et al.*, 1964; Shatia and Hoshika, 1982; Ombolet, 1989; Acharya *et al.*, 1993; Rodriguez and Adamson, 1993; Bahceci and Demirel, 1996; Shimizu and Nakayama, 1997). As with cartilaginous metaplasia, there is often a traceable transition between endometrial stromal cells and osseous cells at the periphery of the bony focus. Osseous metaplasia (Fig. 8.8) tends to occur in a setting of acute or chronic endometritis and is particularly associated with post-miscarriage infections.

The differential diagnosis of osseous metaplasia is, as with cartilaginous metaplasia, from fetal remnants and from bone which is present as a heterologous element in a mixed Müllerian tumour. The criteria for distinguishing these conditions are the same as those outlined above for cartilaginous metaplasia.

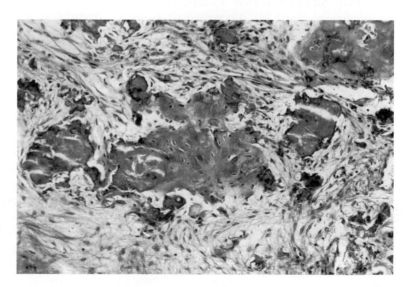

Figure 8.8 Osseous metaplasia. Patchy calcification and focal osteoid metaplasia in the stroma of an endometrium that is extensively fibrosed. Haematoxylin and eosin.

119

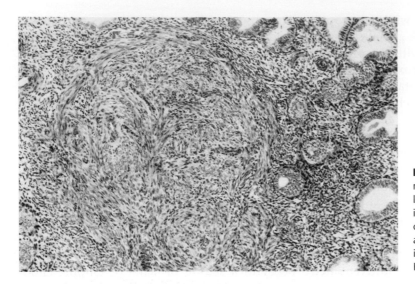

Figure 8.9 Smooth muscle metaplasia. A discrete focus of leiomyomatous metaplasia is present in the endometrium and is compressing the surrounding glands and stroma. The focus was identified in a patient with menorrhagia. Haematoxylin and eosin.

8.3.2.3 Smooth muscle metaplasia

The endometrial stroma can contain small nodules of smooth muscle, which compress the surrounding tissue and are not connected to the underlying superficial myometrium (Fig. 8.9). These have been classed as intra-endometrial leiomyomas but are more probably a result of stromal smooth muscle metaplasia (Bird and Willis, 1965).

Nodular smooth muscle metaplasia in the endometrium must be distinguished from a stromal nodule and this can only be achieved by recognizing that the constituent cells are of smooth muscle type rather than stromal type. The distinction between smooth muscle and stromal tumours, in both morphological and immunocytochemical terms, is discussed in Chapter 11 and it must be emphasized that this differentiation is critically important in biopsies. Both stromal nodules and nodular smooth muscle metaplasia are benign conditions but the presence of a stromal lesion, no matter how apparently banal, necessitates hysterectomy to exclude a low-grade endometrial stromal sarcoma, while smooth muscle metaplasia merits no treatment.

8.4 CYTOLOGICAL ABNORMALITIES

8.4.1 Surface syncytial-like change

The cells of the endometrial surface epithelium may, on occasion, show papillary proliferation (Hendrickson and Kempson, 1980): this change is seen most commonly in association with endometrial shedding. The papillae consist of cytologically bland cells with ovoid, rounded or pyknotic nuclei, indistinct margins and a moderate amount of eosinophilic cytoplasm (Fig. 8.10). The papillae are devoid of any stromal support and the lack of definition of the cell margins gives them a syncytial-like appearance. This papillary syncytial-like change may extend into the superficial portion of adjacent glands and, characteristically, the papillary aggregates are focally or diffusely infiltrated by polymorphonuclear leucocytes. It is probable that this change represents a very early stage of surface squamous metaplasia.

Surface syncytial-like change can, when encountered in curettings, bear some resemblance to a papillary adenocarcinoma of the endometrium. Disastrous overdiagnosis of this

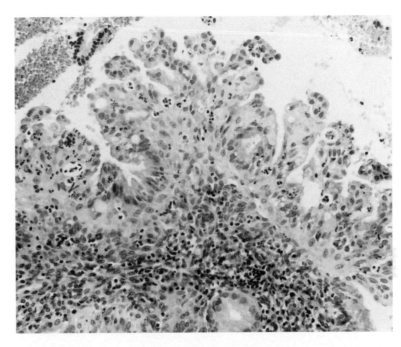

Figure 8.10 Syncytial papillary metaplasia. The endometrial surface is covered by epithelial cells that form a syncytial-like mass with indistinct cell borders. The nuclei are bland. The underlying stroma is chronically inflamed. Haematoxylin and eosin. Photograph kindly supplied by Dr R.L. Kempson.

clinically unimportant abnormality can be averted by noting the bland nature of the cells in surface syncytial-like change.

Syncytial change is to be distinguished from the recently described 'hyperplastic papillary proliferation' of the endometrium in which the papillae have a stromal core (Lehman and Hart, 2001). This papillary change is possibly metaplastic in nature.

8.4.2   Eosinophilic change

Epithelial cells in an endometrium occasionally have small, round, basophilic nuclei and markedly eosinophilic cytoplasm. The oncocytic nature of these cells has been confirmed by electron microscopy (Bergeron and Ferenczy, 1988). Their presence has no clinical significance.

8.5   FETAL REMNANTS

Following either spontaneous miscarriage or termination of pregnancy, fetal tissue can remain embedded in the endometrium (Newton and Abell, 1972; Tyagi *et al.*, 1979). Bleeding, after a period of months or even years, may complicate the implantation of such fetal tissues and curettage under these circumstances will yield endometrium admixed with a melange of fetal tissues such as cartilage, bone, glial tissue, kidney, liver, skin and retina.

Clearly, these findings may give rise to a suspicion of a uterine teratoma and, indeed, it is almost certain that many of the reported cases of teratomatous neoplasms of the uterus were in fact examples of fetal remnants. A distinction of fetal remnants from a teratoma rests upon the usually intimate admixture of the fetal tissues with endometrium and upon the pattern of the implanted tissues, which usually differs markedly from that seen in a teratoma.

In some cases, fetal remnants within the endometrium are represented only by glial tissue (Niven and Stansfeld, 1973; Zettergren, 1973; Roca *et al.*, 1980), a condition sometimes known as endometrial gliomatosis (Fig. 8.11).

121

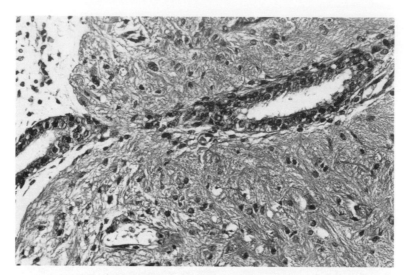

Figure 8.11 Endometrial gliomatosis. The endometrial stroma is almost completely replaced by glial tissue. The distinctly fibrillar structure of the tissue is apparent and the endometrial gland which traverses the field is of normal appearance. Haematoxylin and eosin.

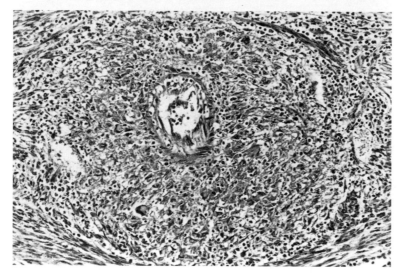

Figure 8.12 Granulomatous arteritis. The wall of this artery, which lies at the junction of the basalis and myometrium, is diffusely infiltrated by non-caseating granulomatous tissue in which macrophage giant cells are seen. The arterial wall is disrupted. Haematoxylin and eosin.

The glial tissue usually forms well-defined islands, may become polypoid and occasionally bears a slight resemblance to decidua. Staining for glial fibrillary, acidic protein will resolve any doubts as to the nature of the tissue.

8.6   VASCULITIS

Giant cell arteritis can affect the vasculature of the uterus (Pirozynski, 1976; Petrides *et al.*, 1979; Ganesan *et al.*, 2000). The vascular lesions may be limited to the arteries within the myometrium (Fig. 8.12) but can extend to involve the spiral arteries in the endometrium, and thus be apparent in curettage specimens. Endometrial arteries involved show replacement of their walls by granulomatous tissue and their appearance may at first sight resemble that of a tuberculous granuloma. Elastic stains will, however, demonstrate the presence

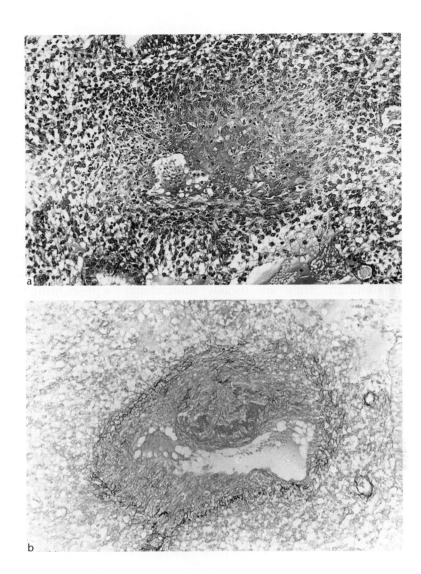

Figure 8.13 **(a)** An acute necrotizing arteritis with intravascular thrombosis. **(b)** An elastic stain demonstrates the interruption to the elastic lamina.

of a vessel in the centre of the inflammatory focus, even when the disease is well advanced, with marked vascular destruction. In patients with a giant cell arteritis a systemic disease, such as temporal arteritis or polymyalgia rheumatica, should be suspected. A necrotizing arteritis of the medium and small muscular arteries of the uterus can occur as a localized lesion and is sometimes encountered in women suffering from polyarteritis nodosa (Fig. 8.13).

8.7 ENDOMETRIAL POLYPS

8.7.1 Simple polyps

The term 'polyp' is purely descriptive and does not, in itself, denote any specific histological process; thus, an endometrial neoplasm or a submucous leiomyoma may well present as a polypoid mass within the uterus. By convention, however, the term 'endometrial polyp' is generally taken as referring to a focal, circumscribed

123

overgrowth of the mucosa, usually but far from always the basal portion, which protrudes into the uterine cavity and is classed as a 'simple polyp'. Simple endometrial polyps are often asymptomatic but can cause abnormal bleeding. Endocrine factors appear to play a role in the pathogenesis of simple polyps. They do not occur before the menarche but increase in frequency thereafter, reaching a peak incidence during the fifth decade; they occur with undue frequency in women receiving oestrogen-containing hormone replacement therapy and have an unusually high incidence in women exposed to tamoxifen (van Bogaert, 1988; Nuovo *et al.*, 1989; Ismail, 1994; Reslova *et al.*, 1999). Interestingly, they are usually monoclonal (Jovanovic *et al.*, 1996) and frequently show karyotypic abnormalities that are not present in the non-polypoid endometrium from which they have developed (Speleman *et al.*, 1991; Dal Cin *et al.*, 1992, 1995).

As seen in curettings, simple endometrial polyps are formed of endometrial glands set in a stroma that is at least partially fibrous (Fig. 8.14). Those originating from the isthmic area may contain an admixture of endometrial and endocervical glands. The endometrial glands in a polyp do not usually share in the normal cyclical activity of the endometrium and are often either inactive or only weakly proliferative. Simple hyperplasia, focal complex hyperplasia or focal atypical hyperplasia, limited to the glands in the polyp, are occasionally seen. In postmenopausal women, the glands are inactive and can show senile cystic change; this latter phenomenon probably reflects more the tendency of foci of senile cystic change to become polypoid rather than the development of cystic change in the glands of a pre-existing polyp. Glandular secretory activity is seen in a small proportion of polyps but is usually patchy, weak and irregular.

The stroma of a simple polyp, as already remarked, invariably contains at least some fibrous tissue, whereas in some the stroma is predominantly fibrous; these latter types are often known as adenofibromatous polyps. In some polyps, however, the stroma is predominantly

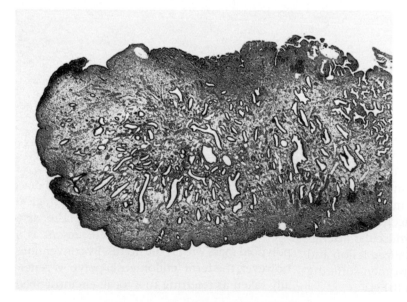

Figure 8.14 Endometrial polyp. A typical, benign polyp composed of functional and basal endometrium. There is a mild degree of glandular architectural atypia. Haematoxylin and eosin.

endometrial type, while in yet others a mixed fibrous–endometrial stromal pattern is seen (Hattab *et al.*, 1999). The stromal cells often show mild nuclear atypia while very exceptionally quite striking atypia is seen in the stromal component of a polyp (Creagh *et al.*, 1995). Stromal mitotic figures are commonly either absent or very sparse but a modest number of mitoses may be seen in those polyps with an endometrial-type stroma (Hattab *et al.*, 1999). A highly characteristic feature is the presence of a leash, or cluster, of small thick-walled vessels (Fig. 8.15), usually in the base or stalk but sometimes seen in the body of the polyp.

Tamoxifen-associated endometrial polyps (see Chapter 5) tend to be unusually large and are often multiple: they often show mitotic activity, periglandular stromal condensation (cambium layer) and diverse, florid epithelial metaplasias, these including ciliated cell, papillary syncytial, oncocytic, hob-nail, mucinous, squamous and clear cell forms (Nuovo *et al.*, 1989; Corley *et al.*, 1992; Berezowsky *et al.*, 1994; Ismail, 1994, 1999; Schlesinger *et al.*, 1998; Kennedy *et al.*, 1999). The glands in these polyps are often polarized to appear orientated along the long axis of the polyp and may have a staghorn appearance; a variable degree of decidual-like change may be seen in the stroma. There are no individual features present in tamoxifen-associated polyps that are not also found in non-tamoxifen related polyps but the particular combination of features in tamoxifen-associated polyps is highly characteristic.

The presence of stromal fibrosis is of considerable diagnostic value in recognizing a polyp in curettings. Reliance for making this diagnosis should not be placed on the presence of surface epithelium on three or all sides of a tissue fragment as a similar appearance can be seen in polypoidal pieces of normal endometrium.

A simple polyp may undergo haemorrhage, infarction or apical ulceration but there is usually a sufficient retention of the histological pattern to allow diagnosis. The cardinal characteristics of stromal fibrous tissue and the presence of thick-walled vessels distinguish a simple polyp from a polypoidal piece of normal endometrium, while the Müllerian adenofibroma, with which a simple polyp can be confused, usually has club-shaped papillary projections

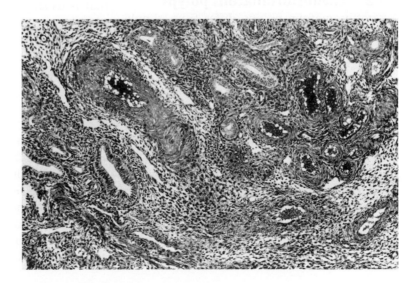

Figure 8.15 Endometrial polyp. A cluster of thick-walled arteries is seen in the core of the polyp. Haematoxylin and eosin.

125

into cystic spaces (Fig. 11.8). Because of the periglandular stromal condensation, or cambium layer, found in tamoxifen-associated polyps, these can be, and indeed probably have been, mistaken for an adenosarcoma from which, however, a distinction can be drawn by the absence of any sarcomatous features, the lack of heterologous tissues and the presence of metaplastic epithelia.

Adenocarcinomatous change in non-tamoxifen-associated polyps is very uncommon, and many reported examples of the phenomenon are instead adenocarcinomas growing in a polypoidal fashion (Salm, 1972). To establish that an adenocarcinoma has arisen in a pre-existing polyp, it is necessary to demonstrate that the malignant tissue is separated from normal endometrium by the base and stalk of the polyp, these latter showing no malignant features. It is commonly not possible to make a topographic analysis of this nature in curettage material. A rather high incidence of adenocarcinomatous change has, however, been described in tamoxifen-associated polyps (Ismail, 1994, 1999).

8.7.2   Adenofibromatous polyps

Adenofibromatous polyps differ from simple polyps only in the fact that their stroma consists solely of fibrous tissue.

8.7.3   Adenomyomatous polyps

These uncommon polyps contain an admixture of endometrial type stroma and bands of smooth muscle in their stroma, with the latter component usually predominating. The glands are lined by a bland endometrial type epithelium; tubal or mucinous metaplasia may be present but squamous metaplasia is very uncommon. The endometrial type stroma is periglandular in site and is, in turn, surrounded by the smooth muscle component, the latter

occasionally showing hypercellularity or containing bizarre nuclei (Gilks *et al.*, 2000). It is not clear whether these muscular elements represent superficial myometrium that was originally admixed with the basal endometrium or smooth muscle metaplasia in the stroma of a simple polyp. Adenomyomatous polyps are distinguished from atypical polypoid adenomyomas by their lack of glandular crowding and epithelial atypia and by their usual lack of intraglandular squamous metaplasia.

8.7.4   Atypical polypoid adenomyoma

This term has been applied to adenomyomatous polyps (Fig. 8.16) in which the glandular component, which is of endometrial type, shows a variable degree of architectural and cytological atypia (Mazur, 1981; Young *et al.*, 1986; Clement and Young, 1987; Rollason and Redman, 1988; Fukunaga *et al.*, 1995; Longacre *et al.*, 1996). The average age at which these occur is 40 years. The glands are irregularly dispersed among bundles of smooth muscle and commonly show a complex architectural pattern together with multilayering and atypia that is usually mild or moderate but is sometimes severe. Squamous metaplasia (or differentiation) is very common within the glands and often takes the form of morules.

These polyps can, in curettings, be mistaken for endometrioid adenocarcinomas that are infiltrating myometrium or endometrioid adenocarcinomas with a prominent stroma. The stromal smooth muscle of the atypical polypoid adenomyoma rarely has, however, the fasciculated pattern of true myometrium, the fibres tending to be arranged in a haphazard fashion. Furthermore, the smooth muscle fibres are commonly admixed with fibrous tissue and there may be a minor endometrial stromal component. It has been suggested that positive

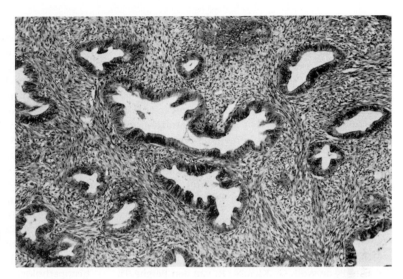

Figure 8.16 Atypical adenomyomatous polyp. The glands are irregular in contour exhibiting in-foldings, epithelial budding and out-pouchings. The stroma is formed predominantly of smooth muscle. Haematoxylin and eosin.

staining of the stroma of an atypical polypoid adenomyoma for smooth muscle actin and desmin distinguishes this lesion from a well-differentiated adenocarcinoma with a stromal reaction (Di Palma *et al.*, 1989; Mazur and Kurman, 1995). However, it has been shown that the stroma of well-differentiated adeno-carcinomas commonly shows a similar stain-ing pattern (Soslow *et al.*, 1996).

Despite their slightly alarming appearance, atypical polypoid adenomyomas appear to behave in a benign fashion, although they may regrow if incompletely removed. Adenocarci-nomatous change within atypical polypoid adenomas has been recorded (Kay *et al.*, 1988; Staros and Shilkitus, 1991; Fukunaga *et al.*, 1995; Sugiyama *et al.*, 1998) but is an exceptional phenomenon.

8.7.5 Stromatous polyps

These are exceptionally rare and consist only of endometrial stroma. It is virtually impossible in curettage material to distinguish polyps of this type from an endometrial stromal nodule or sarcoma.

REFERENCES

Acharya, U., Pinion, S.B., Parkin, D.E., Hamilton, M.P.R. (1993) Osseous metaplasias of the endometrium treated by hysteroscopic resection. *Br. J. Obstet. Gynaecol.* **100**, 793–5.

Andersen, W.A., Taylor, P.T., Fechner, R.E., Pinkerton, J.A. (1987) Endometrial metaplasia associated with endo-metrial adenocarcinoma. *Am. J. Obstet. Gynecol.* **157**, 597–604.

Baggish, M.S., Woodruff, J.D. (1967) The occurrence of squamous epithelium in the endometrium. *Obstet. Gynecol. Surv.* **22**, 69–115.

Bahceci, M., Demirel, L.C. (1996) Osseous metaplasia of the endometrium: a rare cause of infertility and its hysteroscopic management. *Hum. Reprod.* **11**, 2537–9.

Berezowsky, J., Chalvardjian, A., Murray, D. (1994) Iatrogenic endometrial megapolyps in women with breast carcinoma. *Obstet. Gynecol.* **84**, 727–30.

Bergeron, C., Ferenczy, A. (1988) Oncocytic metaplasia in endometrial hyperplasia and carcinoma. *Int. J. Gynecol. Pathol.* **7**, 93–5.

Bird, C.C., Willis, R.A. (1965) The production of smooth muscle by the endometrial stroma of the adult human uterus. *J. Pathol. Bacteriol.* **90**, 75–81.

van Bogaert, L.J. (1988) Clinicopathologic findings in endometrial polyps. *Obstet. Gynecol.* **71**, 771–3.

Clement, P.B., Young, R.H. (1987) Atypical polypoid adenomyoma of the uterus associated with Turner's syndrome: a report of three cases, including a review of 'estrogen-associated' endometrial neoplasms and neoplasms associated with Turner's syndrome. *Int. J. Gynecol. Pathol.* **6**, 104–13.

Corley, D., Rowe, J., Curtis, M.T., Hogan, W.M., Noumoff, J.S., Livolsi, V.A. (1992) Postmenopausal bleeding from unusual endometrial polyps in women on chronic tamoxifen therapy. *Obstet. Gynecol.* **79**, 111–16.

Courpas, A.S., Morris, J.D., Woodruff, J.D. (1964) Osteoid tissue *in utero*: report of three cases. *Obstet. Gynecol.* **24**, 636–40.

Creagh, T.M., Krausz, T., Flanagan, A.M. (1995) Atypical stromal cells in a hyperplastic endometrial polyp. *Histopathology* **27**, 386–7.

Dal Cin, P., de Wolf, G., Klerckx, P., van den Berghe, H. (1992) The 6p21 chromosome is nonrandomly involved in endometrial polyps. *Gynecol. Oncol.* **46**, 393–6.

Dal Cin, P., Vanni, R., Marras, S. *et al.* (1995) Four cytogenetic subgroups can be identified in endometrial polyps. *Cancer Res.* **55**, 1565–8.

Desmopoulos, R.I., Greco, M.A. (1983) Mucinous metaplasia of the endometrium: ultrastructural and histochemical characteristics. *Int. J. Gynecol. Pathol.* **1**, 383–90.

Di Palma, S., Santini, D., Martinelli, G. (1989) Atypical polypoid adenomyoma of the uterus: an immunohistochemical study of a case. *Tumori* **75**, 292–5.

Dutra, F. (1959) Intraglandular morules of the endometrium. *Am. J. Clin. Pathol.* **31**, 60–5.

Fechner, R.E. (1968) Endometrium with pattern of mesonephroma (report of a case). *Obstet. Gynecol.* **31**, 485–90.

Fruin, A.H., Tighe, J.R. (1967) Tubal metaplasia of the endometrium. *J. Obstet. Gynaecol. Br. Cwlth.* **74**, 93–7.

Fukunaga, M., Endo, Y., Ushigome, S., Ishikawa, E. (1995) Atypical polypoid adenomyomas of the uterus. *Histopathology* **27**, 35–42.

Ganem, K.J., Parsons, L., Friedell, G. (1962) Endometrial ossification. *Am. J. Obstet. Gynecol.* **83**, 1592–4.

Ganesan, R., Ferryman, S.R., Meier, L., Rollason, P. (2000) Vasculitis of the female genital tract with clinicopathologic correlation: a study of 46 cases with follow-up. *Int. J. Gynecol. Pathol.* **19**, 258–65.

Gilks, C.B., Clement, P.B., Hart, W.R., Young, R.H. (2000) Uterine adenomyomas excluding atypical polypoid adenomyomas and adenomyomas of endocervical

type: a clinicopathologic study of 30 cases of an underemphasized lesion that may cause diagnostic problems with brief consideration of adenomyomas of other female genital tract sites. *Int. J. Gynecol. Pathol.* **19**, 195–205.

Hattab, E.M., Allam-Nandyala, P., Rhatigan, R.M. (1999) The stromal component of large endometrial polyps. *Int. J. Gynecol. Pathol.* **18**, 332–7.

Hendrickson, M.R., Kempson, R.L. (1980) Endometrial epithelial metaplasias: report of 89 cases and proposed classification. *Am. J. Surg. Pathol.* **4**, 525–42.

Ismail, S.M. (1994) Pathology of the endometrium treated with tamoxifen. *J. Clin. Pathol.* **47**, 827–33.

Ismail, S.M. (1999) Gynaecological effects of tamoxifen. *J. Clin. Pathol.* **52**, 83–8.

Jovanovic, A.S., Boynton, K.A., Mutter, G.L. (1996) Uteri of women with endometrial carcinoma contain a histopathological spectrum of monoclonal putative pre-cancers, some with micro-satellite instability. *Cancer Res.* **56**, 1917–21.

Kaku, T., Tsukamoto, N., Tsuruchi, N., Sugihara, K., Kamura, T., Nakano, H. (1992) Endometrial metaplasia associated with endometrial carcinoma. *Obstet. Gynecol.* **80**, 812–16.

Kaku, T., Silverberg, S.G., Tsukamoto, N. *et al.* (1993) Association of endometrial epithelial metaplasias with endometrial carcinoma and hyperplasia in Japanese and American women. *Int. J. Gynecol. Pathol.* **12**, 297–300.

Kay, S., Frable, W.J., Goplerud, D.R. (1988) Endometrial carcinoma arising in a large polypoid adenomyoma of the uterus. *Int. J. Gynecol. Pathol.* **7**, 391–9.

Kennedy, M.M., Baigrie, C.F., Manek, S. (1999) Tamoxifen and the endometrium: review of 102 cases and comparison with HRT-related and non-HRT-related endometrial pathology. *Int. J. Gynecol. Pathol.* **18**, 130–7.

Lehman, M.B., Hart, W.R. (2001) Simple and complex papillary proliferations of the endometrium: a report of nine cases of apparently localized papillary lesions with fibrovascular stromal cores and endothelial metaplasia. *Am. J. Surg. Pathol.* **25**, 1347–54.

Longacre, T.A., Chung, M.H., Rouse, R.V., Hendrickson, M.R. (1996) Atypical polypoid adenofibromas (atypical polypoid adenomyomas) of the uterus: a clinicopathologic study of 55 cases. *Am. J. Surg. Pathol.* **20**, 1–20.

Mazur, M.T. (1981) Atypical polypoid adenomyomas of the endometrium. *Am. J. Surg. Pathol.* **5**, 473–82.

Mazur, M.T., Kurman, R.J. (1995) *Diagnosis of Endometrial Biopsies and Curettings: A Practical Approach.* New York: Springer-Verlag.

Newton, C.W., Abell, M.R. (1972) Iatrogenic fetal implants. *Obstet. Gynecol.* **40**, 686–91.

Niven, P.A.R. and Stansfeld, A.C. (1973) 'Glioma' of the uterus: a fetal homograft. *Am. J. Obstet. Gynecol.* **115**, 534–8.

Nucci, M.R., Prasad, C.J., Crum, C.P., Mutter, G.L. (1999) Mucinous endometrial epithelial proliferations: a morphologic spectrum of changes with diverse clinical significance. *Mod. Pathol.* **12**, 1137–42.

Nuovo, M.A., Nuovo, G.J., McCaffrey, R.M., Levine, R.U., Baron, B., Winkler, B. (1989) Endometrial polyps in postmenopausal patients receiving tamoxifen. *Int. J. Gynecol. Pathol.* **8**, 125–31.

Ombelet, W. (1989) Endometrial ossification, an unusual finding in an infertility clinic: a case report. *J. Reprod. Med.* **34**, 303–6.

Petrides, M., Robertson, I.C., Fox, H. (1979) Giant cell arteritis of the female genital tract. *Br. J. Obstet. Gynaecol.* **86**, 148–51.

Pirozynski, W.J. (1976) Giant cell arteritis of the uterus: report of two cases. *Am. J. Clin. Pathol.* **65**, 308–13.

Reslova, T., Tosner, J., Resl, M., Kugler, R., Vavrova, I. (1999) Endometrial polyps: a clinical study of 245 cases. *Arch. Gynecol. Obstet.* **262**, 133–9.

Roca, A.N., Guarjardo, M., Estrada, W.J. (1980) Glial polyp of the cervix and endometrium. *Am. J. Clin. Pathol.* **73**, 718–20.

Rodriguez, B.Z., Adamson, G.D. (1993) Hysteroscopic treatment of ectopic intrauterine bone: a case report. *J. Reprod. Med.* **38**, 515–20.

Rollason, T.P., Redman, C.W. (1988) Atypical polypoid adenomyoma – clinical, histological and immunocytochemical findings. *Eur. J. Gynaecol. Oncol.* **9**, 444–51.

Roth, E., Taylor, H.B. (1966) Heterotopic cartilage in uterus. *Obstet. Gynecol.* **27**, 838–44.

Salm, R. (1972) The incidence and significance of early carcinomas in endometrial polyps. *J. Pathol.* **108**, 47–54.

Shatia, N.N., Hoshika, M.G. (1982) Uterine osseous metaplasia. *Obstet. Gynecol.* **60**, 256–9.

Schlesinger, C., Kamoi, S., Ascher, S.M., Kendell, M., Lage, J.M., Silverberg, S.G. (1998) Endometrial polyps: a comparison study of patients receiving tamoxifen with two control groups. *Int. J. Gynecol. Pathol.* **17**, 302–11.

Shumizu, M., Nakayama, M. (1997) Endometrial ossification in a postmenopausal woman. *J. Clin. Pathol.* **50**, 171–2.

Soslow, R.A., Chung, M.H., Rouse, R.V., Hendrickson, M.R., Longacre, T.A. (1996) Atypical polypoid adenofibroma (APA) versus well-differentiated endometrial carcinoma with prominent stromal matrix: an immunohistochemical study. *Int. J. Gynecol. Pathol.* **15**, 209–16.

Speleman, F., Dal Cin, P., van Roy, N. *et al.* (1991) Is t(6;20) (p21;q13) a characteristic chromosomal change in endometrial polyps? *Genes Chromosomes Cancer* **3**, 318–19.

Staros, E.B., Shilkitus, W.F. (1991) Atypical polypoid adenomyoma with carcinomatous transformation: a case report. *Surg. Pathol.* **4**, 157–66.

Sugiyama, T., Ohta, S., Nishida, T., Okura, N., Tanabe, K., Yakushiji, M. (1998) Two cases of endometrial adenocarcinoma arising from atypical polypoid adenomyoma. *Gynecol. Oncol.* **71**, 141–4.

Tyagi, S.P., Saxena, K., Rizvi, R. and Langley, F.A. (1979) Foetal remnants in the uterus and their relation to other uterine heterotopias. *Histopathology* **3**, 339–45.

Wells, M. and Tiltman, A. (1989) Intestinal metaplasia of the endometrium. *Histopathology* **15**, 431–3.

Young, R.H., Treger, T., Scully, R.E. (1986) Atypical polypoid adenomyomas of the uterus: a report of 27 cases. *Am. J. Clin. Pathol.* **86**, 139–45.

Zettergren, L. (1973) Glial tissue in the uterus. *Am. J. Pathol.* **71**, 419–26.

9 Endometrial hyperplasias and intra-endometrial adenocarcinoma

9.1 CLASSIFICATION OF ENDOMETRIAL HYPERPLASIAS

A pathologist confronted with the task of recognizing and categorizing the various forms of endometrial hyperplasia, as seen in curettage material, must work within the framework of a classification of these conditions. Unfortunately, no generally agreed classification of hyperplastic abnormalities of the endometrium exists and, indeed, the entire topic has become confused almost to the point of anarchy by a plethora of proposed classifications and by a complicated and inconsistent nomenclature.

The only important distinction, in both prognostic and therapeutic terms, between the various forms of endometrial hyperplasia is between those that are associated with a significant risk of evolving into an endometrial adenocarcinoma and those devoid of any such risk. There is now quite widespread agreement that the defining (and only) feature of an endometrial hyperplasia that is indicative of a potential for malignant change is cytological atypia (Welch and Scully, 1977; Fox and Buckley, 1982; Kurman *et al.*, 1985; Norris *et al.*, 1986; Huang *et al.*, 1988; Ferenczy and Bergeron, 1992). Hence, the fundamental subdivision of the endometrial hyperplasias is into those with cytological atypia and those lacking this feature. From a prognostic viewpoint, this is a fully adequate classification, but one that is possibly too stark for diagnostic purposes in so far as hyperplasias without cytological atypia may involve both glands and stroma, or may be confined solely to the glands and may or may not show architectural abnormalities.

The recommended classification of the endometrial hyperplasias is therefore that shown in Table 9.1 in which hyperplasia with cytological atypia is classed as 'atypical hyperplasia' and hyperplasias lacking cytological atypia are subdivided into 'simple' and 'complex' forms. This classification differs from that of World Health Organization (WHO) (Scully *et al.*, 1994) in that the term 'adenomatous hyperplasia' is

Table 9.1 Classification of endometrial hyperplasias

Simple hyperplasia
Complex hyperplasia
Atypical hyperplasia

not used as a synonym for complex hyperplasia and hyperplasia with cytological atypia is not subdivided into simple and complex forms. The term 'adenomatous hyperplasia' should have no place in any contemporary classification of endometrial hyperplasias since this diagnostic label has been used so indiscriminately that it have lost any meaning it may once have had and is, furthermore, indefensible in both conceptual and semantic terms. There seems no good reason for dividing hyperplasia with cytological atypia into simple and complex forms, especially as we are far from convinced that there is such an entity as simple atypical hyperplasia.

The classification suggested here is straightforward, uncomplicated and prognostically valid. The condition of simple hyperplasia corresponds with that which was sometimes called 'cystic glandular hyperplasia': the latter term is, however, inappropriate since this type of hyperplasia is not restricted to the glandular component of the endometrium and the glands are not necessarily cystic in appearance.

A complex hyperplasia corresponds to glandular hyperplasia with architectural atypia. Some authors define a complex hyperplasia in terms of both glandular crowding and architectural atypia (Norris et al., 1986) but, while agreeing that glandular crowding is usually present, we accept architectural atypia as the defining feature of this form of endometrial hyperplasia.

Any apparently hyperplastic condition in which there is cytological atypia is classed as an atypical hyperplasia, although pathologists differ as to the criteria for the recognition of atypia and it is a diagnosis subject to considerable inter-observer variation (Skov et al., 1997; Kendall et al., 1998; Bergeron et al., 1999). We have elaborated elsewhere (Fox and Buckley, 1982; Fox, 1994) our reasons for believing that the endometrial abnormality usually classed as a hyperplasia with cytological atypia is a form of intra-endometrial neoplasia rather than a true hyperplasia. This belief has been strengthened by the demonstration that atypical hyperplasias, but not other forms of endometrial hyperplasia, are usually monoclonal (Jovanovic et al., 1996). It is important to stress that under the term 'intra-endometrial neoplasia' we include both atypical hyperplasia and lesions that would be considered by many as well-differentiated endometrioid adenocarcinomas that are confined to the endometrium, and in which stromal invasion is not clearly apparent.

There has been increasing acceptance of the view that atypical hyperplasia merits classification as a form of neoplasia (Ferenczy and Bergeron, 1992; Bergeron et al., 1999; Mutter and the Endometrial Collaborative Group, 2000) but no real agreement about nomenclature or about whether atypical hyperplasia should be combined with well-differentiated adenocarcinoma as a diagnostic entity. Thus, Ferenczy and Bergeron (1992) use the term 'endometrial intra-epithelial neoplasia' in the same sense as we use 'intra-endometrial neoplasia', while Mutter and the Endometrial Collaborative Group (2000) also use the term 'endometrial intra-epithelial neoplasia' but exclude any form of adenocarcinoma from this diagnosis. In contrast, Bergeron et al. (1999) propose that both atypical hyperplasia and well-differentiated endometrioid adenocarcinoma should, in curettage or biopsy material, be classed as 'endometrioid neoplasia'. All this seems, and indeed is, confusing but boils down to the increasing belief that atypical hyperplasia is a neoplastic rather than a hyperplastic process. Time and further studies will more clearly define an acceptable nomenclature and conceptual approach. However, it must be stressed that the term 'endometrial intraepithelial carcinoma' is applied to a quite different entity which is associated with, and believed to be a precursor of, serous papillary carcinoma of the endometrium (Ambros *et al.*, 1995) and which is totally unrelated to atypical hyperplasia or well-differentiated endometrioid adenocarcinoma (see Chapter 10).

Although the concept of atypical hyperplasia as a neoplastic process is winning wider support, it is still far from being universally accepted (Zaino, 2000), despite there being overwhelming scientific evidence for its validity. The term 'intra-endometrial neoplasia' is therefore still not widely used in diagnostic histopathology and hence we will, albeit with some reluctance, use the term 'atypical hyperplasia' in this text while adding (IEN) to the descriptive and diagnostic label.

Secretory change may be superimposed on any form of hyperplasia if, for instance, a progestagen is given or if ovulation occurs after a series of anovulatory cycles. We do not recognize, however, any specific condition of 'secretory hyperplasia'.

9.2 HISTOLOGICAL APPEARANCES OF THE VARIOUS FORMS OF ENDOMETRIAL HYPERPLASIA

9.2.1 Simple hyperplasia

This condition represents the physiological response of the endometrium to prolonged, unopposed oestrogenic stimulation, whether this is of endogenous (repeated anovulatory cycles, oestrogenic ovarian tumour or polycystic ovary syndrome) or exogenous (administration of oestrogens without a progestagen) origin. It is a true hyperplasia with an increase in endometrial bulk and hence curettings from women with this condition tend to be bulky and sometimes polypoid. The tissue often has a somewhat velvety appearance and tiny cystic spaces may be apparent even on naked-eye examination. Simple hyperplasia is a diffuse process that involves the entire endometrium, with resulting loss of the distinction between basal and functional zones. This will not, of course, be apparent in curettage material but the biopsied tissue will show the appearance throughout of a simple hyperplasia, there being no admixture of hyperplastic and non-hyperplastic endometrium and no basal type endometrium. In a simple hyperplasia, the stroma shares in the hyperplastic process and hence the gland-to-stroma ratio is not uncommonly normal. In many cases, however, the stroma is less stimulated than the glands and the gland to stroma ratio will be increased, with the glands appearing crowded.

The endometrial glands show a proliferative pattern but vary markedly in calibre (Fig. 9.1), with some being unusually large, others being of approximately normal diameter and others unduly small. It is this variability in size, rather than just the presence of glands which appear dilated, that is the characteristic feature of this form of endometrial hyperplasia. The glands often have a smooth rounded contour, although some degree of budding into the stroma is not uncommon. The glandular epithelium (Fig. 9.2) is formed by plump, regular, tall cuboidal or low columnar cells, which have strongly basophilic cytoplasm and round, basally or centrally sited nuclei. There is commonly a minor or moderate degree of multilayering but no intraluminal tufting, loss of polarity or cytological atypia are seen.

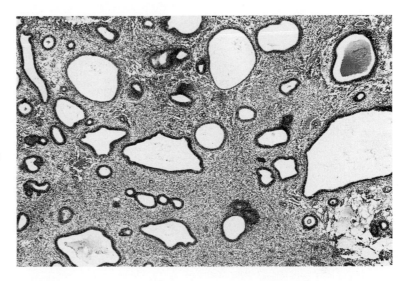

Figure 9.1 Simple hyperplasia. This is characterized by great variability in glandular size. Some glands are large and cystically dilated while others are of normal or even unusually small size. The stroma is cellular. The normal gland to stroma ratio is maintained. Haematoxylin and eosin.

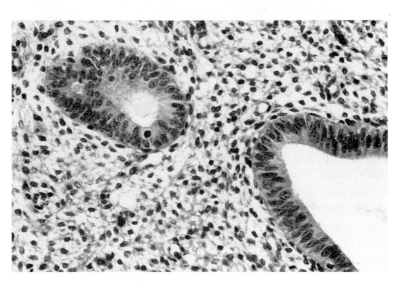

Figure 9.2 Simple hyperplasia. The stroma is cellular and of the type seen in the normal follicular phase. The glands are lined by an epithelium that is pseudostratified, contains occasional mitoses, resembles that seen in the proliferative phase and shows no evidence of cytological atypia. Haematoxylin and eosin.

The glands may show quite well-marked tubal or squamous metaplasia, the latter often taking the form of morules. Eosinophilic cell change is not uncommon.

The stroma usually appears hypercellular and often shows the 'naked nuclei' appearance characteristic of a proliferative phase endometrium. Focal areas of necrosis may be present in the stroma (Fig. 9.3) and these are often infiltrated by inflammatory cells; small collections of foamy stromal histiocytes are not uncommon. Dilated subepithelial sinusoidal vascular spaces are a characteristic feature of a simple hyperplasia but these will rarely be apparent in biopsy specimens.

Mitotic figures, both in the glands and in the stroma, may be abundant or sparse but are invariably of normal form.

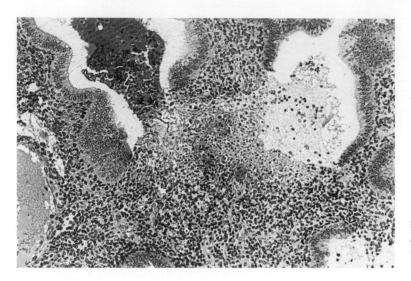

Figure 9.3 Simple hyperplasia. An area of necrosis which is infiltrated by polymorphonuclear leucocytes. Haematoxylin and eosin.

Episodic bleeding, often severe and prolonged, occurs in women with a simple endometrial hyperplasia. It is assumed, perhaps rather simplistically, that this is due either to an intermittent waning of oestrogen levels or to the endometrium reaching a bulk that surpasses the supportive capacity of the oestrogens. Curettage in such cases may reveal a surprisingly undisturbed picture of simple hyperplasia or may show a necrotic, haemorrhagic endometrium with a shrunken stroma and collapsed glands. The circumference of the latter may suggest, however, that some of these had been cystically dilated.

9.2.2 Complex hyperplasia

This endometrial abnormality may occur under the same conditions as does a simple hyperplasia, i.e. in the endometrium exposed to unopposed oestrogenic stimulation, but it can also develop in normally cycling or atrophic endometria. A complex hyperplasia is restricted to the glandular component of the endometrium and does not involve the stroma.

Furthermore, the hyperplastic process is almost invariably focal rather than generalized, hence curettings from cases of complex hyperplasia are not usually unduly bulky and commonly contain an admixture of hyperplastic and normal endometrium. The hyperplastic glands are variable in size but are often larger and more numerous than normal, with consequent crowding and a reduction in the amount of intervening stroma. By definition, there is an abnormal pattern of glandular growth with 'outpouchings', or budding, of the glandular epithelium into the surrounding stroma (Fig. 9.4) to produce the 'finger-in-glove' pattern. In biopsies, the glands may be cut longitudinally and multiple outpouchings can impart a serrated pattern that may be confused with that of a normal late secretory endometrium (Fig. 9.5). Papillary projections of cells, with connective tissue cores, into the glandular lumina are not uncommon and tangential cutting of these may give an impression of solid buds of cells extending into the glands (Fig. 9.6). The glandular epithelium is regular (Fig. 9.7) and formed of tall cuboidal or low

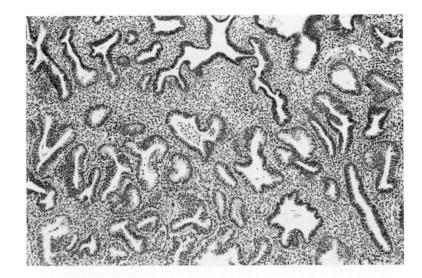

Figure 9.4 Complex hyperplasia. The glands are rather crowded, irregular in contour and exhibit budding and outpouchings. Haematoxylin and eosin.

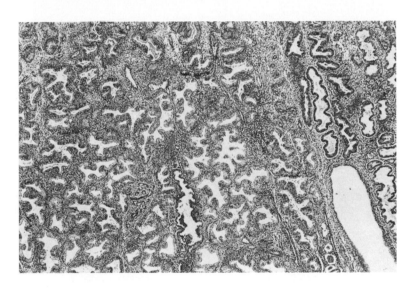

Figure 9.5 Complex hyperplasia. The endometrial glands to the left of the field are closely packed and resemble those of the late secretory phase, having irregular contours, infolding of the epithelium and outpouchings. Haematoxylin and eosin.

columnar cells with ovoid or, less commonly, rounded basal or central nuclei. Nucleoli are inconspicuous, cellular atypia is absent, multilayering is minimal and there is no loss of nuclear polarity. The stroma between the hyperplastic glands is commonly compressed but is not hypercellular. Mitotic figures may be numerous in the glandular epithelium and are of normal form.

9.2.3 Atypical hyperplasia (IEN)

This form of hyperplasia is restricted to the endometrial glands and is always focal in nature, often very sharply so, hence, again, biopsy specimens may include both hyperplastic and normal endometrium. In the hyperplastic areas there is always crowding of the glands, with a reduction in the amount of intervening stroma and in severe cases the

135

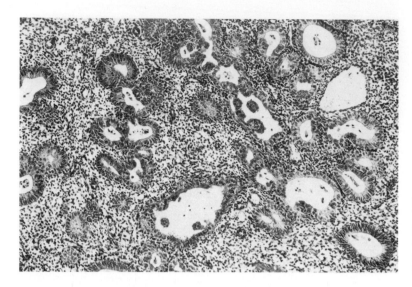

Figure 9.6 Complex hyperplasia. The glands to the right exhibit prominent budding of their epithelium and there is some loss of nuclear polarity. Haematoxylin and eosin.

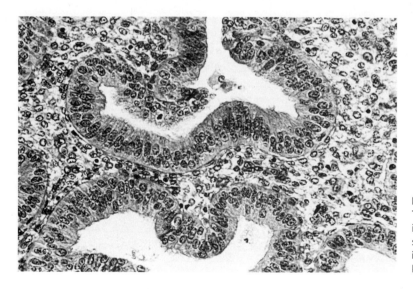

Figure 9.7 Complex hyperplasia. The cells lining the glands are similar in appearance to those seen in simple hyperplasia (Fig. 9.2). There is no evidence of cytological atypia. Haematoxylin and eosin.

glands show a back-to-back pattern (Fig. 9.8) with the interglandular stroma being reduced either to a thin wisp, often detectable only by reticulin stains, or completely obliterated. The glands may have an outline similar to that seen in a complex hyperplasia but are usually markedly irregular in shape, showing a degree of deformity that goes beyond that explicable solely in terms of multiple outbuddings. The cells lining the hyperplastic glands tend to be larger than those seen in a normal proliferative endometrium and show varying degrees of both cytological and nuclear atypia (Fig. 9.9). In the milder forms of atypical hyperplasia, the nuclei are ovoid or sausage-shaped, the nucleo–cytoplasmic ratio is normal or only

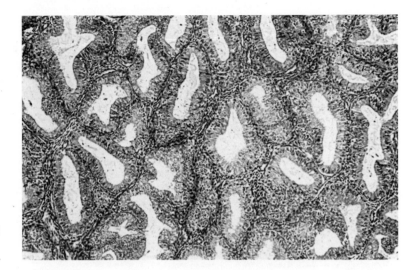

Figure 9.8 Atypical hyperplasia. Intense crowding of the glands which have assumed a 'back-to-back' pattern. The lining epithelium is stratified and exhibits a mild loss of polarity. Haematoxylin and eosin.

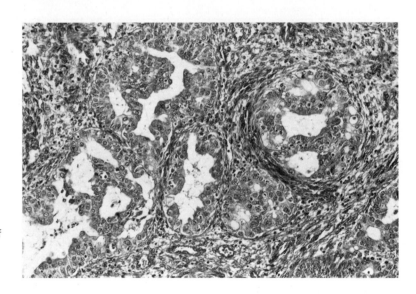

Figure 9.9 Atypical hyperplasia. Focal cytological atypia in a cluster of closely packed glands. The glandular epithelium exhibits loss of nuclear polarity, stratification and forms bridges across the lumina. Haematoxylin and eosin.

slightly increased, nuclear polarity is retained, the nucleoli are not enlarged and there is a normal nuclear chromatin pattern. In more severe cases of atypical hyperplasia the nucleo–cytoplasmic ratio is increased, the nuclei tend to be enlarged and rounded, nuclear polarity is disturbed or lost, nucleoli are increased in size and nuclear chromatin may be either clumped or cleared. If clearing of nuclear chromatin occurs, the nuclear membrane is often very prominent. The cytoplasm may be relatively sparse in the milder forms of atypical hyperplasia but can, rather curiously, be relatively abundant in some cases of severe atypia.

There is commonly, but not invariably, some pseudostratification of the cells lining

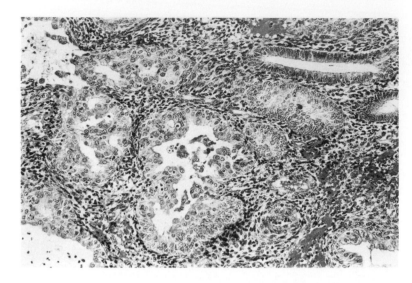

Figure 9.10 Atypical hyperplasia. The glands to the lower left of the field are lined by a stratified epithelium in which nuclear polarity is lost and in which intraluminal budding and bridging are apparent. Haematoxylin and eosin.

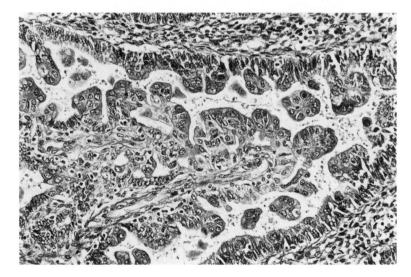

Figure 9.11 Atypical hyperplasia. Marked intraluminal budding in one of a group of glands showing atypical hyperplasia. Haematoxylin and eosin.

the glands in the milder forms of atypical hyperplasia and with progressing severity of the atypia there is an increasing degree of multilayering (Fig. 9.10) and of intraluminal tufting and budding (Fig. 9.11). In severe cases, the intraluminal tufting may be of a complex pattern and the tufts can fuse to give a cribriform pattern within the glands (Fig. 9.12).

These apparent intraglandular epithelial bridges retain a stromal support, albeit one which may only be revealed by a trichrome or reticulin stain. Mitotic figures are uncommon in cases of hyperplasia with mild atypia but tend to be more numerous in the more severely atypical glands, and are usually of normal form.

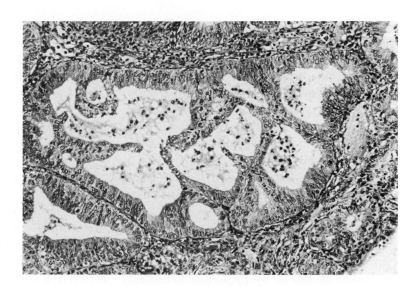

Figure 9.12 Atypical hyperplasia. The glandular epithelium forms bridges across the lumen of a gland in a focus of atypical hyperplasia. Haematoxylin and eosin.

9.3 INTERRELATIONSHIPS OF THE VARIOUS FORMS OF HYPERPLASIA

Each form of endometrial hyperplasia has been described separately but it is not uncommon to encounter, within a single biopsy specimen, various combinations of hyperplastic patterns. Simple hyperplasia commonly exists in a pure form but it is not unusual to encounter a combination of simple hyperplasia with either complex or atypical hyperplasia, or both. Conversely, while a pure complex hyperplasia may be found in isolation, there is often an accompanying simple or atypical hyperplasia. Atypical hyperplasia is commonly associated with a complex hyperplasia or, less frequently, with a simple hyperplasia.

These complicated interrelationships may suggest that the various forms of hyperplasia are either different morphological expressions of a common basic abnormality of growth or that they form a continuous spectrum. However, there is no evidence that a simple hyperplasia is a precursor of a purely glandular hyperplasia, since transitional forms between simple and glandular hyperplasia are not seen. Even when both are present in the same endometrial biopsy, there is almost invariably a sharp and clear boundary between the two abnormal patterns. Conversely, a complex hyperplasia often appears to evolve into an atypical hyperplasia and transitional stages between these two forms of glandular hyperplasia are common.

9.4 ENDOMETRIAL ENDOMETRIOID ADENOCARCINOMA *IN SITU*

Before discussing the histological differentiation of atypical hyperplasia from an endometrial adenocarcinoma of endometrioid type, it is necessary to consider what precisely is meant in this context by the term 'adenocarcinoma'. It is perfectly clear that an endometrioid

139

adenocarcinoma that is invading the myometrium is a true malignant neoplasm but there has been considerable controversy as to the meaning of 'endometrial adenocarcinoma *in situ*'. This term has been used in several different ways in accounts of endometrial pathology (Hertig *et al.*, 1949; Gusberg and Kaplan, 1963; Vellios, 1974). Some have equated adenocarcinoma *in situ* with severe atypical hyperplasia, while others, although drawing a clear distinction between these two entities, have not always specified whether they consider an *in situ* adenocarcinoma to be one that is not invading the endometrial stroma or one that is not invading the myometrium. An adenocarcinoma *in situ* is, by presumed definition, a non-invasive lesion and therefore a true adenocarcinoma *in situ* is one in which the glands have undergone neoplastic change but in which there is no invasion of the endometrial stroma. It is debatable whether an adenocarcinoma of this type exists or if it could be recognized even if it did. Therefore, a form of nomenclature has to be found to describe a lesion, which although thought to be adenocarcinomatous in nature, is confined to the endometrium and does not invade the myometrium. The term 'stage 0 carcinoma' has been applied to a lesion of this type but this is using a clinical staging system to describe a histological finding. The terms 'focal' and 'early' adenocarcinoma have little merit but the term 'intra-endometrial endometrioid adenocarcinoma' seems appropriate if overt evidence of stromal invasion is present. In the absence of evidence of stromal invasion, we would, as already discussed, class such lesions as intra-endometrial neoplasias.

It should be noted that the term 'endometrial carcinoma *in situ*' has also been applied (Spiegel, 1995) to the lesion described by Ambros *et al.* (1995) as the precursor lesion of serous papillary carcinoma of the endometrium and classed as endometrial intraepithelial carcinoma. Confusion about this topic would be decreased if the word 'serous' were introduced into both these terms.

9.5 HISTOLOGICAL DISTINCTION BETWEEN HYPERPLASIA AND ENDOMETRIOID ADENOCARCINOMA

There should not be any difficulty in distinguishing simple or complex hyperplasia from an adenocarcinoma in a curettage specimen. The differentiation in such specimens between a severe atypical hyperplasia and a well-differentiated endometrioid adenocarcinoma does, however, pose a real problem that has not yet been fully solved. Suggested criteria for diagnosing adenocarcinoma, rather than atypical hyperplasia, have included the formation of intraglandular epithelial bridges lacking any stromal support, the presence of polymorphonuclear leucocytes and nuclear debris within glandular lumina, stratification of cells to form a 'gland-within-gland' pattern, loss of nuclear polarity, marked nuclear irregularity, rounding of the nuclei, nucleolar prominence, the finding of numerous mitotic figures, the complete absence of stroma between glands, the piling up of cells into random sheets or masses, the finding of abnormal mitoses and proliferation of metaplastic squamous cells to form solid sheets that replace glands (Silverberg, 1977; Tavassoli and Kraus, 1978; Robertson, 1981; Kurman and Norris, 1982; Hendrickson *et al.*, 1983; Norris *et al.*, 1986). Features suggested as indicating stromal invasion, and therefore implying the malignant nature of the glands, include a desmoplastic reaction in the intervening stroma and focal stromal necrosis (Silverberg, 1977; King *et al.*, 1984).

In practice, many of these features appear to be of relatively little discriminatory value and in some of these studies it has not been clear whether the authors were defining an adenocarcinoma as one which is myoinvasive or not. The real distinction that has to be made is between an atypical hyperplasia (IEN) and a myoinvasive adenocarcinoma; Hendrickson *et al.* (1983) considered that the best predictive features for a myoinvasive lesion were a complex or confluent glandular pattern together with marked cytological abnormalities. Architectural features noted by these workers as indicative of myoinvasion included apposed glands without any intervening stroma, a gland-within-gland pattern, villoglandular areas, papillary infoldings into the glands and epithelial bridging. Cytological criteria included marked nuclear enlargement, striking chromatin changes and prominent nucleoli. The presence of intraluminal polymorphonuclear leucocytes or of areas of necrosis were also considered as pointers towards a diagnosis of invasive adenocarcinoma but evidence of stromal invasion within the endometrium was not considered as being of diagnostic value. In a later study from the same laboratory (Longacre *et al.*, 1995), it was considered that the best indicators of a myoinvasive lesion were a highly complex pattern of glandular growth, marked nuclear pleomorphism and notably prominent nucleoli. This is a summary of a long and complex paper but it is clear from these studies that these workers relied on striking architectural and cytological atypia as guidelines to the diagnosis of a myoinvasive carcinoma.

Kurman and Norris (1982) adopted a quite different and indeed, converse approach to this problem and laid down criteria for the recognition of a myoinvasive carcinoma which were based particularly upon the recognition of stromal invasion as a diagnostic prerequisite. Thus, they required the presence of at least one

of the following features: (1) an irregular infiltration of glands which elicit a desmoplastic response; (2) a confluent pattern of glandular growth in which individual glands are not separated from each other by intervening stroma, and merge to give a cribriform pattern; (3) an extensive papillary pattern; and (4) replacement of the stroma by sheets of squamous cells. The last three changes were required to occupy at least half of a low-power microscopic field 4.2 mm in diameter. Bergeron *et al.* (1999) agreed to a considerable extent with Kurman and Norris (1982) in that they thought that the only feature distinguishing an atypical hyperplasia from a well-differentiated adenocarcinoma in curettage specimens was evidence of stromal invasion: they also found, however, that there was poor inter-observer agreement in the recognition of stromal invasion.

It is our view that there are only a few cardinal, though far from absolute, findings in a biopsy which prompt a diagnosis of well-differentiated adenocarcinoma rather than atypical hyperplasia, using the term 'adenocarcinoma' in this respect to mean a myoinvasive neoplasm. These are:

1. True intraglandular epithelial bridges that are devoid of a stromal support (Fig. 9.13);
2. The random piling up into sheets or masses of cells with rounded, irregular, usually cleared, nuclei and scanty cytoplasm (Fig. 9.14);
3. The presence of abnormal mitotic figures;
4. The presence of polymorphonuclear leucocytes and nuclear debris within glandular lumina (Fig. 9.15).

We are reasonably confident that application of the above criteria will lead to an accurate differentiation between atypical hyperplasia and adenocarcinoma in many, possibly most, cases. We are less certain that we can clearly distinguish, in biopsy material, between a

141

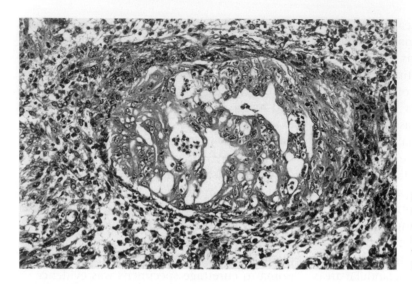

Figure 9.13 Adenocarcinoma. Glandular epithelium forms disorganized proliferations and unsupported epithelial bridges within the lumen of the gland. Haematoxylin and eosin.

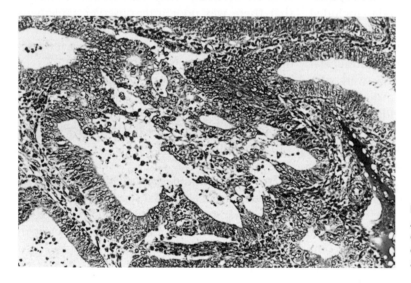

Figure 9.14 Adenocarcinoma. A further example of unsupported epithelial bridges and disorganized epithelial proliferations (epithelial anarchy). Haematoxylin and eosin.

severe atypical hyperplasia and an intra-endometrial adenocarcinoma. Indeed, even in a hysterectomy specimen, the distinction between these two conditions is, unless overt evidence of stromal invasion, such as stromal fibrosis, stromal necrosis and stromal polymorpho-nuclear infiltration is clearly apparent, often a matter of opinion rather than of fact, and hence

the value of a diagnosis of intra-endometrial neoplasia in these circumstances.

While we believe that the discriminatory criteria we use will exclude cases of atypical hyperplasia, we recognize that they will also exclude some cases of very well-differentiated adenocarcinoma. False 'positives' and false 'negatives' are bound to occur when attempting

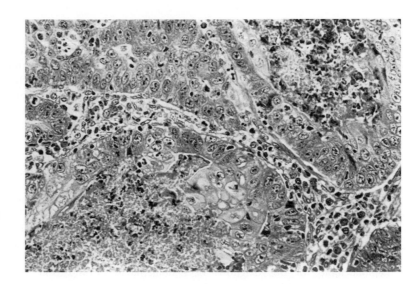

Figure 9.15 Adenocarcinoma. The glands, lined by profoundly atypical epithelium which shows abnormalities of nuclear chromatin dispersion, and contains nucleoli are focally infiltrated by polymorphonuclear leucocytes. Haematoxylin and eosin.

to distinguish between atypical hyperplasia and adenocarcinoma, and pathologists must decide whether the diagnostic criteria they set are more likely to lead to an excess of false positives or to an undue number of false negatives. The natural tendency of a pathologist faced with an equivocal case is towards overdiagnosis in favour of adenocarcinoma, an attitude spurred by the fear of 'missing' a neoplasm and exacerbated by the increasing tendency of the public to resort to litigation. However, the agonizing of pathologists over the histological distinction of atypical hyperplasia and a well-differentiated endometrioid adenocarcinoma is becoming increasingly irrelevant in a clinical context. The crucial factors governing therapy of both these conditions are the patient's age and her desire, or otherwise, to retain her fertility. It is these factors, rather than the niceties of histological diagnosis, which the gynaecologist takes into account when considering management of a woman with a diagnosis of either atypical endometrial hyperplasia or well-differentiated endometrioid adenocarcinoma and the therapeutic decision will be only minimally influenced by the histological diagnosis.

REFERENCES

Ambros, R.A., Sherman, M.E., Zahn, C.M., Bitterman, P., Kurman, R.J. (1995) Endometrial intraepithelial carcinoma: a distinctive lesion specifically associated with tumors displaying serous differentiation. *Hum. Pathol.* **26**, 1260–7.

Bergeron, C., Nogales, F.F., Masseroli, M. *et al.* (1999) A multicentric European study testing the reproducibility of the WHO classification of endometrial hyperplasia with a proposal of a simplified working classification for biopsy and curettage specimens. *Am. J. Surg. Pathol.* **23**, 1102–8.

Ferenczy, A., Bergeron, C. (1992) Endometrial hyperplasia. In Lowe, D., Fox H. (eds), *Advances in Gynaecological Pathology*, Edinburgh: Churchill Livingstone, 207–34.

Fox, H. (1994) Endometrial hyperplasia. *Curr. Diagn. Pathol.* **1**, 151–7.

Fox, H., Buckley, C.H. (1982) The endometrial hyperplasias and their relationship to endometrial neoplasia. *Histopathology* **4**, 493–510.

Gusberg, S.B., Kaplan, A.L. (1963) Precursors of corpus cancer. IV. Adenomatous hyperplasia as Stage 0

143

carcinoma of the endometrium. *Am. J. Obstet. Gynecol.* **87**, 662–76.

Hendrickson, M.R., Ross, J.C., Kempson, R.L. (1983) Towards the development of morphologic criteria for well-differentiated carcinoma of the endometrium. *Am. J. Surg. Pathol.* **7**, 819–38.

Hertig, A.T., Sommers, S.C., Bengloff, H. (1949) Genesis of endometrial carcinoma *in situ*. *Cancer* **2**, 964–71.

Huang, S.J., Amparo, E.G., Fu, Y.S. (1988) Endometrial hyperplasia: histologic classification and behaviour. *Surg. Pathol.* **1**, 215–29.

Jovanovic, A.S., Boynton, K.A., Mutter, G.L. (1996) Uteri of women with endometrial carcinoma contain a histopathological spectrum of monoclonal putative precancers, some with microsatellite instability. *Cancer Res.* **56**, 1917–21.

Kendall, B.S., Ronnet, B.M., Isacson, C. *et al.* (1998) Reproducibility of the diagnosis of endometrial hyperplasia, atypical hyperplasia and well differentiated carcinoma. *Am. J. Surg. Pathol.* **22**, 1012–19.

King, A., Seraj, I., Walner, R.J. (1984) Stromal invasion in endometrial adenocarcinoma. *Am. J. Obstet. Gynecol.* **149**, 10–15.

Kurman, R.J., Katminiski, P.F., Norris, H.J. (1985) The behaviour of endometrial hyperplasia: a long-term study of 'untreated' hyperplasia in 170 patients. *Cancer* **56**, 403–12.

Kurman, R.J., Norris, H.J. (1982) Evaluation of criteria for distinguishing atypical endometrial hyperplasia from well-differentiated adenocarcinoma. *Cancer* **49**, 2547–59.

Longacre, T.A., Chung, M.H., Jensen, D.N., Hendrickson, M.R. (1995) Proposed criteria for the diagnosis of well-differentiated endometrial

carcinoma: a diagnostic test for myoinvasion. *Am. J. Surg. Pathol.* **19**, 371–406.

Mutter, G.L., Endometrial Collaborative Group. (2000) Endometrial intraepithelial neoplasia (EIN): will it bring order to chaos? *Gynecol. Oncol.* **76**, 287–90.

Norris, H.J., Connor, M.P., Kurman, R.J. (1986) Preinvasive lesions of the endometrium. *Clinics Obstet. Gynaecol.* **13**, 725–38.

Robertson, W.B. (1981) *The Endometrium*. London: Butterworths.

Scully, R.E., Bonfiglio, T.A., Kurman, R.J., Silverberg, S.G., Wilkinson, E.J. (1994) *International Histological Classifications and Typing of Female Genital Tract Tumours*. New York: Springer-Verlag.

Silverberg, S.G. (1977) *Surgical Pathology of the Uterus*. New York: John Wiley.

Skov, B.G., Broholm, H., Engel, U. *et al.* (1997) Comparison of the reproducibility of the WHO classifications of 1975 and 1994 of endometrial hyperplasia. *Int. J. Gynecol. Pathol.* **16**, 33–7.

Spiegel, G.W. (1995) Endometrial carcinoma *in situ* in postmenopausal women. *Am. J. Surg. Pathol.* **19**, 417–32.

Tavassoli, F., Kraus, F.T. (1978) Endometrial lesions in uteri resected for atypical endometrial hyperplasia. *Am. J. Clin. Pathol.* **70**, 770–9.

Vellios, F. (1974) Endometrial hyperplasia and carcinoma *in situ*. *Gynecol. Oncol.* **2**, 152–9.

Welch, W.R., Scully, R.E. (1977) Precancerous lesions of the endometrium. *Hum. Pathol.* **8**, 503–12.

Zaino, R. J. (2000) Endometrial hyperplasia: is it time for a quantum leap to a new classification? *Int. J. Gynecol. Pathol.* **19**, 314–21.

10 Carcinoma of the endometrium (endometrial Müllerian epithelial tumours)

The pathologist dealing with a biopsy from a case of suspected carcinoma of the endometrium has first to confirm or refute the presence of a neoplasm. If a carcinoma is diagnosed the pathologist must then proceed to:

1. Identify the precise histological type of the tumour.
2. Assess the grade of the tumour.
3. Distinguish between an endocervical and an endometrial tumour.
4. Judge whether any non-neoplastic endometrium included in the biopsy is normally cycling, atrophic or hyperplastic.

The last three tasks are common to all types of endometrial carcinomas but the problem of grading differs with the histological type.

10.1 CLASSIFICATION OF ENDOMETRIAL CARCINOMAS

The histological classification of endometrial carcinomas shown in Table 10.1 is very similar to that currently recommended by the International Society of Gynecological Pathologists but has been supplemented by a number of relatively newly recognized entities.

The term 'endometrioid adenocarcinoma' merits comment. The vast majority of endometrial adenocarcinomas (80 per cent) show some degree of endometrial differentiation and bear a resemblance, albeit an anarchic one, to normal proliferative endometrium; these are, therefore, 'the usual type of endometrial adenocarcinoma'. However, a more succinct alternative is required for this unwieldy phrase and it is fully acceptable to class such neoplasms as 'endometrioid adenocarcinomas', a term not to everyone's taste but one that is semantically, even pedantically, correct.

It has to be emphasized that a simple diagnosis of endometrial adenocarcinoma represents an inadequate response to the finding of a carcinoma in an endometrial biopsy insofar as some of the histological subtypes in Table 10.1 have a particularly poor prognosis

145

Table 10.1 Classification of primary epithelial neoplasms of the endometrium

1. Endometrioid adenocarcinoma
    Variants
        with squamous differentiation
        papillary (villoglandular)
        secretory
        ciliated cell
        Sertoliform
        signet-ring cell
2. Serous papillary carcinoma
3. Clear cell adenocarcinoma
4. Mucinous adenocarcinoma
5. Microglandular carcinoma
6. Oncocytic carcinoma
7. Squamous cell carcinoma
8. Transitional cell carcinoma
9. Small cell neuroendocrine carcinoma
10. Undifferentiated carcinoma

and their identification in a diagnostic curettage is of great importance in the planning of definitive therapy.

10.2 ENDOMETRIOID ADENOCARCINOMA

All neoplasms in this category show, by definition, some degree of endometrial differentiation. The majority are well differentiated and consist of irregular, complex glandular acini, which are lined by a predominantly cuboidal or low columnar epithelium of recognizably endometrial type (Fig. 10.1). There is a marked shift, in favour of the glandular component, in the gland to stroma ratio and the glandular acini are often separated from each other by only a thin wisp of stroma or show a true back-to-back pattern.

The epithelium lining the neoplastic acini shows a variable degree of multilayering and intra-acinar tufting (Fig. 10.2), while intraglandular epithelial bridges, lacking any stromal support, are a characteristic feature and will, if widespread, impart a cribriform appearance to the neoplasm. The epithelial nuclei may be rather bland and ovoid-shaped but are more commonly rounded with either irregular, jagged condensation or a complete clearing of nuclear chromatin. Perhaps the most characteristic nuclear pattern is that of rounded nuclei with sharply etched limiting membranes and cleared chromatin. This nuclear pattern can, however, be induced simply by inadequate fixation (Longacre *et al.*, 1995) and hence it should be noted whether the nuclei of stromal or inflammatory cells in the biopsy specimen also show this appearance (Fig. 10.3). The cleared, rounded nuclei are often aggregated into syncytial-like intra-acinar masses ('cellular anarchy') while mitotic figures, almost invariably of normal form, are usually present – their absence indicates considerable diagnostic caution. Clear cell areas may be seen in endometrioid adenocarcinomas and there may be oncocytic change of variable extent (Pitman *et al.*, 1994; Fukuoka *et al.*, 1998).

Foci of necrosis are common, even in very well-differentiated tumours, and these are often infiltrated by polymorphonuclear leucocytes. Even more characteristic is the presence of such cells within glandular acini in non-necrotic areas of the tumour. The presence of foamy cells in the stroma (Fig. 10.4), either singly or in clumps, is a characteristic, but by no means diagnostic, feature of endometrioid adenocarcinomas (Dalwagne and Silverberg, 1982).

A minority of endometrioid adenocarcinomas are less well differentiated and have a partly acinar and a partly solid pattern. In such neoplasms the degree of cytological atypia is greater than in the well-differentiated tumours

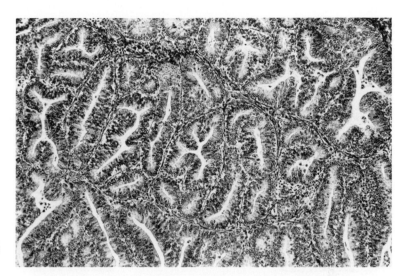

Figure 10.1 Well-differentiated endometrioid adenocarcinoma (Histological Grade 1). The tumour is composed of closely packed, well-formed glandular acini, lined by a stratified columnar epithelium, set in a fibrous stroma. Haematoxylin and eosin.

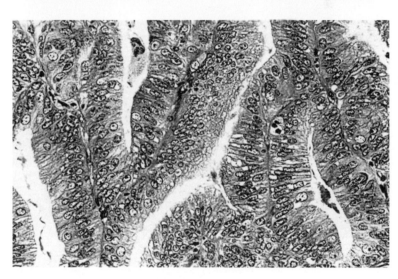

Figure 10.2 Well-differentiated endometrioid adenocarcinoma (Histological Grade 1). The glandular acini are lined by stratified columnar epithelium. The nuclei are round to oval, some contain nucleoli, and there is some loss of nuclear polarity. Note the finely dispersed nuclear chromatin in this biopsy fixed in Bouin's fixative. Haematoxylin and eosin.

while nuclear abnormalities are more marked; mitotic figures are abundant and some will be of abnormal form.

Poorly differentiated endometrioid adenocarcinomas are relatively rare, have a predominantly solid growth pattern and usually show marked atypia. They can only be recognized as being of endometrioid type if there is, in some areas at least, a tentative attempt at formation of endometrial-like glandular acini.

10.2.1 Grading of endometrioid adenocarcinoma

Grading of endometrioid adenocarcinoma in curettings may, rather obviously, be less than satisfactory because of the limited sampling of the neoplasm. Nevertheless, a provisional grading should be attempted because tumour grade is an important consideration when planning therapy. The traditional grading of endometrioid adenocarcinomas into well,

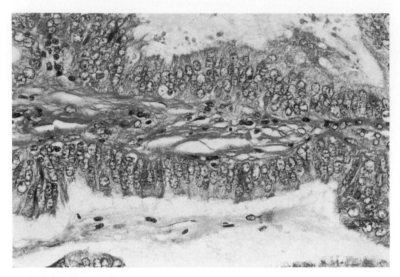

Figure 10.3 Well-differentiated endometrioid adenocarcinoma. This tumour is morphologically similar to that shown in Figure 10.2, but the tissue has been fixed more slowly in formalin. The nuclei of both the malignant epithelium and, importantly, the nuclei in the stromal cells appear 'cleared' and the nuclear membranes are therefore relatively more prominent. This is an artefact. Haematoxylin and eosin.

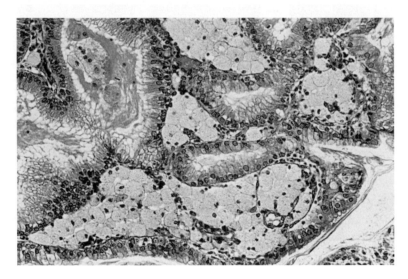

Figure 10.4 Aggregates of foamy histiocytes in the stroma of a well-differentiated endometrioid adenocarcinoma. Haematoxylin and eosin.

moderately and poorly differentiated adenocarcinomas is highly subjective and a modified FIGO grading system is recommended:

- Grade 1 – 5 per cent or less of the tumour shows a solid growth pattern (Fig. 10.1);
- Grade 2 – between 5 and 50 per cent of the tumour is growing in a solid fashion (Fig. 10.5);
- Grade 3 – more than 50 per cent of the tumour shows a solid growth pattern (Fig. 10.6).

In making this grading, solid sheets of cells in an endometrioid adenocarcinoma should be regarded as glandular unless definitive evidence of squamous differentiation is present. Any squamous element present is not included

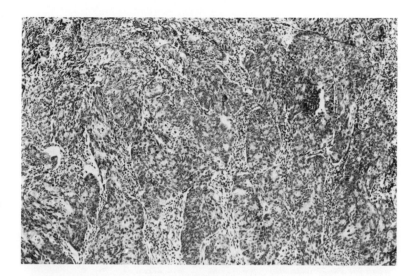

Figure 10.5 Moderately well-differentiated endometrioid adenocarcinoma (Histological Grade 2). Glandular acini are poorly formed, though approximately 50 per cent of the neoplasm has a glandular/acinar pattern. Haematoxylin and eosin.

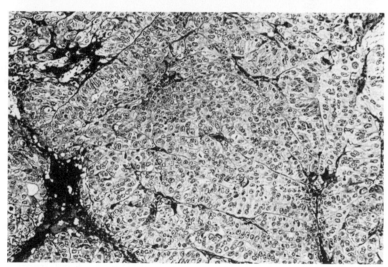

Figure 10.6 Poorly-differentiated/undifferentiated carcinoma (Histological Grade 3). The neoplasm is composed of sheets and nests of large, round to oval cells with vesicular nuclei in which there are prominent nucleoli. Haematoxylin and eosin.

in the grading. Recently, it has been suggested that a two-tier rather than a three-tier system be used for grading endometrioid adenocarcinomas (Taylor *et al.*, 1999) using 20 per cent solid growth pattern as the cut-off point between the two grades; it is argued that such a system is more effective in assessing prognosis. It may well prove to be the case that this system has clear advantages over the presently used FIGO system but, clearly, a great deal

more experience is required before advising a change in the current grading system.

The above grading system takes account only of the architectural pattern of the tumour and neglects cytological features. In order to rectify this deficiency a rider is added 'notable nuclear atypia, inappropriate for the architectural grade, raises the grade of a Grade 1 or Grade 2 tumour by 1'. FIGO did not define in any precise manner the degree of nuclear

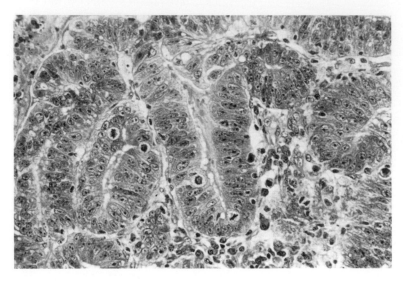

Figure 10.7 Endometrioid adenocarcinoma (Histological Grade 2). Despite the presence of well-formed glandular acini, the degree of cytological atypia in this tumour is severe. Mitotic activity is prominent, nucleocytoplasmic ratios are high and there is loss of cellular polarity. Haematoxylin and eosin.

atypia meriting an assignation of 'notable' but Zaino *et al*. (1995) have defined three nuclear grades:

- Grade 1 – rounded to oval nuclei with evenly distributed chromatin and inconspicuous nucleoli;
- Grade 2 – irregular oval nuclei with chromatin clumping and moderate-sized nucleoli;
- Grade 3 – large pleomorphic nuclei with coarse chromatin and large irregular nucleoli (Fig. 10.7).

If a carcinoma is Grade 1 or 2 on the FIGO grading system, it should be raised a Grade if it shows Grade 3 nuclear abnormalities.

Generally, the FIGO grading system correlates well with prognosis but there are a number of practical difficulties. It can be difficult to tell whether solid growth is non-squamous or squamous, there remains a degree of subjectivity in nuclear grading and a distinction between less than 5 per cent solid growth and more than 5 per cent solid growth is often arbitrary. In an effort to overcome these difficulties, Lax *et al*. (2000) have proposed a binary architectural grading system for endometrioid adenocarcinomas in which the tumours are graded either as high grade or low grade. An adenocarcinoma is classified as high grade if at least two of the following architectural features are present:

1. More than 50 per cent solid growth, with no distinction being made between squamous and non-squamous differentiation;
2. Tumour cell necrosis;
3. A diffusely infiltrative, as opposed to an expansive, growth pattern.

For tumours confined to the endometrium, only the percentage of solid growth and the presence of necrosis are noted and if both these features are present, the neoplasm is classed as high grade.

This grading system appears to have a similar prognostic value to that of the FIGO grading system but has greater reproducibility, partly because it is relatively easy to assess if a tumour has a majority solid growth pattern and partly because the system takes no note of nuclear atypia. Whether or not this system gains wide acceptance will depend on further and wider experience of its use.

10.2.2 Differential diagnosis

The problem of distinguishing between a well-differentiated endometrioid adenocarcinoma and an atypical hyperplasia of the endometrium has been fully discussed in Chapter 9 and the arguments outlined there will not be repeated in this chapter.

A menstrual endometrium is sometimes misconstrued as an endometrioid adenocarcinoma but this solecism can be avoided if the disproportionate degree of haemorrhage and necrosis and, most importantly, the lack of cytological atypia in a menstrual endometrium are recognized.

A very poorly differentiated adenocarcinoma can resemble an endometrial stromal sarcoma, but a careful search for tentative gland formation, the noting of periodic acid–Schiff (PAS)-positive mucus, the finding of reticulin fibres surrounding groups of cells (rather than individual cells) and the demonstration of positive staining reactions for both epithelial membrane antigen and cytokeratins, and a negative reaction for vimentin will usually allow for the recognition of an adenocarcinoma. It should, however, be noted that a proportion of endometrial adenocarcinomas co-express both cytokeratins and vimentin (Dabbs *et al.*, 1986), thus posing a diagnostic trap for those placing undue reliance on immunohistochemical techniques.

A malignant lymphoma of the endometrium can also resemble a poorly differentiated adenocarcinoma. Lymphomas, however, often envelop normal endometrial glands, have a different nuclear pattern from that of an adenocarcinoma and are characterized by a positive staining reaction for leucocyte common antigen and a negative reaction for epithelial markers.

10.3 HISTOLOGICAL VARIANTS OF ENDOMETRIOID ADENOCARCINOMA

10.3.1 Endometrioid adenocarcinoma with squamous differentiation

We have long felt that a clear distinction can be made between endometrioid adenocarcinomas showing squamous metaplasia, in which the squamous component appears benign, and adenosquamous carcinomas, which appear to contain both malignant glandular and malignant squamous components (Ng *et al.*, 1973; Haqqani and Fox, 1976; Alberhasky *et al.*, 1982). We considered these as different lesions with vastly differing prognoses. Others have not concurred with this view (Zaino and Kurman, 1988) and a number of large studies have now shown, with considerable conviction, that the prognosis of endometrioid adenocarcinomas with squamous differentiation depends almost entirely on the grade of the glandular component; this gives a better prognostic assessment than does either grading of the squamous element or separating the tumours into endometrioid carcinomas showing squamous metaplasia and adenosquamous carcinomas (Zaino *et al.*, 1991; Abeler and Kjorstad, 1992). It therefore seems reasonable to accept that the two previously separately described lesions of endometrioid adenocarcinoma with squamous metaplasia and adenosquamous carcinoma should now be considered as a single entity of endometrioid adenocarcinoma with squamous differentiation. By definition, at least 10 per cent of the neoplasm must show squamous differentiation for it to fall into this category.

Histologically endometrioid carcinomas showing squamous differentiation are often well differentiated but can be Grade 2 or 3. The squamous component may appear histologically benign, may show atypical features not

151

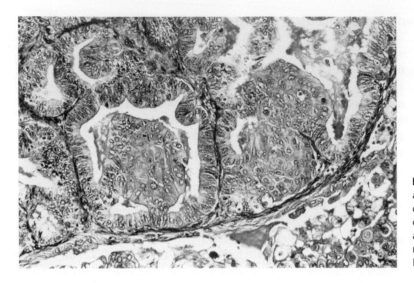

Figure 10.8 Endometrioid adenocarcinoma with squamous differentiation. The glandular component is well differentiated and the squamous tissue is morphologically benign. Haematoxylin and eosin.

amounting to carcinoma or may appear frankly malignant. Histologically benign-appearing squamous differentiation is usually found in Grade 1 endometrioid adenocarcinomas and can be a conspicuous feature. It can occur as foci of bland, well-differentiated squamous tissue, as morules or as masses of keratin. Foci of well-differentiated squamous tissue are usually seen within glandular acini (Fig. 10.8), appear to blend with the epithelial cells lining the acini, have a fully benign appearance and show typical squamous features, such as keratinization, intercellular bridges, sharp cell margins and eosinophilic cytoplasm. Morules (Chapter 8) consist of nests of cells, often spindly in shape, with bland, relatively small uniform nuclei and moderately abundant, sometimes eosinophilic, cytoplasm (Hendrickson and Kempson, 1995). Occasional foci of overt squamous differentiation may be seen in some of these cell nests and large morules can, on occasion, show central necrosis. The morules lie within glandular acini and sometimes expand to compress, and mask or even obliterate, the surrounding glandular cells. Occasionally

squamous differentiation in an endometrioid adenocarcinoma is manifest only by the presence of masses of keratinous material. These are sometimes hyalinized, may evoke a foreign-body giant cell reaction (Fig. 10.9) and can be so abundant as to obscure the underlying adenocarcinoma.

Most endometrioid adenocarcinomas with extensive histologically benign-appearing squamous differentiation are, as already remarked, Grade 1 and thus have a good prognosis. There has been a tendency in the past to class such neoplasms as 'adenoacanthomas' but endometrioid adenocarcinomas showing a striking degree of squamous differentiation are associated with a prognosis that does not differ significantly from endometrioid adenocarcinomas of similar grade showing no squamous metaplasia (Barrowclough and Jaarsma, 1980). Hence, there is no justification for considering the adenoacanthoma as a distinct nosological entity and this diagnostic term should be abandoned.

Endometrioid carcinomas with squamous differentiation showing malignant features are

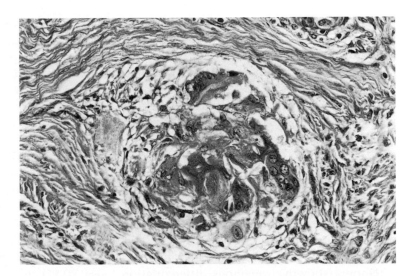

Figure 10.9 Foreign-body reaction to the presence of keratin produced by an endometrioid adenocarcinoma in which there was extensive squamous differentiation. The granuloma contains several macrophage giant cells surrounding irregular aggregates of keratin. Haematoxylin and eosin.

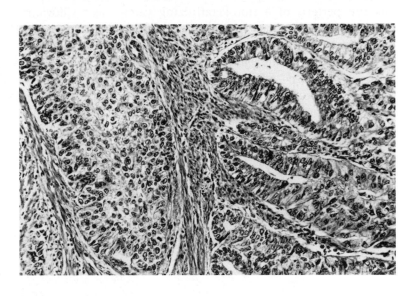

Figure 10.10 Endometrioid adenocarcinoma with squamous differentiation. The squamous element has the features of a non-keratinizing large cell squamous carcinoma. In this area, the glandular and squamous components appear separate from each other. Haematoxylin and eosin.

usually Grade 2 or Grade 3 and the squamous component often appears as a well-differentiated non-keratinizing large cell carcinoma. The two histologically malignant components may be intermixed or can appear to be quite discrete from each other (Fig. 10.10). In a proportion of these neoplasms, the squamous element may show, to a variable extent, a 'glassy-cell' pattern with very distinct cell margins and eosinophilic, slightly granular cytoplasm (Christopherson *et al.*, 1982c).

Because endometrioid adenocarcinomas showing extensive benign-appearing squamous differentiation are usually Grade 1, the presence of the squamous tissue often makes the task of distinguishing between a complex hyperplasia and an adenocarcinoma in a biopsy more difficult. The principles already

153

outlined for differentiating these two entities are not, however, altered by the presence of the squamous tissue.

As endometrioid adenocarcinomas with squamous differentiation are graded solely on the features of their glandular component, a problem may be encountered if morules are mistaken for solid foci of carcinoma – an error that can lead to inaccurate grading. Again, however, the distinction is based on the bland nature of the morules, their small uniform nuclei contrasting sharply with the large, atypical nuclei seen in solid masses of carcinomatous cells. The problem of grading also arises if the squamous component of an endometrioid carcinoma showing squamous differentiation has the pattern of a non-keratinizing carcinoma for this also may be difficult to distinguish from a focus of solid adenocarcinoma. The presence of intercellular bridges and of cells with sharp margins, eosinophilic or 'glassy' cytoplasm and a relatively low nucleo–cytoplasmic ratio suggest the squamous nature of a solid group of cells.

In assessing biopsy material it is necessary to bear in mind that a tumour showing both malignant glandular and squamous elements could represent a 'collision' of a cervical squamous carcinoma with an endometrial adenocarcinoma or a cervical adenosquamous carcinoma. The exclusion of these possibilities is commonly dependent on accurate clinical information.

10.3.2 Papillary variant of endometrioid adenocarcinoma (villoglandular carcinoma)

Many otherwise typical endometrioid adenocarcinomas of the endometrium have a papillary pattern in some areas. This pattern predominates in a small proportion of such neoplasms (Fig. 10.11) and tumours of this type are known as 'villoglandular endometrioid adenocarcinomas' (Hendrickson and Kempson, 1995) or as 'well differentiated papillary adenocarcinomas' (Chen *et al.*, 1985). The papillae in this variant of endometrioid adenocarcinoma are fine and non-complex with a thin fibrovascular core. The covering epithelium is formed by relatively uniform cuboidal or low columnar cells of endometrial type with ovoid, basally situated nuclei showing only a minor degree of pleomorphism and

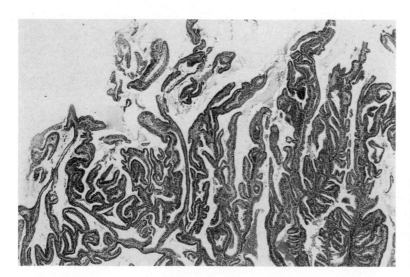

Figure 10.11 Endometrioid adenocarcinoma with papillary pattern. The superficial layers of this neoplasm are composed of fine fibrous tissue papillae covered by neoplastic epithelium. Haematoxylin and eosin.

hyperchromasia. Stratification of the covering epithelial cells is an inconspicuous feature while tufting is not seen. Psammoma bodies are usually absent and mitotic figures are scanty and of normal form. In most tumours of this type, there is a transition, in some areas at least, to the more conventional acinar pattern of an endometrioid adenocarcinoma, but this may not be apparent in a biopsy specimen.

There has been some dispute about the prognostic significance of a papillary pattern in endometrioid adenocarcinomas. Some have considered that these neoplasms have exactly the same prognosis as endometrioid carcinomas not showing a papillary pattern (Chen *et al.*, 1985; Ward *et al.*, 1990). Others have claimed that this form of papillary neoplasm behaves in a manner intermediate between that of an endometrioid adenocarcinoma and that of a papillary serous adenocarcinoma (Sutton *et al.*, 1987; O'Hanlan *et al.*, 1990). In a recent large series, however, it has been clearly shown that the prognosis for the papillary (villoglandular) form of endometrioid carcinoma is the same as that for a conventional endometrioid adenocarcinoma (Zaino *et al.*,

1998). It is therefore critically important that the villoglandular endometrioid carcinomas are distinguished from the highly aggressive serous papillary carcinoma of the endometrium (see Section 10.4). The distinction between these two neoplasms of vastly differing prognosis rests upon the fine nature of the papillae in the endometrioid carcinoma, on the endometrioid rather than serous nature of the covering epithelium and, most importantly, on the relatively low-grade atypia in the epithelial cells.

10.3.3 Secretory variant of endometrioid adenocarcinoma

This term is applied to those endometrioid adenocarcinomas in which the neoplastic epithelial cells show either supranuclear or infranuclear vacuolation (Tobon and Watkins, 1985); luminal secretion is also apparent in most of such neoplasms (Fig. 10.12). A positive PAS staining of both the cytoplasm of the epithelial cells and the luminal secretions, the former being rendered negative after diastase digestion, and a negative reaction with Best's carmine stain are characteristic of these

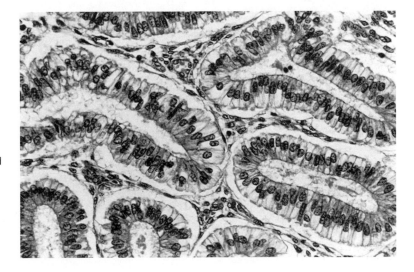

Figure 10.12 Secretory changes in a well-differentiated endometrioid adenocarcinoma. The subnuclear vacuoles seen in virtually all the epithelial cells are due to the fact that the patient had been treated with progestagens for postmenopausal bleeding. Haematoxylin and eosin.

neoplasms. The luminal secretions, but not the cytoplasm of the epithelial cells, tend to stain positively with Alcian blue.

These tumours appear to be well-differentiated endometrioid adenocarcinomas with superimposed secretory change. In premenopausal women, the secretory change is probably induced by the cyclical secretion of progesterone and hence neoplasms showing a secretory pattern in curettings may not show such activity at the time of subsequent hysterectomy. In postmenopausal women, the stimulus to neoplastic secretory activity is obscure if treatment with an exogenous progestagen is excluded.

Secretory endometrioid adenocarcinomas are graded in exactly the same way as are similar neoplasms lacking secretory activity; as the vast majority are Grade 1, they have a good prognosis. Secretory adenocarcinomas must, however, be distinguished from endometrial hyperplasias showing secretory change, from an Arias-Stella reaction and from a clear-cell endometrial carcinoma. The distinction of a secretory endometrioid adenocarcinoma

from hyperplasia with superimposed secretory change is based on the same principles as the distinction between the non-secretory forms of these two entities while an Arias-Stella reaction can be recognized by its setting within a hypersecretory pregnancy-type endometrium. The distinction between the secretory variant of an endometrioid adenocarcinoma and the much more sinister clear cell adenocarcinoma of the endometrium (see Section 10.5), though not always drawn in reported series, is quite clear-cut. Secretory endometrioid adenocarcinomas do not show the mixed tubulocystic, papillary and solid patterns of a clear cell adenocarcinoma, do not contain hobnail nuclei and show a relatively minor degree of atypia.

10.3.4 Ciliated cell variant of endometrioid adenocarcinoma

Endometrioid adenocarcinomas often contain a few ciliated cells but occasionally such neoplasms are formed predominantly (Fig. 10.13), or even exclusively, of ciliated cells (Hendrickson

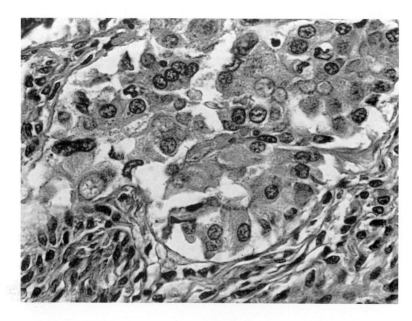

Figure 10.13 Ciliated cell carcinoma. The glandular acini are lined by cells with round to oval nuclei and copious cytoplasm. The cell surface is covered by cilia which protrude into the acinar lumen. Haematoxylin and eosin. Photograph kindly supplied by Dr R.L. Kempson.

and Kempson, 1983). These very rare tumours have a distinctive histological appearance and tend to consist of sheets of cells to which a cribriform pattern is imparted by scattered extracellular lumina. The cells limiting the lumina have prominent cilia, which project into the luminal space. Many of the cells elsewhere contain sharply delineated intra-cytoplasmic vacuoles that contain tangled or matted eosinophilic cilia. The cells in these tumours have nuclei showing typically malignant features and, very characteristically, strongly eosinophilic cytoplasm. Many of these neoplasms contain areas of more typical endometrioid adenocarcinoma.

Grading of ciliated cell adenocarcinomas presents difficulties and it is probable that most reliance should be placed on nuclear, rather than architectural, grade; most are nuclear Grade 1 or 2 and have a reasonably good prognosis.

It is necessary to differentiate a ciliated cell carcinoma from ciliated cell metaplasia in an endometrial hyperplasia. Again, the general principles of differentiation of a hyperplasia from an adenocarcinoma still apply.

10.3.5 Sertoliform variant of endometrioid adenocarcinoma

Very rarely an endometrioid adenocarcinoma is composed in part, or almost wholly, of tubular structures that resemble those seen in a Sertoli cell tumour (Fig. 10.14) of the ovary (Fox and Brander, 1988; Eichhorn *et al.*, 1996). This should not cause confusion if, in curettage material, there is an admixture of Sertoliform tubules and conventional endometrioid adenocarcinoma. If the tumour tissue in a biopsy shows only a Sertoliform pattern it may be difficult to distinguish a Sertoliform adenocarcinoma from a stromal sarcoma showing a sex-cord-like pattern. Both lesions necessitate hysterectomy and, therefore, an inability to make a definitive diagnosis in these circumstances is of little practical importance.

10.3.6 Signet-ring cell carcinoma

A single example of a primary signet-ring cell carcinoma of the endometrium has been described (Mooney *et al.*, 1997). This can be regarded as a variant of an endometrioid

Figure 10.14 Sertoliform endometrioid adenocarcinoma. The tumour is composed of narrow, remarkably regular tubules lined by a tall columnar epithelium with well-orientated basal nuclei. There is an acute resemblance to a Sertoli cell tumour of the ovary. Elsewhere, there was a transition to a more conventional endometrioid pattern. Haematoxylin and eosin.

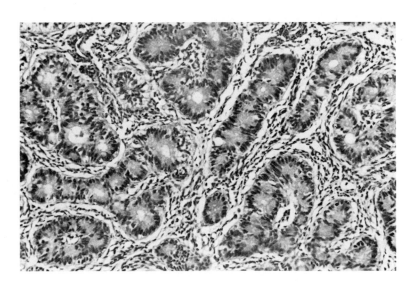

carcinoma because it showed a transition in one area to a conventional endometrioid carcinomatous pattern. The signet-ring cells stained positively for mucin and in many areas showed a pattern of infiltration of the stroma around normal endometrial glands. The significance of this variant form of endometrioid carcinoma is that both a signet-ring cell pattern and infiltration of stroma around normal glands are usually considered as characteristics of a metastatic carcinoma in the endometrium from a primary site outside the genital tract (see Chapter 12). If a signet-ring cell neoplasm is observed in an endometrial biopsy, it is most likely to be from a metastatic tumour but the remote possibility of a primary endometrial neoplasm has to be borne in mind.

10.4 SEROUS PAPILLARY CARCINOMA

These endometrial tumours, which usually occur in elderly women and typically arise from an inactive or atrophic endometrium, are histologically identical to papillary serous adenocarcinomas of the ovary (Lauchlan, 1981; Christopherson *et al.,* 1982b; Walker and Mills, 1982; Hendrickson *et al.,* 1982; Chen *et al.,* 1985).

Serous papillary carcinomas commonly have, as their name indicates, a predominantly papillary architecture (Fig. 10.15), sometimes simple but more commonly complex, with broad, coarse fibrovascular cores covered by pleomorphic epithelial cells; the papillary cores may be hyalinized or oedematous. The cells covering the papillae (Fig. 10.16) are of serous type and show marked atypia. Their nuclei tend to be large with sharp limiting membranes, irregularly condensed chromatin and prominent eosinophilic nucleoli. The epithelial cells often show irregular pseudostratification and tufting while the development of secondary papillary structures and formation of interconnecting arches are common features. Clumps of cells often exfoliate – a feature not commonly apparent in biopsy specimens – while mitotic figures are numerous and frequently of abnormal form. Although their architecture is generally papillary, these neoplasms frequently show a solid

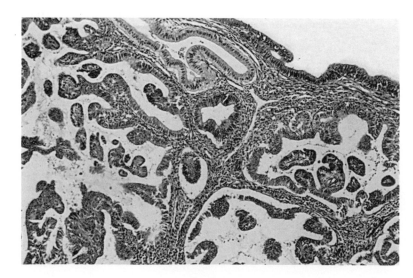

Figure 10.15 Serous papillary carcinoma. The endometrium is infiltrated by a morphologically well-differentiated papillary adenocarcinoma. Haematoxylin and eosin.

growth pattern in some areas, with large undifferentiated cells growing in sheets that show foci of necrosis; a glandular pattern is also seen with some frequency. Typical psammoma bodies are present in 30–50 per cent of serous papillary carcinomas.

In the current FIGO staging system it is recommended that papillary serous carcinomas are graded solely on the basis of their nuclear characteristics but it is doubtful if grading is of any real value since, almost by definition, these neoplasms invariably show high-grade nuclear atypia. The vast majority of papillary serous carcinomas stain positively for *p53* (Sherman *et al.*, 1995; Moll *et al.*, 1996) and *p53* mutations are detectable by molecular techniques (Tashiro *et al.*, 1997): they lack demonstrable oestrogen and progesterone receptors (Sasano *et al.*, 1990).

Serous papillary carcinomas of the endometrium are aggressive tumours that tend to permeate, in a very extensive fashion, uterine and adnexal lymphatic and vascular channels at an early stage in their evolution, and are associated with a particularly gloomy prognosis (Silverberg, 1984; Abeler and Kjorstad, 1990a; Lee and Belinson, 1992; Sherman *et al.*, 1992;

Rosenberg *et al.*, 1993; Goff *et al.*, 1994; Gitsch *et al.*, 1995; Kato *et al.*, 1995; Tay and Ward, 1999). It is generally thought that even tumours apparently limited to the endometrium or confined to an endometrial polyp have a poor prognosis (Silva and Jenkins, 1990; Carcangui and Chambers, 1992, 1997). However, Wheeler *et al.* (2000) have recently shown that serous papillary carcinomas, which are not invading the myometrium and do not show lymphovascular invasion, have an excellent prognosis in the absence of extrauterine disease. It is vitally important that serous papillary carcinomas are distinguished from the relatively banal papillary variant of an endometrioid adenocarcinoma; the grounds for making this distinction are outlined in Section 10.3.2. A papillary serous adenocarcinoma can also resemble closely an endometrial clear cell carcinoma showing a papillary pattern but since both neoplasms share the same wretched prognosis, their differentiation is of little practical importance. Syncytial metaplasia of the endometrium may show a papillary pattern but lacks malignant cytological features, in particular high-grade nuclear atypia is not a feature of this metaplastic change.

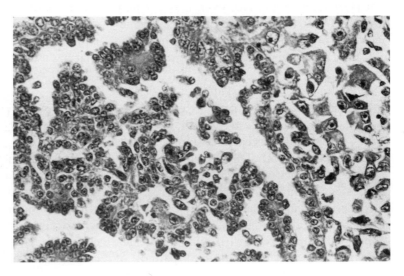

Figure 10.16 Serous papillary carcinoma. The well-formed papillary processes of the carcinoma contrast sharply with the profound cytological atypia characterized by loss of nuclear polarity, high nucleocytoplasmic ratios and, particularly in the pleomorphic cells to the right, prominent nucleoli. Haematoxylin and eosin.

159

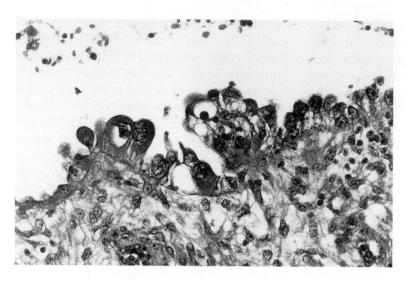

Figure 10.17 A focus of endometrial intraepithelial carcinoma in the endometrial surface epithelium. This was discrete from a serous papillary carcinoma that was also present. Haematoxylin and eosin.

Serous papillary tumours may be admixed with an endometrioid adenocarcinoma and it is thought that if the serous component accounts for more than 25 per cent of such a mixed tumour the neoplasm will have a prognosis that approximates to that of a serous papillary carcinoma (Lee and Belinson, 1992; Sherman *et al.*, 1992; Williams *et al.*, 1994). In biopsy material it would clearly be difficult, and probably impossible, to give any realistic estimate of the proportion of a mixed tumour that is of serous type. However, it is crucially important that the presence of such a component in a neoplasm that otherwise shows the appearances of an endometrioid adenocarcinoma is noted.

Serous adenocarcinomas are not associated with antecedent or accompanying endometrial hyperplasia but are very frequently associated with a presumed antecedent lesion classed as endometrial intraepithelial carcinoma (Ambros *et al.*, 1995; Spiegel, 1995). This is characterized by focal or multifocal replacement of surface or superficial glandular epithelial cells by single-layered or stratified malignant polygonal or hobnail-shaped cells with enlarged nuclei, large nucleoli and an abnormal pattern of nuclear chromatin (Fig. 10.17). There may be a micropapillary growth pattern and, by definition, there is no invasion of the endometrial stroma or of vessels. These foci of intra-epithelial carcinoma stain positively for *p53* (Sherman *et al.*, 1995; Zheng *et al.*, 1998). A focus of endometrial intra-epithelial carcinoma in curettings in which a tissue from a papillary serous adenocarcinoma is also present is likely to be overlooked or ignored. However, if such a focus is seen in curettage material in which no obvious tumour is present the pathologist should comment that there might be an associated papillary serous tumour of the endometrium that has escaped the sampling procedure.

10.5 CLEAR CELL ADENOCARCINOMA

Endometrial tumours of this type commonly occur in relatively elderly women and although most develop in an inactive or atrophic endometrium, a few are associated with an endometrial hyperplasia. Endometrial clear cell carcinomas are histologically identical to clear cell carcinomas of the ovary and

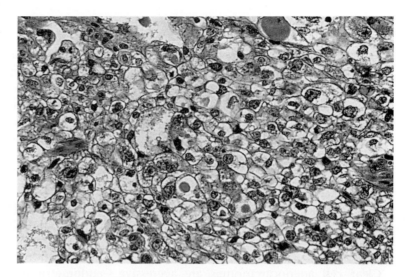

Figure 10.18 Clear cell adenocarcinoma. In this field the tumour has a solid pattern and is composed of large cells with prominent, well-defined cell margins, large nuclei and clear cytoplasm. Eosinophilic globules lie between the stromal cells. Haematoxylin and eosin.

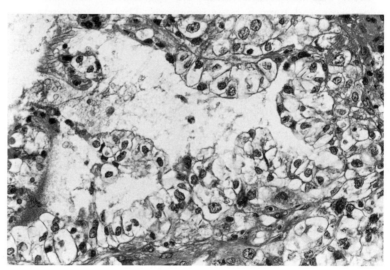

Figure 10.19 Clear cell adenocarcinoma. The glandular acini are lined by large cells with sharply defined cell margins, clear cytoplasm and prominent nuclei which, in many cells, lie at the apex of the cell, protrude into the glandular lumen and are described as having a hob-nailed appearance. Haematoxylin and eosin.

vagina (Silverberg and DeGiorgi, 1973; Kurman and Scully, 1976; Crum and Fechner, 1979; Photopoulos *et al.*, 1979; Christopherson *et al.*, 1982a; Abeler and Kjorstad, 1991; Abeler *et al.*, 1996). In a significant proportion of cases, they are combined with, or show areas of, papillary serous tumour or endometrioid adenocarcinoma (Lax *et al.*, 1998). Clear cell carcinomas show a complex permutation of solid, papillary, tubulocystic and glandular patterns (Fig. 10.18),

although in any individual neoplasm one of these patterns may be predominantly, or even exclusively, seen. The constituent cells have abundant clear, or slightly eosinophilic, cytoplasm and large irregular nuclei with distinct, sharply angulated contours, dense chromatin and prominent irregular nucleoli. Cells lining tubular or glandular spaces often have scanty cytoplasm and large nuclei, which protrude into the lumen (hobnail pattern; Fig. 10.19).

161

In papillary areas of these neoplasms the papillae have a broad fibrovascular core and are covered by cells showing marked pleomorphism, tufting and budding. Occasional psammoma bodies may be present while PAS-positive diastase resistant, intracytoplasmic or intraluminal rounded hyaline bodies are frequently seen (Christopherson, 1986). The neoplasms contain abundant glycogen and often a little mucus. Oncocytic cells are present in a high proportion of clear cell carcinomas and these may form a prominent feature. The tumours are usually oestrogen and progesterone receptor negative and only about 25 per cent stain positively for *p53* (Lax *et al.*, 1998).

Clear cell adenocarcinomas are aggressive neoplasms and have a poor prognosis. Their histological pattern is not of prognostic importance and they can be graded only on their nuclear characteristics, though it has not been clearly shown that nuclear grading in these neoplasms correlates well with prognosis (Christopherson, 1986; Kanbour-Shakir and Tobon, 1991).

The clear cell carcinoma of the endometrium should be distinguished from an endometrioid adenocarcinoma with clear cell areas and from the secretory variant of the endometrioid adenocarcinoma. The overall architectural pattern of these last two tumours differs considerably from that of a clear cell carcinoma whilst they show a much lesser degree of cytological and nuclear atypia. Confusion between an Arias-Stella reaction and a clear cell carcinoma can be avoided by observing the setting of the former in a typical pregnancy-type endometrium which shows no cytological atypia and by noting the lack of mitotic figures in an Arias-Stella reaction. Distinguishing between a predominantly papillary clear cell carcinoma and a serous papillary carcinoma can be a difficult if not almost impossible task in biopsy specimens but, as previously remarked, an inability to differentiate between these two neoplasms of similarly poor prognosis is of no practical importance. It also has to be borne in mind that a metastasis from a renal carcinoma can mimic almost exactly the appearance of a clear cell adenocarcinoma of the endometrium. The only clue available for suspecting a metastasis is that renal adenocarcinomas usually show a somewhat blander nuclear pattern.

10.6 MUCINOUS ADENOCARCINOMA

Many endometrioid adenocarcinomas of the endometrium contain a scattering of cells with demonstrable intracytoplasmic mucin. A small proportion of endometrial neoplasms consist predominantly of mucus-containing cells (Fig. 10.20). It is suggested that the term 'mucinous adenocarcinoma' is justified when more than 50 per cent of the cells of an endometrial adenocarcinoma contain intracytoplasmic mucin (Ross *et al.*, 1983). It should be noted that luminal border staining for mucin, without intracytoplasmic staining, is not considered evidence of mucinous differentiation.

Mucinous adenocarcinomas are usually virtually identical histologically to endocervical adenocarcinomas (Ross *et al.*, 1993; Melhem and Tobon, 1987). They are commonly well differentiated, formed of columnar cells with apical cytoplasmic mucin, show relatively mild atypia and have a predominantly acinar pattern, although a papillary architecture is often present in some areas; some tumours contain goblet cells. The mucin, best demonstrated by PAS/Alcian blue staining after diastase digestion, often forms intra-acinar and stromal pools that appear to attract, and are infiltrated by, polymorphonuclear leucocytes.

Mucinous adenocarcinomas have a prognosis similar to that of endometrioid adenocarcinomas

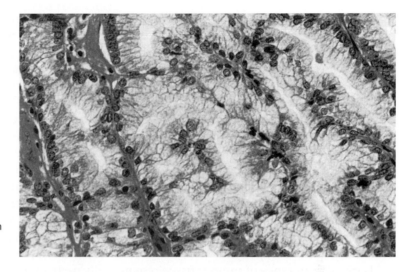

Figure 10.20 Mucinous adenocarcinoma. The glandular acini are lined by a tall mucus-secreting epithelium with well-orientated basal nuclei. The absence of cytological atypia in these neoplasms may cause diagnostic problems in a small biopsy and care should be exercised in distinguishing these tumours from mucinous metaplasia. Haematoxylin and eosin.

of the same grade and, since most are Grade 1, are associated with an excellent 5-year survival rate. The often acute problem of distinguishing these adenocarcinomas from an endocervical adenocarcinoma is considered in Section 10.13. Mucinous adenocarcinomas must also be differentiated from atypical endometrial hyperplasias with mucinous metaplasia, from clear cell carcinomas of the endometrium and from endometrioid adenocarcinomas with superimposed secretory change. The distinction from an atypical hyperplasia with mucinous metaplasia is based on the same general principles as that between an atypical hyperplasia and an endometrioid adenocarcinoma, though this task is more difficult with mucinous lesions and can be almost impossible in curettage material.

Differentiation of a mucinous carcinoma from both a clear cell carcinoma and an endometrioid adenocarcinoma with secretory change is usually obvious on histological grounds but in occasional cases the employment of a PAS/Alcian blue stain, both before and after diastase digestion, may be helpful. Because the last two neoplasms contain an abundance of glycogen and a paucity of mucin, such findings are the reverse of those typical for a mucinous

adenocarcinoma. Finally, a uterine metastasis from a colonic adenocarcinoma can be histologically identical in biopsy material, with a primary adenocarcinoma (Fig. 12.7). The sharpness of this diagnostic dilemma is lessened if the adenocarcinoma is admixed with, and appears to be arising from, hyperplastic endometrium while a negative reaction for carcinoembryonic antigen (CEA) virtually rules out the possibility of a metastasis from the colon, a positive staining reaction being however, of no discriminatory value. The use of a panel of cytokeratin stains, such as those used for discriminating between primary and metastatic mucinous tumours of the ovary, may be of value in distinguishing a primary endometrial mucinous neoplasm from a colonic metastasis but there have been no reported studies of their use in this particular diagnostic dilemma.

10.7 MICROGLANDULAR ADENOCARCINOMA

A rare form of endometrial adenocarcinoma is one that morphologically resembles microglandular carcinoma of the endocervix (Young and

163

Scully, 1992; Zaloudek *et al.*, 1997). In this neoplasm, microcystic spaces are lined by flattened, cuboidal or columnar cells while solid nests of tumour cells surround glands in some areas. The tumour cells are uniform and bland and mitotic figures are few; there is usually a well-marked inflammatory cell infiltrate, predominantly polymorphonuclear, within the tumour cells and within gland lumina. Staining for CEA, B72.3 and mucus are positive. The tumours may show this microglandular pattern throughout or may be admixed in part with either a mucinous or an endometrioid adenocarcinoma; the frankly adenocarcinomatous element usually forms only a relatively minor component.

Clearly, the presence of tumour tissue resembling microglandular hyperplasia in curetted material will usually lead to a conclusion that the material is non-neoplastic in nature and has been derived from the endocervix. A suspicion of the correct diagnosis may only be roused if it is certain that the tissue is from the endometrial cavity or if there is an admixture with a minor component of more conventional mucinous or endometrioid adenocarcinoma. Even if the tissue is known with certainty to be derived from the uterine cavity, confusion can still arise between a microglandular adenocarcinoma and a conventional endometrioid adenocarcinoma that shows surface epithelial changes mimicking those of microglandular hyperplasia (Jacques *et al.*, 1995). In this latter circumstance the curetted material will usually, unless only very little material is present, show a predominance of the typical endometrioid adenocarcinoma.

10.8 ONCOCYTIC CARCINOMA

Oncocytic change can occasionally be seen in both clear cell and endometrioid adenocarcinomas of the endometrium, but a small number of pure oncocytic carcinomas of the endometrium, which differ significantly from endometrioid adenocarcinomas with oncocytic change have been described (Silver *et al.*, 1999). These neoplasms occur in postmenopausal women and are composed exclusively of oncocytic cells showing a solid, glandular or tubo-papillary growth pattern. The tumour cells show the typical oncocytic features of eosinophilic granular cytoplasm and distinct cell borders but also show pleomorphism, an increased nucleo–cytoplasmic ratio and prominent nucleoli: a moderate number of mitotic figures (an average of 3 per 10 high-power fields) are usually present. These neoplasms are usually oestrogen- and progesterone-receptor negative and stain positively for *p53*.

Oncocytic carcinomas not uncommonly show deep invasion and appear to behave in a more malignant fashion than endometrioid adenocarcinomas showing oncocytic change from which they can be distinguished by their receptor negativity and their positive staining for *p53*. A distinction from oncocytic metaplasia rests, in biopsy material, upon the presence of nuclear atypia and pleomorphism.

10.9 SQUAMOUS CELL CARCINOMA

Primary squamous cell carcinomas (Fig. 10.21) of the endometrium are extremely rare (Lifshitz *et al.*, 1981; Yamashima and Kobara, 1986; Simon *et al.*, 1988; Abeler and Kjorstad, 1990b; Gedikoglu *et al.*, 1991; Jeffers *et al.*, 1991; Adelson and Strumpf, 1992; Yamamoto *et al.*, 1995; Goodman *et al.*, 1996). The traditional belief, which was propagated in older reports, that they occur most commonly in women with either a chronic pyometra or ichthyosis uteri seems less valid now; the tumour occurs predominantly in older women, with the mean

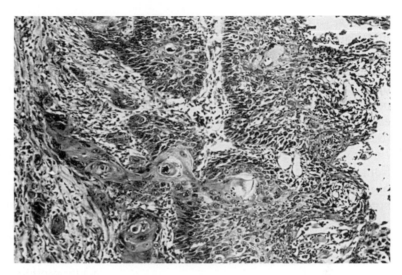

Figure 10.21 Squamous carcinoma of the endometrium. The uterus in this hysterectomy specimen is lined by squamous epithelium with features of intraepithelial neoplasia and a well-differentiated infiltrating squamous carcinoma arises from its deep surface. Haematoxylin and eosin.

age being in the seventh decade. The finding of malignant squamous epithelium in uterine curettings will inevitably suggest that the tissue has come from a cervical squamous cell carcinoma and differentiation between a cervical and an endometrial lesion will clearly rest largely on clinical evidence. In this respect, it should be noted that a squamous cell carcinoma involving both the cervix and the endometrium is, by convention, regarded as having originated in the cervix. If a biopsy specimen showing squamous cell carcinoma is known definitely to be derived from the endometrium it is necessary to try to exclude, preferably by step-sectioning of the entire biopsy, the possibility of an endometrioid carcinoma showing squamous differentiation. Some squamous carcinomas of the endometrium are highly differentiated and the malignant nature of squamous epithelium in curettings from such neoplasms may be overlooked unless particular care is taken to look for minor degrees of atypia.

Verrucous carcinoma of the endometrium can occur (Ryder, 1982; Hussain, 1988), while a verrucous carcinoma of the cervix may extend upwards to involve the endometrium (Tiltman

and Atad, 1982). The diagnosis of a verrucous carcinoma rests not only on its cytological features but also on the nature of its 'pushing' base. Therefore, this tumour cannot be diagnosed in curettings, especially as very similar squamous tissue in endometrial biopsies may be derived from flat condylomatous lesions of the cervix that have extended into the uterine cavity (Venkatasesham and Woo, 1985; Roberts and Carrow-Brown, 1985). A squamous cell carcinoma of the uterine cavity can arise from an extensive condylomatous lesion of this type.

It should be noted that cervical intraepithelial neoplasia can also extend up into the endometrium (Salm, 1969; Kambour and Stock, 1978; Sworn *et al.*, 1995; Pins *et al.*, 1997; Sherwood *et al.*, 1997) and atypical epithelium of this type, covering the endometrial surface and extending into glands, may be seen in curettings.

10.10 TRANSITIONAL CELL CARCINOMA

Transitional cell carcinomas of the endometrium are extremely rare (Lininger *et al.*,

1997): they occur in a relatively old age group (mean age 61 years) and have an aggressive pattern of behaviour. These neoplasms can exist in a pure form but more commonly the transitional cell component is admixed with another pattern, most often squamous but sometimes endometrioid or serous papillary. When a pure transitional cell carcinoma is encountered in curettage material it must be distinguished from a metastatic carcinoma of the bladder: the primary endometrial tumours are CK7 positive but CK20 negative.

10.11 SMALL CELL CARCINOMA

Although often included under the portmanteau heading of undifferentiated carcinoma of the endometrium, the small cell neuroendocrine carcinoma does merit special consideration. These are aggressive neoplasms that usually occur in postmenopausal women and are histologically identical to small cell (oat cell) carcinomas of the bronchus. The tumour cells grow in dense sheets of monotonous small to intermediate sized round cells, sometimes with focal areas of spindle cells (Paz et al., 1985; Manivel et al., 1986; Campo et al., 1992; Huntsman et al., 1994; van Hoeven et al., 1995; Tsujioka et al., 1997; Verschraegen et al., 1999). They usually stain positively for epithelial markers such as Cam 5.2 or epithelial membrane antigen (EMA), give a positive reaction for chromogranin, may stain positively for one or more neuropeptides and are seen on electron microscopy to contain dense-core secretory granules. Neoplasms of this type clearly represent a distinct nosological entity, though they are quite commonly intermingled with adenocarcinomas or with endometrioid adenocarcinomas showing squamous differentiation. It is important to note that the mere presence of cells staining positively for chromogranin

within an endometrial neoplasm does not imply a diagnosis of small cell carcinoma: such cells may be present, in small or large numbers, in any type of endometrial adenocarcinoma. The presence of such cells is of no diagnostic or prognostic importance in such neoplasms (Ueda et al., 1979; Bannatyne et al., 1983; Sivridis et al., 1984).

Small cell neuroendocrine tumours differ from the extremely rare primitive neuroectodermal tumours of the endometrium (Daya et al., 1992; Molyneux et al., 1992) in their lack of foci of neural, ependymal, glial or medulloepithelial differentiation and by their negative reaction staining reaction for glial fibrillary acidic protein. Small cell carcinomas admixed with an adenocarcinoma may be mistaken histologically for a carcinosarcoma. However, they can be distinguished by their positive staining for neuroendocrine markers.

10.12 UNDIFFERENTIATED CARCINOMA

Undifferentiated endometrial carcinomas lack evidence of glandular, papillary, squamous or neuroendocrine differentiation and are usually formed of relatively large cells growing in sheets with foci of necrosis. They tend to pursue an aggressive course (Abeler et al., 1991). The recognition of an undifferentiated carcinoma, and its distinction from a lymphoma or sarcoma, rests upon demonstration of a positive staining reaction for epithelial membrane antigen and cytokeratins and a negative reaction for leucocyte common antigen, vimentin and desmin.

Undifferentiated endometrial carcinomas may show foci of multinucleated trophoblast-like differentiation (Civantos and Rywlin, 1972; Pesce et al., 1991) and such tumours must be distinguished from choriocarcinoma. The biphasic pattern of cytotrophoblast and syncytiotrophoblast typical of a choriocarcinoma is absent from these neoplasms, while carcinomas showing trophoblast-like differentiation usually occur in postmenopausal patients, in contrast to choriocarcinomas, which arise in women of reproductive age.

Instances of undifferentiated endometrial carcinomas with an intense infiltrate of lymphocytes and plasma cells have been described and classed as lymphoepithelioma-like carcinomas (Vargas and Merino, 1998). Whether or not such cases truly represent a distinct clinicopathological nosological entity will only be revealed by the reporting of further examples.

10.13 DIFFERENTIATION BETWEEN ENDOMETRIAL AND ENDOCERVICAL ADENOCARCINOMAS

In curettage material containing adenocarcinomatous tissue, it may be far from clear whether the tumour is of endometrial or endocervical origin. This problem is at its most acute with a mucinous adenocarcinoma but can be encountered with any type of endometrial epithelial neoplasm. In many cases the clinical findings will leave little doubt as to the site of origin of the tumour while, in theory at least, fractional curettage should go a long way towards resolving the dilemma in clinically debatable cases. It has been our experience, however, that fractional curettage, although of diagnostic value in some cases, often yields equivocal results, thus leaving the decision as to site of origin in the hands of the pathologist.

In attempting to make a distinction between an endometrial and an endocervical neoplasm the pathologist must rely mainly on clues gleaned from a study of the non-neoplastic tissue present in the biopsy specimen. Thus, features such as a fibrotic stroma, a merging with

typical endocervical epithelium or the concomitant presence of tissue showing cervical adenocarcinoma *in situ*, atypical endocervical glandular epithelium or cervical squamous intraepithelial neoplasia would all hint at an endocervical adenocarcinoma. Conversely, the presence of stromal foam cells and a merging with either normal or hyperplastic endometrium would suggest that the tumour is endometrial in nature.

It has been claimed that staining for CEA is of some value in differential diagnosis, since endocervical adenocarcinomas tend to stain positively for this antigen and endometrial tumours usually give a negative reaction (Wahlstrom *et al.*, 1979; Ueda *et al.*, 1983). However, others have found a CEA stain to be of little or no discriminatory value (Cohen *et al.*, 1982; Cooper *et al.*, 1987). The use of various mucin stains to distinguish these two neoplasms also appears to be unhelpful (Cooper *et al.*, 1987; Longacre *et al.*, 1995; Maes *et al.*, 1998). It has been claimed that positive vimentin staining is helpful in distinguishing endometrial from endocervical adenocarcinomas, the former tending to be vimentin positive and the latter vimentin negative (Dabbs *et al.*, 1986). This, although true to a significant extent, is not invariably the case and greater precision can be obtained by combining staining for vimentin with staining for CEA: vimentin-positive, CEA-negative endometrioid tumours are usually of endometrial origin and vimentin-negative, CEA-positive neoplasms of similar histological type usually originate in the endocervix (Dabbs *et al.*, 1996).

10.14 ASSESSMENT OF NON-NEOPLASTIC ENDOMETRIUM

In curettage material containing an endometrial adenocarcinoma, it is of value to assess and comment upon any non-neoplastic endometrium included in the biopsy specimen. It was thought that adenocarcinomas arising from a background of atypical endometrial hyperplasia are associated with a much better 5-year survival rate than are those developing in an endometrium that shows a normal cycling pattern, is atrophic or shows simple hyperplasia (Beckner *et al.*, 1985). This is indeed true but only because a high proportion of tumours arising from an atrophic endometrium are serous papillary, clear cell or Grade 3 endometrioid adenocarcinomas while most neoplasms occurring in a hyperplastic endometrium are Grade 1 endometrioid adenocarcinomas. A Grade 1 endometrioid adenocarcinoma developing from an atrophic endometrium has, however, the same prognosis as does an endometrioid adenocarcinoma of similar grade arising in a hyperplastic endometrium (Sivridis *et al.*, 1998) and hence the state of the non-neoplastic endometrium is not, in itself, of any prognostic interest. Nevertheless, histologically identical tumours developing from atrophic or hyperplastic endometria probably arise through different genetic mechanisms and, hence, documentation of the nature of the non-neoplastic endometrium may eventually be of molecular epidemiological significance.

REFERENCES

Abeler, V.M., Kjorstad, K.E. (1990a) Serous papillary carcinoma of the endometrium: a histopathological study of 22 cases. *Gynecol. Oncol.* **39**, 266–71.

Abeler, V.M., Kjorstad, K.E. (1990b) Endometrial squamous cell carcinoma: report of three cases and review of the literature. *Gynecol. Oncol.* **39**, 321–6.

Abeler, V.M., Kjorstad, K.E. (1991) Clear cell carcinoma of the endometrium: a histopathological and clinical study of 97 cases. *Gynecol. Oncol.* **40**, 207–17.

Abeler, V.M., Kjorstad, K.E. (1992) Endometrial adenocarcinoma with squamous cell differentiation. *Cancer* **69**, 488–95.

Abeler, V.M., Kjorstad, K.E., Nesland, J.M. (1991) Undifferentiated carcinoma of the endometrium: a histopathologic and clinical study of 31 cases. *Cancer* **68**, 98–105.

Abeler, V.M., Vergore, I.B., Kjorstad, K.E., Trope, C.G. (1996) Clear cell carcinoma of the endometrium: prognosis and metastatic pattern. *Cancer* **78**, 1740–7.

Adelson, M.D., Strumpf, K.B. (1992) Squamous cell carcinoma of the endometrium presenting as peritonitis with small bowel obstruction. *Gynecol. Oncol.* **45**, 214–18.

Alberhasky, R.C., Connelly, P.J., Christopherson, W.M. (1982) Carcinoma of the endometrium. IV. Mixed adenosquamous carcinoma: a clinico-pathological study of 68 cases with long-term follow-up. *Am. J. Clin. Pathol.* **77**, 655–64.

Ambros, R.A., Sherman, M.E., Zahn, C.M., Bitterman, P., Kurman, R.J. (1995) Endometrial intraepithelial carcinoma: a distinctive lesion specifically associated with tumors showing serous differentiation. *Hum. Pathol.* **26**, 1260–7.

Bannatyne, P., Russell, P., Wills, E. (1983) Argyrophilia and endometrial carcinoma. *Int. J. Gynecol. Pathol.* **2**, 235–54.

Barrowclough, H., Jaarsma, K.W. (1980) Adenoacanthoma of the endometrium: a separate entity or a histological curiosity? *J. Clin. Pathol.* **33**, 1064–7.

Beckner, M.E., Mori, I., Silverberg, S.G. (1985) Endometrial carcinoma: nontumor factors in prognosis. *Int. J. Gynecol. Pathol.* **4**, 131–45.

Campo, E., Brunier, M.N., Merino, M.J. (1992) Small cell carcinoma of the endometrium with associated ocular paraneoplastic syndrome. *Cancer* **69**, 2283–8.

Carcangui, M.L., Chambers, J.T. (1997) Early pathologic stage clear cell carcinoma and uterine papillary serous carcinoma of the endometrium. *Int. J. Gynecol. Pathol.* **14**, 30–8.

Carcangui, M.L., Chambers, J.T. (1992) Uterine papillary serous carcinoma: a study of 108 cases with emphasis on the prognostic significance of associated endometrioid adenocarcinoma, absence of invasion, and concomitant ovarian carcinoma. *Gynecol. Oncol.* **47**, 298–305.

Chen, J.L., Trost, D.C., Wilkinson, E.J. (1985) Endometrial papillary adenocarcinomas: two clinico-pathological types. *Int. J. Gynecol. Pathol.* **4**, 279–88.

Christopherson, W.M. (1986) The significance of the pathological findings in endometrial cancer. *Clinic. Obstet. Gynecol.* **13**, 673–93.

Christopherson, W.M., Alberhasky, R.C., Connelly, P.J. (1982a) Carcinoma of the endometrium. I. A clinicopathologic study of clear cell carcinoma and secretory carcinoma. *Cancer* **69**, 1511–23.

Christopherson, W.M., Alberhasky, R.C., Connelly, P.J. (1982b) Carcinoma of the endometrium. II. Papillary adenocarcinoma: a clinical-pathological study of 46 cases. *Am. J. Clin. Pathol.* **77**, 534–40.

Christopherson, W.M., Alberhasky, R.C., Connelly, P.J. (1982c) Glassy cell carcinoma of the endometrium. *Hum. Pathol.* **13**, 418–21.

Civantos, F., Rywlin, A.M. (1972) Carcinoma with trophoblastic differentiation and secretion of chorionic gonadotrophins. *Cancer* **29**, 789–98.

Cohen, C., Shulman, C., Budgeon, L.R. (1982) Endocervical and endometrial adenocarcinoma: an immunoperoxidase and histochemical study. *Am. J. Surg. Pathol.* **6**, 151–7.

Connelly, P.J., Alberhasky, R.C., Christopherson, W.M. (1982) Carcinoma of the endometrium. III. Analysis of 865 cases of adenocarcinoma and adenoacanthoma. *Obstet. Gynecol.* **59**, 569–75.

Cooper, P., Russell, G., Wilson, B. (1987) Adenocarcinoma of the endocervix – a histochemical study. *Histopathology* **11**, 1321–30.

Crum, P., Fechner, R.E. (1979) Clear cell adenocarcinoma of the endometrium: a clinicopathologic study of 11 cases. *Am. J. Diagn. Gynecol. Obstet.* **1**, 261–7.

Dabbs, D.J., Celsinger, K.R., Norris, H.T. (1986) Intermediate filaments in endometrial and endocervical carcinomas: the diagnostic utility of vimentin pattern. *Am. J. Surg. Pathol.* **10**, 568–75.

Dalwagne, M.P., Silverberg, S.G. (1982) Foam cells in endometrial carcinoma: a clinicopathologic study. *Gynecol. Oncol.* **13**, 67–75.

Daya, D., Lukka, H., Clement, P.B. (1992) Primitive neuroectodermal tumors of the uterus: a report of four cases. *Hum. Pathol.* **23**, 1120–9.

Eichhorn, J.H., Young, R.H., Clement, P.B. (1996) Sertoliform endometrial adenocarcinoma: a study of four cases. *Int. J. Gynecol. Pathol.* **15**, 119–26.

Fox, H., Brander, S. (1988) Sertoliform adenocarcinoma of the endometrium. *Histopathology* **13**, 584–6.

Fukuoka, K., Hirokawa, M., Shimizu, M. *et al.* (1998) Oxyphilic cell variant of endometrioid adenocarcinoma. *Pathol. Int.* **48**, 754–6.

Gedikoglu, G., Demirel, D., Gunhan, O., Finci, R. (1991) Endometrial squamous cell carcinoma. *Acta Obstet. Gynecol. Scand.* **70**, 619–21.

Goff, B.A., Kato, D.T., Schmidt, R.A., *et al.* (1994) Uterine papillary serous carcinoma: patterns of metastatic spread. *Gynecol. Oncol.* **54**, 264–8.

Gitsch, G., Friedlander, M.L., Wain, G.V., Hacker, N.F. (1995) Uterine papillary serous carcinoma: a clinical study. *Cancer* **75**, 2239–43.

Goodman, A., Zukerberg, L.R., Rice, L.W., Fuller, A.F., Scully, R.E. (1996) Squamous cell carcinoma of the endometrium: a report of eight cases and a review of the literature. *Gynecol. Oncol.* **61**, 54–60.

Haqqani, M.T., Fox, H. (1976) Adenosquamous carcinoma of the endometrium. *J. Clin. Pathol.* **29**, 959–66.

Hendrickson, M., Kempson, R.L. (1983) Ciliated carcinoma – a variant of endometrial adenocarcinoma: a report of 10 cases. *Int. J. Gynecol. Pathol.* **2**, 13–27.

Hendrickson, M.R., Kempson, R.L. (1995) Endometrial hyperplasia, metaplasia and carcinoma. In: Fox, H. (ed.), *Haines and Taylor: Obstetrical and Gynaecological Pathology*, 4th edn. Edinburgh: Churchill Livingstone, 421–510.

Hendrickson, M., Ross, J., Eiffel, P., Martinez, A., Kempson, R. (1982) Uterine papillary serous carcinoma: a highly malignant form of endometrial carcinoma. *Am. J. Surg. Pathol.* **6**, 93–108.

van Hoeven, K.H., Hudock, J.A., Woodruff, J.M., Suhrland, M.J. (1995) Small cell neuroendocrine carcinoma of the endometrium. *Int. J. Gynecol. Pathol.* **14**, 21–9.

Huntsman, D., Clement, P., Gilks, C., Scully, R.E. (1994) Small cell carcinoma of the endometrium: a clinicopathological study of sixteen cases. *Am. J. Surg. Pathol.* **18**, 364–75.

Hussain, S.F. (1988) Verrucous carcinoma of the endometrium: a case report. *Acta Pathol. Microbiol. Immunol. Scand.* **96**, 1075–8.

Jacques, S.M., Qureshi, F., Lawrence, W.D. (1995) Surface epithelial changes in endometrial adenocarcinoma: diagnostic pitfalls in curettage specimens. *Int. J. Gynecol. Pathol.* **14**, 191–7.

Jeffers, M.D., McDonald, G.S., McGuinness, E.P. (1991) Primary squamous carcinoma of the endometrium. *Histopathology* **19**, 177–9.

Kambour, A.J., Stock, R.I. (1978) Squamous cell carcinoma *in situ* of the endometrium and Fallopian tube as superficial extension of invasive cervical carcinoma. *Cancer* **42**, 570–80.

Kanbour-Shakir, A., Tobon, H. (1991) Primary clear cell carcinoma of the endometrium: a clinicopathologic study of 20 cases. *Int. J. Gynecol. Pathol.* **10**, 67–78.

169

Kato, D.T., Ferry, J.A., Goodman, S. *et al.* (1995) Uterine papillary serous carcinoma (UPSC): a clinicopathologic study of 30 cases. *Gynecol. Oncol.* **59**, 384–9.

Kurman, R.J., Scully, R.E. (1976) Clear cell carcinoma of the endometrium: an analysis of 21 cases. *Cancer* **37**, 872–82.

Lauchlan, S.C. (1981) Tubal (serous) carcinoma of the endometrium. *Arch. Pathol. Lab. Med.* **105**, 615–18.

Lax, S.F., Pizer, E.S., Ronnett, B.M., Kurman, R.J. (1998) Clear cell carcinoma of the endometrium is characterized by a distinctive profile of p53, Ki-67, estrogen and progesterone receptor expression. *Hum. Pathol.* **29**, 551–8.

Lax, S.F., Kurman, R.J., Pizer, E.S., Wu, L., Ronnett, B.M. (2000) A binary architectural grading system for uterine endometrial endometrioid carcinoma has superior reproducibility compared with FIGO grading and identifies subsets of advance-stage tumors with favourable and unfavourable prognosis. *Am. J. Surg. Pathol.* **24**, 1201–8.

Lee, K.R., Belinson, J.L. (1992) Papillary serous adenocarcinoma of the endometrium: a clinicopathologic study of 19 cases. *Gynecol. Oncol.* **46**, 51–4.

Lifshitz, S., Schauberger, C.W., Platz, C.A., Roberts, J.A. (1981) Primary squamous cell carcinoma of the endometrium. *J. Reprod. Med.* **26**, 25–7.

Lininger, R.A., Ashfaq, R., Albores-Saavedra, J., Tavassoli, F.A. (1997) Transitional cell carcinoma of the endometrium and endometrial carcinoma with transitional cell differentiation. *Cancer* **79**, 1933–43.

Longacre, T.A., Kempson, R.L., Hendrickson, M.R. (1995) Endometrial hyperplasia, metaplasia and carcinoma. In Fox, H. (ed.), *Haines and Taylor: Obstetrical and Gynaecological Pathology*, 4th edn. Edinburgh: Churchill Livingstone, 421–510.

Maes, G., Fleuren, G., Bara, J., Nap, M. (1988) The distribution of mucins, carcinoembryonic antigen, and mucus-associated antigens in endocervical and endometrial adenocarcinomas. *Int. J. Gynecol. Pathol.* **7**, 112–22.

Manivel, C., Wick, M.R., Sibley, R.K. (1986) Neuroendocrine differentiation in Müllerian neoplasms: an immunohistochemical study of a 'pure' endometrial small cell carcinoma and a mixed Müllerian tumor containing small cell carcinoma. *Am. J. Clin. Pathol.* **86**, 438–43.

Melhem, M.F., Tobon, H. (1987) Mucinous adenocarcinoma of the endometrium: a clinico-pathological review of 18 cases. *Int. J. Gynecol. Pathol.* **6**, 347–55.

Moll, U.M., Chalas, E., Auguste, M., Meaney, D., Chumas, J. (1996) Uterine papillary serous carcinoma evolves via a p53-driven pathway. *Hum. Pathol.* **27**, 1295–1300.

Molyneux, M.J., Deen, S., Sundaresan, V. (1992) Primitive neuroectodermal tumour of the uterus. *Histopathology* **21**, 584–5.

Mooney, E.E., Robboy, S.J., Hammond, C.B., Berchuk, A., Bentley, R.C. (1997) Signet-ring cell carcinoma of the endometrium: a primary tumor masquerading as a metastasis. *Int. J. Gynecol. Pathol.* **16**, 169–72.

Ng, A.B.P., Reagan, J.W., Storaasli, J.P., Wentz, W.G. (1973) Mixed adenosquamous carcinoma of the endometrium. *Am. J. Clin. Pathol.* **59**, 765–81.

O'Hanlan, K.A., Levine, P.A., Harbatkin, D., Feiner, C., Goldberg, G.L., Jones, J.G. (1990) Virulence of papillary endometrial carcinoma. *Gynecol. Oncol.* **37**, 112–19.

Paz, R., Frigerio, B., Sundblad, A., Eusebi, V. (1985) Small cell (oat cell) carcinoma of the endometrium. *Arch. Pathol. Lab. Med.* **109**, 270–72.

Photopoulos, G.J., Carney, C.N., Edelman, D.A., Hughes, R.R., Fowler, W.C., Walton, R.A. (1979) Clear cell carcinoma of the endometrium. *Cancer* **43**, 1448–56.

Pesce, C., Merino, M.J., Chambers, J.T., Nogales, F. (1991) Endometrial carcinoma with trophoblastic differentiation: an aggressive form of uterine cancer. *Cancer* **68**, 1799–1802.

Pins, M.R., Young, R.H., Crum, C.P., Leach, I.H., Scully, R.E. (1997) Cervical squamous cell carcinoma *in situ* with intraepithelial extension to the upper genital tract and invasion of tubes and ovaries: report of a case with human papilloma virus analysis. *Int. J. Gynecol. Pathol.* **16**, 272–8.

Pitman, M.B., Young, R.H., Clement, P.B., Dickersin, G.R., Scully, R.E. (1994) Endometrioid carcinoma of the ovary and endometrium, oxyphilic cell type: a report of nine cases. *Int. J. Gynecol. Pathol.* **13**, 290–301.

Roberts, P.F., Carrow-Brown, J. (1985) Condylomatous atypia of the endometrial cavity. *Br. J. Obstet. Gynaecol.* **42**, 535–8.

Rosenberg, P., Blom, R., Hogberg, T., Simonsen, E. (1993) Death rate and recurrence pattern among 841 clinical stage I endometrial cancer patients with special reference to uterine papillary serous carcinoma. *Gynecol. Oncol.* **51**, 311–15.

Ross, J.C., Eifel, P.J., Cox, R.S., Kempson, R.L., Hendrickson, M.R. (1983) Primary mucinous adenocarcinoma of the endometrium: a clinicopathologic and histochemical study. *Am. J. Surg. Pathol.* **7**, 715–29.

Ryder, D.A. (1982) Verrucous carcinoma of the endometrium: a unique neoplasm with long survival. *Obstet. Gynecol.* **59**, 78s–80s.

Salm, R. (1969) Superficial intra-uterine spread of intraepithelial cervical carcinoma. *J. Pathol.* **97**, 261–8.

Sasano, H., Cormerford, J., Wilkinson, D.S., Schwartz, A., Garrett, C.T. (1990) Serous papillary carcinoma of the endometrium: analysis of proto-oncogene amplification, flow cytometry, estrogen and progesterone receptors, and immunohistochemistry. *Cancer* **65**, 1545–51.

Sherman, M.E., Bitterman, P., Rosenhein, N.B., Delgado, G., Kurman, R.J. (1992) Uterine serous carcinoma: a morphologically diverse neoplasm with unifying clinicopathologic features. *Am. J. Surg. Pathol.* **16**, 600–10.

Sherman, M.E., Bur, M.E., Kurman, R.J. (1995) p53 in endometrial cancer and its putative precursors: evidence for diverse pathways of tumorigenesis. *Hum. Pathol.* **26**, 1268–74.

Sherwood, J.B., Carlson, J.A., Gold, M.A., Chou, T.Y., Isacson, C., Talerman, A. (1997) Squamous metaplasia of the endometrium associated with HPV 6 and 11. *Gynecol. Oncol.* **66**, 141–5.

Silva, E.G., Jenkins, R. (1990) Serous carcinoma in endometrial polyps. *Mod. Pathol.* **3**, 120–8.

Silver, S., Cheung, A.N.Y., Tavassoli, F.A. (1999) Oncocytic metaplasia and carcinoma of the endometrium: an immunohistochemical and ultrastructural study. *Int. J. Gynecol. Pathol.* **18**, 12–19.

Silverberg, S.G. (1984) New aspects of endometrial carcinoma. *Clin. Obstet. Gynaecol.* **11**, 189–208.

Silverberg, S.G., DeGiorgi, L.S. (1973) Clear cell carcinoma of the endometrium: clinical, pathologic and ultrastructural findings. *Cancer* **31**, 1127–40.

Simon, A., Kopolovic, J., Beyth, Y. (1988) Primary squamous cell carcinoma of the endometrium. *Gynecol. Oncol.*, **31**, 454–61.

Sivridis, E., Buckley, C.H., Fox, H. (1984) Argyrophil cells in normal, hyperplastic and neoplastic endometrium. *J. Clin. Pathol.* **27**, 378–81.

Sivridis, E., Fox, H., Buckley, C.H. (1998) Endometrial carcinoma: two or three entities? *Int. J. Gynecol. Cancer* **8**, 183–88.

Spiegel, G.W. (1995) Endometrial carcinoma *in situ* in postmenopausal women. *Am. J. Surg. Pathol.* **19**, 417–32.

Sworn, M.J., Jones, H., Letchworth, H.J., Herrington, C.S., McGee, J. (1995) Squamous intraepithelial neoplasia in an ovarian cyst, cervical intraepithelial neoplasia and human papillomavirus. *Hum. Pathol.* **26**, 344–7.

Sutton, G.P., Brull, L., Michael, H., Stehman, F.B., Ehrlich, C.E. (1987) Malignant papillary lesions of the endometrium. *Gynecol. Oncol.* **27**, 294–304.

Tashiro, H., Isaacson, C., Levine, R., Kurman, R.J., Cho, K.R., Hedrick, L. (1997) *p53* gene mutations are common in uterine serous carcinomas and occur early in their pathogenesis. *Am. J. Pathol.* **150**, 177–85.

Tay, E.H., Ward, B.G. (1999) The treatment of uterine papillary serous carcinoma (UPSC): are we doing the right thing? *Int. J. Gynecol. Cancer* **9**, 463–9.

Taylor, R.R., Zeller, J., Libermann, R.W., O'Connor, D.M. (1999) An analysis of two versus three grades for endometrial carcinoma. *Gynecol. Oncol.* **74**, 3–6.

Tiltman, A.J., Atad, J. (1982) Verrucous carcinoma of the cervix with endometrial involvement. *Int. J. Gynecol. Pathol.* **1**, 221–6.

Tobon, H., Watkins, G.J. (1985) Secretory adenocarcinoma of the endometrium. *Int. J. Gynecol. Pathol.* **4**, 328–35.

Tsujioka, H., Eguchi, F., Emoto, M., Hachisuga, T., Kawarabayashi, T., Shirakawa, K. (1997) Small cell carcinoma of the endometrium: an immunohistochemical and ultrastructural analysis. *J. Obstet. Gynaecol. Res.* **23**, 9–16.

Ueda, G., Yamasaki, M., Indue, M., Kurachi, K. (1979) A clinicopathologic study of endometrial carcinomas with argyrophil cells. *Gynecol. Oncol.* **7**, 223–32.

Ueda, S., Tsubara, A., Izumi, H., Sasaki, M., Morii, S. (1983) Immuno-histochemical studies of carcinoembryonic antigen in adenocarcinoma of the uterus. *Acta Pathol. Jpn.* **33**, 59–69.

Vargas, M.P., Merino, M.J. (1998) Lymphoepithelioma-like carcinoma: an unusual variant of endometrial cancer: a report of two cases. *Int. J. Gynecol. Pathol.* **17**, 272–6.

Venkatasesham, V.S., Woo, T.H. (1985) Diffuse viral papillomatosis (condyloma) of the uterine cavity. *Int. J. Gynecol. Pathol.* **4**, 370–77.

Verschraegen, C.F., Matei, C., Loyer, E. *et al.* (1999) Ocreotide induced remission of a refractory small cell carcinoma of the endometrium. *Int. J. Gynecol. Cancer* **9**, 80–5.

Wahlstrom, I., Lindgren, J., Korhonen, M., Seppala, M. (1979) Distinction between endocervical and endometrial adenocarcinoma with immuno-peroxidase staining of carcinoembryonic antigen in routine histological tissue specimens. *Lancet* **ii**, 1159–60.

Walker, A.N., Mills, S.E. (1982) Serous papillary carcinoma of the endometrium: a clinicopathologic study of 11 cases. *Diagn. Gynecol. Obstet.* **4**, 261–7.

Ward, B.G., Wright, R.G., Free, K. (1990) Papillary carcinomas of the endometrium. *Gynecol. Oncol.* **39**, 347–51.

Wheeler, D.T., Bell, K.A., Kurman, R.J., Sherman, M.E. (2000) Minimal uterine serous carcinoma: diagnosis and clinicopathologic correlation. *Am. J. Surg. Pathol.* **24**, 797–806.

Williams, K.E., Waters, E.D., Woolas, R.P., Hammond, I.G., McCartney, A.J. (1994) Mixed serous-endometrioid carcinoma of the uterus: pathologic and cytopathologic analysis of a high-risk endometrial carcinoma. *Int. J. Gynecol. Cancer* **4**, 7–18.

Yamamoto, Y., Izumi, K., Otsuka, H., Mimura, T., Okitsu, O. (1995) Primary squamous cell carcinoma of the endometrium: a case report and a suggestion of new histogenesis. *Int. J. Gynecol. Pathol.* **14**, 75–80.

Yamashima, M., Kobara, T.Y. (1986) Primary squamous cell carcinoma with its spindle cell variant in the endometrium: a case report and review of the literature. *Cancer* **57**, 340–45.

Young, R.H., Scully, R.E. (1992) Uterine carcinomas simulating microglandular hyperplasia: a report of six cases. *Am. J. Surg. Pathol.* **16**, 1092–7.

Zaloudek, C., Hayashi, G.M., Ryan, I.P., Powell, C.B., Miller, T.R. (1997) Microglandular adenocarcinoma of the endometrium: a form of mucinous adenocarcinoma that may be confused with microglandular hyperplasia of the cervix. *Int. J. Gynecol. Pathol.* **16**, 52–9.

Zaino, R., Kurman, R.J. (1988) Squamous differentiation in carcinoma of the endometrium: a critical appraisal of adenoacanthoma and adenosquamous carcinoma. *Semin. Diagn. Pathol.* **5**, 154–71.

Zaino, R., Kurman, R.J., Herbold, D. *et al.* (1991) The significance of squamous differentiation in endometrial adenocarcinoma: data from a Gynecologic Oncology Group study. *Cancer* **68**, 2293–2302.

Zaino, R., Kurman, R.J., Diana, K., Morrow, C. (1995) The utility of the revised International Federation of Gynecology and Obstetrics histologic grading of endometrial adenocarcinoma using a defined nuclear grading system. *Cancer* **75**, 81–6.

Zaino, R., Kurman, R.J., Brunetto, V.L. *et al.* (1998) Villoglandular adenocarcinoma of the endometrium: a clinicopathologic study of 61 cases: a Gynecologic Oncology Group study. *Am. J. Surg. Pathol.* **22**, 1379–85.

Zheng, W., Khurana, R., Farahmand, S., Wang, Y., Zhang, Z.F., Felix, J.C. (1998) p53 immunostaining as a significant adjunct diagnostic method for uterine surface carcinoma: precursor of uterine papillary serous carcinoma. *Am. J. Surg. Pathol.* **22**, 1463–73.

11 Non-epithelial and mixed endometrial tumours of Müllerian origin

Endometrial stem cells of Müllerian origin have a potential to differentiate into epithelial cells, mesenchymal cells or both. Tumours derived from such cells may therefore be purely epithelial, solely non-epithelial or mixed. Furthermore, cells developing along a non-epithelial pathway may differentiate not only into endometrial stromal cells but also into mesenchymal elements not normally found in the uterus, such as cartilage, bone or striated muscle.

Non-epithelial endometrial neoplasms of Müllerian origin are therefore categorized either as pure, containing only non-epithelial cells, or mixed, containing both non-epithelial and epithelial components. The tumours are further subdivided on the basis of whether they consist only of homologous components, i.e. those normally present in the uterus, or whether they contain, or consist solely of heterologous tissues that are normally alien to the uterus. A full classification of these neoplasms is given in Table 11.1. This may at first appear complex but is, if the above comments are taken into account, both logical and simple. All these neoplasms are, with the exception of leiomyomas, uncommon; those encountered least infrequently being the endometrial stromal sarcomas and the carcinosarcomas.

It will be appreciated that the classification shown in Table 11.1 refers only to tumours thought to be of Müllerian origin. It is possible for non-epithelial neoplasms to arise also from non-Müllerian tissues such as the blood vessels or neural elements and these rare tumours are considered in Chapter 12.

11.1 PURE NON-EPITHELIAL NEOPLASMS OF ENDOMETRIAL STROMAL TYPE

Endometrial stromal neoplasms are rare, occur over a wide age range but are most common in the fifth and sixth decades and usually present with abnormal vaginal bleeding.

173

Table 11.1 Classification of uterine non-epithelial and mixed epithelial/non-epithelial tumours of Müllerian origin

	Non-epithelial tumours	Mixed tumours

Homologous	*Of endometrial stromal type*
	    Stromal nodule
	    Endometrial stromal sarcoma
	Of smooth muscle type
	    Leiomyoma
	    Leiomyosarcoma
		Benign
		    Adenofibroma
		Of low-grade malignancy
		    Adenosarcoma
		    Carcinofibroma
		Of high-grade malignancy
		    Carcinosarcoma

Heterologous	Rhabdomyosarcoma
	Chondrosarcoma
	
	Osteosarcoma
		Of low-grade malignancy
		    Adenosarcoma with heterologous
		    components
		Of high-grade malignancy
		    Carcinosarcoma with heterologous
		    elements

11.1.1 Histological features

The defining feature of all endometrial stromal neoplasms is that they are formed of cells that, to a greater or lesser degree, resemble the stromal cells of the normal endometrium during the proliferative phase of the cycle. It must be stressed, at the risk of repetition, that a tumour can only be classed as an endometrial stromal neoplasm if it bears a recognizable resemblance to proliferative-phase endometrial stroma.

The categorization of endometrial stromal neoplasms is a matter of dispute. The classical subdivision is into a benign lesion (the endometrial stromal nodule), a low-grade malignant lesion (the low-grade endometrial stromal sarcoma) and a lesion of high-grade malignancy (the high-grade endometrial stromal sarcoma) (Norris and Taylor, 1966a; Tavassoli and Norris, 1981). The endometrial stromal nodule persists

as an undisputed entity but there is disagreement as to whether endometrial stromal sarcomas can be subdivided into low- and high-grade categories. The conventional dividing line between these two grades of malignancy has been a mitotic count of 10 mitotic figures per 10 high-power fields (Hendrickson and Kempson, 1980; Fekete and Vellios, 1984). Most tumours that have a mitotic count of over 10 per 10 high-power fields do not, however, have morphology reminiscent of proliferative phase stroma and are composed of very poorly differentiated or anaplastic cells. It has been argued, quite correctly, that such neoplasms should be regarded as high-grade undifferentiated uterine sarcomas of indeterminate origin and removed from the category of endometrial stromal sarcoma (Evans, 1982). If such neoplasms, which are very aggressive and associated with a poor

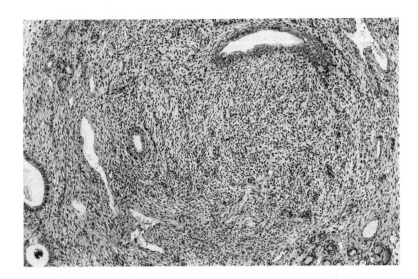

Figure 11.1 A stromal nodule. A discrete nodule of stromal cells occupies the centre of the field. There is no cytological atypia or mitotic activity. Haematoxylin and eosin.

prognosis, are taken out of the category of endometrial stromal neoplasms, does there remain a basis for a classification into high- and low-grade endometrial stromal sarcomas? A study of a large number of malignant neoplasms that met the diagnostic criteria of an endometrial stromal tumour showed that, in Stage 1 cases, neither the mitotic count nor the degree of atypia were prognostic features (Chang *et al.*, 1990). This indicates that the classical distinction drawn between low-grade and high-grade endometrial stromal sarcomas is not valid. This question is not, however, fully settled since some feel that tumours with high mitotic rates have a relatively poor prognosis, even when there is little cytological atypia (De Nictolis *et al.*, 1994), while others consider that tumours with marked cytological atypia tend to behave more aggressively than do those with bland cytological features (Silverberg and Kurman, 1992; Zaino, 1996). This latter claim indicates that there is some difficulty in defining exactly how much atypia is necessary before changing a diagnosis of endometrial stromal sarcoma to that of undifferentiated sarcoma

and suggests that cases showing marked atypia should probably be regarded with some caution.

It does seem reasonable, however, to conclude that there are really only two stromal neoplasms, the benign endometrial stromal nodule and the endometrial stromal sarcoma, which usually pursues an indolently malignant course. The endometrial stromal nodule (Fig. 11.1) is a well-circumscribed benign lesion (Norris and Taylor, 1966a; Tavassoli and Norris, 1981), while the endometrial stromal sarcoma of low-grade malignancy (previously known either as 'uterine stromatosis' or as 'endolymphatic stromal myosis') is an infiltrative neoplasm that also tends to invade blood vessels (Baggish and Woodruff, 1972; Hart and Yoonessi, 1977; Hendrickson and Kempson, 1980). A distinction between these two neoplasms rests solely upon whether the tumour margin is smooth and pushing or is infiltrating and hence can only be made on examination of a hysterectomy specimen.

Endometrial stromal nodules vary in size from 5 mm to 15 cm in diameter but average

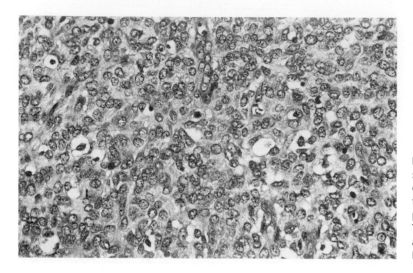

Figure 11.2 Endometrial stromal sarcoma. The neoplasm is composed of sheets of cells that are similar to those of the stroma of a proliferative-phase endometrium. There is no significant cytological atypia and mitotic activity is sparse. Haematoxylin and eosin.

about 4 cm in diameter (Tavassoli and Norris, 1981). They may be polypoid and protrude into the endometrial cavity but some are entirely intramyometrial. Endometrial stromal sarcomas may also be polypoidal but are more commonly largely intramural and poorly circumscribed. The biopsy appearances of the two lesions are identical and they cannot be distinguished in curettage material. Both are formed of sheets of generally uniform cells with darkly staining, small, round or ovoid nuclei, scanty cytoplasm and ill-defined limiting membranes (Fig. 11.2). Occasional cells may have fusiform nuclei and in rare instances this pattern predominates. Nuclear pleomorphism and cytological atypia are variable but commonly minimal, necrosis is rarely seen and any mitotic figures are invariably of normal form. Focal hyaline change is common and is sometimes a prominent feature with extensive areas of hyalinized tissue compressing the tumour cells into trabeculae or cords. There is a rich, ramifying vascular framework within these neoplasms, the vessels sometimes resembling spiral arterioles (Fig. 11.3). A reticulin stain is of considerable value for revealing the abundance of the vasculature. Not infrequently, the tumour cells condense around the blood vessels and in the 'pericytic' variant of the endometrial stromal sarcoma there is an exaggeration of this perivascular pattern.

All cases of possible endometrial stromal neoplasm should be stained for reticulin as they demonstrate a very characteristic pattern of reticulin fibres surrounding individual cells or, at the most, small groups of cells. A periodic acid–Schiff (PAS) stain is also mandatory and will show that stromal tumours are devoid of both glycogen and mucus. Immunocytochemical stains reveal a somewhat confusing pattern because these tumours not only stain positively, as would be expected, for vimentin but often also for desmin, actin, myosin, α-l-antitrypsin and α-l-chymotrypsin (Bonazzi del Poggetto *et al.*, 1983; Marshall and Braye, 1985; Binder *et al.*, 1991; Farhood and Abrams, 1991; Franquemont *et al.*, 1991). The tumours are almost invariably diploid on flow cytometry and express oestrogen and progesterone receptors (Katz *et al.*, 1987; Hitchcock and Norris, 1992; Blom *et al.*, 1999).

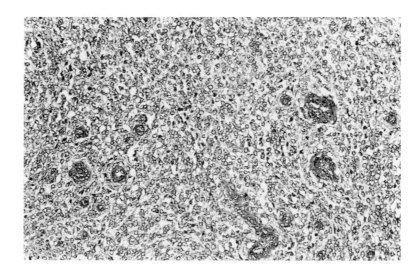

Figure 11.3 Endometrial stromal sarcoma. These neoplasms have a rich ramifying vascular supply, the vessels resembling spiral arterioles. Haematoxylin and eosin.

11.1.2 Differential diagnosis between stromal nodule and stromal sarcoma

As already noted, a distinction between these two entities cannot usually be made in biopsy material. The endometrial stromal nodule has a pushing margin that compresses the surrounding tissues, while the stromal sarcoma has an infiltrating margin and invades blood vessels. However, the distinction is not quite as simple as that, as focal, finger-like projections of up to 3 mm into the adjacent tissues does not exclude a diagnosis of stromal nodule (Zaino, 1996) and the diagnosis of a stromal sarcoma rests upon the presence of an irregular pattern of infiltration and clear evidence of vascular invasion. Hence, in biopsy specimens, it is usually unwise to diagnose anything more than 'Stromal neoplasm: ?Stromal nodule ?Stromal sarcoma'.

11.1.3 Histological variants of stromal neoplasms

A number of histological variants of stromal neoplasms, usually sarcomas rather than nodules, may be encountered. Occasionally, a minor degree of glandular differentiation is apparent within an otherwise typical pure stromal neoplasm. Such glandular elements are usually of endometrioid type, appear fully benign and are usually few. Occasionally, however, epithelial differentiation may be a prominent, florid feature and in one such case, the epithelial glands showed a markedly atypical pattern (Clement and Scully, 1992).

Some endometrial stromal tumours, of any degree of malignancy, contain epithelial-like elements arranged in trabecular cords, nests or tubules (Fig. 11.4) and in occasional neoplasms, this pattern is the predominant or even sole feature. Such tumours bear a quite striking similarity to an ovarian sex cord stromal neoplasm (Clement and Scully, 1976) to the extent that neoplasms in which this feature is a dominant one are often known as 'uterine tumours resembling sex cord tumours of the ovary'. These neoplasms, perhaps not surprisingly, have a considerable potential for causing confusion when encountered in curettage material. The nature of these epithelial-like elements is unknown, though they usually stain positively for actin and desmin, and sometimes also for

177

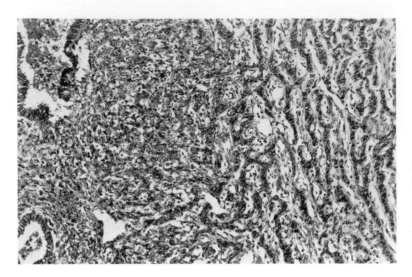

Figure 11.4 Endometrial stromal sarcoma with sex cord pattern. The endometrium is infiltrated by a stromal sarcoma in which epithelial-like elements form well-ordered trabeculae that resemble those seen in sex cord tumours of the ovary. Haematoxylin and eosin.

keratin (Farhood and Abrams, 1991; Lillemoe *et al.*, 1991; McCluggage *et al.*, 1993). It has been widely thought that true sex cord differentiation does not occur in uterine tumours: this belief may need to be reconsidered in view of the recent demonstration that the sex cord-like cells often, though not invariably, stain positively for the two markers of ovarian sex cord tumours, α-inhibin and the *MIC2* gene product (Krishnamurthy *et al.*, 1998; Baker *et al.*, 1999; McCluggage, 1999).

Stromal tumours often show actin positivity in the absence of any recognizable smooth muscle differentiation but some contain foci of overt smooth muscle differentiation and occasionally smooth muscle is a prominent feature of a stromal neoplasm (Oliva *et al.*, 1998). Stromal neoplasms may also show prominent fibrous or myxoid change (Oliva *et al.*, 1999).

Rhabdoid differentiation, characterized by the presence of cells with eccentric vacuolated nuclei, large nucleoli and eosinophilic cytoplasm, in which hyaline globules are often seen, has been noted in occasional endometrial stromal sarcomas (Fitko *et al.*, 1990; Kim *et al.*, 1996; McCluggage *et al.*, 1996: Rosty *et al.*,

1998). The rhabdoid cells stain positively for vimentin but show a rather variable and inconsistent pattern of staining for cytokeratins and epithelial membrane antigen.

11.1.4 Differential diagnosis of stromal neoplasms

In curettage material, it is occasionally necessary to differentiate stromal neoplasms from an anaplastic endometrial carcinoma, malignant lymphoma or leukaemic infiltration of the endometrium and, perhaps surprisingly, a severe chronic endometritis. The finding of tentative attempts at glandular differentiation, of PAS-positive mucus, of reticulin fibres surrounding alveolar masses of cells and of a positive staining reaction for common epithelial membrane antigen and cytokeratin, together with a negative stain for vimentin will all favour a diagnosis of adenocarcinoma rather than endometrial stromal sarcoma. Malignant lymphoma and leukaemic infiltrates commonly tend to surround included normal endometrial glands, and are often of recognizably histiocytic or granulocytic nature. In doubtful cases the demonstration of non-specific esterase, common leucocyte antigen or B- and T-cell markers may be of diagnostic value. A very severe endometritis, of the type sometimes seen in chlamydial infections (Chapter 7) can evoke a diffuse cellular infiltrate that destroys endometrial glands and is sufficiently dense as to suggest a neoplastic process. The inflammatory nature of the infiltrate is usually revealed by the presence of ill-formed germinal centres, by the finding of tingible body macrophages and by the recognition of the lymphoplasmocytic nature of the cellular infiltrate.

The relatively few endometrial stromal sarcomas with predominantly fusiform nuclei can be confused with a leiomyosarcoma, although in most such neoplasms there is usually a transition, in at least some areas of the tumour, to a more characteristic rounded nuclear pattern. The cells in a leiomyosarcoma have more abundant cytoplasm than do those of an endometrial stromal sarcoma, a distinction made more clear with a trichrome stain, and, after staining with PTAH, may be shown to contain demonstrable myofibrils. Immunocytochemical stains are of value in distinguishing between malignant smooth muscle and endometrial stromal neoplasms in that, while both stain positively for desmin and vimentin, only the latter give a positive reaction for α-1-antitrypsin, though, admittedly, not in all cases, and CD10 (Toki *et al.*, 2002).

Endometrial stromal sarcomas, particularly those showing a pericytic pattern, can closely resemble a haemangiopericytoma. Many will dispute that this presents a diagnostic problem, claiming that all apparent uterine haemangiopericytomas are incorrectly diagnosed endometrial stromal sarcomas. We agree, however, with those who maintain that uterine haemangiopericytomas are a genuine entity and believe that such neoplasms can usually be recognized by their content of branching, 'staghorn' vessels (Chapter 12).

Stromal tumours showing a sex cord-like pattern must be distinguished from a Sertoliform endometrioid adenocarcinoma (see Chapter 10), while those with a prominent epithelial glandular component can be differentiated from an adenosarcoma by the absence of a frond-like pattern and of a cambium layer and the presence of vascular invasion. Tumours showing prominent muscular differentiation can be distinguished from pure smooth muscle neoplasms by the fact that there are usually admixed areas of typical stromal tumour, while those with extensive myxoid change can be differentiated, on the same grounds, from a myxoid leiomyosarcoma.

11.2 PURE NON-EPITHELIAL NEOPLASMS OF SMOOTH MUSCLE TYPE

Pure smooth muscle tumours of the uterus are considered here largely for the sake of completeness, since being of myometrial rather than endometrial origin they lie outside the scope of this book. Those wanting a detailed discussion and analysis of these neoplasms are referred to Kempson and Hendrickson (1995).

Despite the above avowal, smooth muscle neoplasms can be encountered in curettage material, albeit rather uncommonly. Tissue may be obtained from a submucous leiomyoma, especially one that is polypoid, while it is far from unusual for a leiomyosarcoma to ulcerate through the endometrium and grow into the uterine cavity.

Recognition of a leiomyomatous or leiomyosarcomatous neoplasm in a biopsy rests upon finding evidence of smooth muscle differentiation. Most leiomyomas show evident smooth muscle differentiation, being composed of elongated cells with abundant eosinophilic cytoplasm and bland cigar-shaped nuclei.

Longitudinal myofibrils may be clearly seen in haematoxylin and eosin stained sections and are, in equivocal cases, more readily recognized in PTAH stained sections. A minority of leiomyosarcomas show equally clear evidence of smooth muscle differentiation but many, at the other end of the spectrum, are very poorly differentiated and are formed of a mixture of spindle and polygonal cells that lack any obvious myofibrils.

Smooth muscle neoplasms of the uterus fall into one of three categories: benign, of uncertain malignant potential and malignant. Placement of a particular neoplasm into one of these groups depends upon a consideration of the degree and extent of cytological atypia, the number of mitotic figures and the presence or absence of coagulative tumour cell necrosis. It is important when analysing a smooth muscle neoplasm to consider all these factors and not to rely on one finding and neglect the others.

Cellular, epithelioid, bizarre ('symplastic') and neurilemmoma-like variants of the usual leiomyoma may all be encountered in biopsies and for each of these histological types the criteria for categorization as malignant vary (Kempson and Hendrickson, 1995). Recognition of a neoplasm showing overtly sarcomatous features, such as marked atypia, a high mitotic figures content and extensive tumour cell necrosis, as malignant is easy but some leiomyosarcomas are diagnosed solely on careful histological analysis. In curettage material the only real problem in differential diagnosis presented by smooth muscle tumours is the distinction of poorly differentiated leiomyosarcomas from undifferentiated uterine sarcomas and from poorly differentiated endometrial carcinomas. The distinction of a leiomyosarcoma from an undifferentiated sarcoma is based, in theory at least, on the former having more elongated cells and retaining some semblance of a fascicular pattern; in practice,

however, distinction may be impossible. A combination of a PAS stain, a stain for reticulin fibres and immunocytochemical stains for epithelial membrane antigen, vimentin and desmin will usually allow a distinction to be drawn between poorly differentiated leiomyosarcomas and carcinomas. It should be noted that a proportion of leiomyosarcomas also give a positive staining reaction for cytokeratins (Brown et al., 1987; Norton et al., 1987). This apparently paradoxical finding should not be allowed to detract from a diagnosis of leiomyosarcoma.

A final point to consider is that leiomyosarcomatous tissue in a curetting could come from either a pure neoplasm or from a mixed Müllerian tumour. It may be impossible to decide between these two possibilities in a biopsy specimen and, as both conditions necessitate a hysterectomy, it is fruitless to worry about this diagnostic dilemma.

11.3 PURE HETEROLOGOUS NON-EPITHELIAL NEOPLASMS

These are extremely rare and generally take the form of a rhabdomyosarcoma (Donkers et al., 1972; Hart and Craig, 1978; Vakiani et al., 1982; Siegal et al., 1983; Podczaski et al., 1990; Ordi et al., 1997; Holcomb et al., 1999), osteosarcoma (Crum et al., 1980; Emoto et al., 1994) or chondrosarcoma (Clement, 1978). Rhabdomyosarcomas are usually of the pleomorphic variety (Fig. 11.5) but alveolar (Chiarle et al., 1997) and embryonic (Montag et al., 1996) types have also been described.

The histological features of all these neoplasms are identical to those of their counterparts arising in sites that are more conventional: they are usually clearly malignant with considerable pleomorphism, atypia and mitotic activity. When encountered in

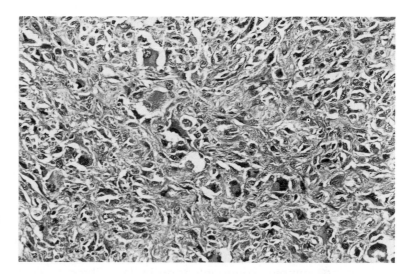

Figure 11.5 Endometrial rhabdomyosarcoma. The tumour is composed of pleomorphic cells some of which are very large and have copious eosinophilic cytoplasm with one or more eccentrically placed nuclei. Haematoxylin and eosin.

biopsy material, however, it is not usually possible to tell whether material from a heterologous sarcoma is from a pure neoplasm or is part of the mesenchymal component of a mixed Müllerian tumour of high-grade malignancy. A heterologous sarcoma that has enveloped normal endometrial glands may be confused with an adenosarcoma but in such a neoplasm, there will not be the characteristic condensation around the included glands to form a cambium layer.

In practice, the drawing of a distinction between a pure heterologous sarcoma and a mixed tumour is of no importance since both lesions necessitate hysterectomy. It is, however, crucially important not to confuse osseous or cartilaginous metaplasia in the endometrial stroma with an osteosarcoma or a chondrosarcoma. Usually, the clearly malignant nature of the sarcomatous neoplasm contrasts sharply with the benign pattern shown by metaplastic cartilage or bone. Furthermore, it can often be seen, even in biopsy material, that the metaplastic tissue arises from, and blends smoothly with, normal endometrial stroma. Fetal remnants may also enter into the differential diagnosis of an osteosarcoma or a chondrosarcoma. Any retained fetal bone or cartilage lacks malignant features and is often admixed with other fetal elements, such as neural tissue (Chapter 8).

11.4 MIXED TUMOURS

Mixed tumours contain both epithelial and non-epithelial elements, both of which may be benign (adenofibroma) or both of which may be malignant (carcinosarcoma). Between these two extremes are those neoplasms in which either the mesenchymal element is malignant and the epithelial component benign (adenosarcoma) or the epithelial element is malignant and the stromal component benign (carcinofibroma); these two neoplasms are grouped together as mixed tumours of low-grade malignancy (Östör and Fortune, 1980; Östör and Rollason, 1995).

Mixed tumours develop most frequently in postmenopausal women, though occasional cases have been reported in children and young women (Chumas *et al.*, 1983; Amr *et al.*, 1986; Solder *et al.*, 1995). Although there appears to be little evidence that adenosarcomas and carcinosarcomas are hormone dependent, there has been a surprisingly large number of reports of such neoplasms developing in women receiving tamoxifen therapy (Bocklage *et al.*, 1992; Altaras *et al.*, 1993; Clarke, 1993; Seoud *et al.*, 1993; Evans *et al.*, 1995; Clement *et al.*, 1996; McCluggage *et al.*, 1997, 2000; Mouritz *et al.*, 1998). Some, but by no means all, of these reports have been of single cases and there has undoubtedly been an element of selective reporting: nevertheless, they cannot be simply ignored and should be borne in mind when examining biopsy material from women receiving tamoxifen.

The mixed tumours commonly form bulky polypoid masses that fill the uterine cavity and may project through the cervical os. The patients usually present with a complaint of vaginal bleeding, though sometimes a vaginal discharge or the passage of tissue fragments per vaginum is noted.

11.4.1 Histological features

Adenofibromas (Fig. 11.6) are rare and contain an admixture of benign mesenchymal and epithelial components (Vellios *et al.*, 1973; Grimalt *et al.*, 1975; Zaloudek and Norris, 1981). The epithelial element covers broad papillary fronds that project both from the surface (Fig. 11.7) and into cystic spaces within the neoplasm and forms a lining to glandular acini, clefts and cysts that are set in the mesenchymal component. The epithelial cells are cytologically bland and may be of endometrial, tubal, endocervical, squamous or nondescript cuboidal type. In many adenofibromas, there is a melange of different epithelia but in some, only one type, usually an endometrioid epithelium, is present. The mesenchymal component of an adenofibroma consists of endometrial–stromal-like cells, fusiform cells or a mixture of these two components. The mesenchymal tissue tends to be condensed around or beneath the epithelial component, is histologically benign, does not contain heterologous components and has a mitotic count of less than 2 per 10 high-power fields (Clement and Scully, 1990a; Östör and Rollason, 1995). Although adenofibromas are benign, they may recur if incompletely excised (Seltzer *et al.*,

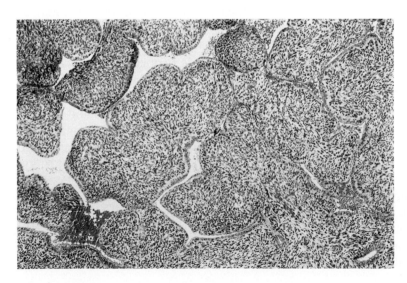

Figure 11.6 Müllerian adenofibroma. The neoplasm is composed of closely packed, somewhat moulded, coarse papillae with fibrous and endometrial stromal cores covered by a cubo-columnar epithelium of endometrial type. There is a minor degree of stromal condensation deep to the surface epithelium but this is much less marked than is the case in an adenosarcoma. Haematoxylin and eosin.

1990) and are therefore usually treated by hysterectomy.

The adenosarcoma contains a benign epithelial element and a low-grade malignant mesenchymal component (Clement and Scully, 1974; Fox *et al.*, 1979; Martinelli *et al.*, 1980; Östör and Fortune, 1980; Zaloudek and Norris, 1981; Chen, 1985; Clement and Scully, 1990b). At first sight, these neoplasms closely resemble an adenofibroma with an epithelial component covering papillae on the surface, within clefts and lining cysts or glands embedded in the stroma (Fig. 11.8). The epithelium may be of any Müllerian type, as in the adenofibroma, but the most common pattern is for it to be predominantly endometrioid with a minor admixture of endocervical and squamous elements. The epithelium may show a minor

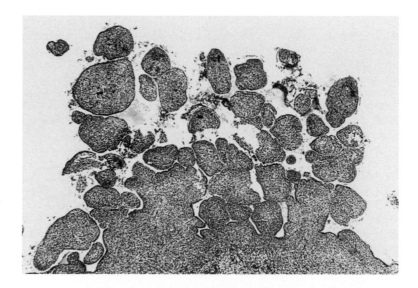

Figure 11.7 Müllerian adenofibroma. The surface of the neoplasm has a prominent papillary pattern, the papillae being covered most commonly by endometrial-type epithelium or a flattened epithelium of indeterminate type. Haematoxylin and eosin.

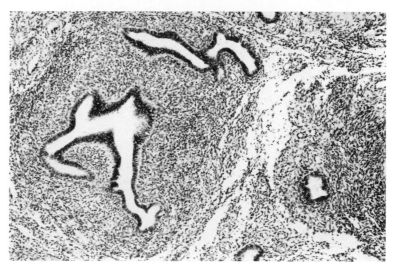

Figure 11.8 Müllerian adenosarcoma. Neoplastic glandular elements, lined by epithelium of endometrial type, are set in a cellular stroma. Haematoxylin and eosin.

degree of multilayering and irregularity and there may be, focally, a minor degree of cytological atypia. The mesenchymal component of these neoplasms tends to be predominant and is usually formed by cells with round, ovoid or fusiform nuclei, scanty cytoplasm and indistinct margins (Fig. 11.9), their appearance closely resembles that of an endometrial stromal sarcoma or, less commonly, the features are those of a fibrosarcoma. The sarcomatous tissue tends to be of variable cellularity and compactness but is, characteristically, condensed beneath the surface epithelium and around the contained glands or cysts (Fig. 11.10) to form a distinct 'cambium' layer. The stromal elements show pleomorphism and atypia, though this is rarely of a striking degree, and contain more than 2 mitotic figures per 10 high-power fields but

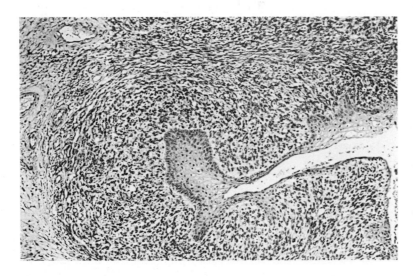

Figure 11.9 Müllerian adenosarcoma. A glandular acinus is lined by stratified squamous epithelium, which shows a very minor degree of cytological atypia. The stroma is highly cellular, mildly pleomorphic and contains a moderate number of mitoses. Haematoxylin and eosin.

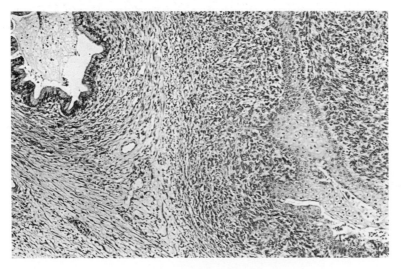

Figure 11.10 Müllerian adenosarcoma. Condensation of the sarcomatous stroma to form a cambium layer is particularly marked around the neoplastic gland to the right, which is lined by stratified squamous epithelium. The gland to the left is lined by a single layer of mucus-secreting epithelium of endocervical type and, here, the cambium layer, although clearly present, is less striking. Haematoxylin and eosin.

less than 20. Heterologous elements, such as rhabdomyoblasts, cartilage or fat, are present in the stroma in about one-third of cases (Clement and Scully, 1990b; Kaku *et al.* 1992) while a sex-cord like pattern with epithelial-type cells arranged in nests, trabeculae or tubules is seen in a small minority of cases (Hirschfield *et al.*, 1986; Clement and Scully, 1989). In rare cases, an adenosarcoma may be overgrown by a high-grade sarcoma (Clement, 1989). Adenosarcomas are of low-grade malignancy and rarely metastasize but about 20 per cent recur after hysterectomy. The prognosis for cases with overgrowth of a high-grade sarcoma is very poor (Verschraegen *et al.*, 1998).

Carcinofibromas, in which a malignant glandular component is supported by a prominent but benign stroma are extremely rare (Östör and Fortune, 1980; Thompson and Husemeyer, 1981; Engdahl and Wolfhagen, 1988) and, indeed, not everyone is convinced that such an entity truly exists. The epithelial component is usually an endometrioid adenocarcinoma, while the stromal element resembles normal endometrial stroma; heterologous elements may be present (Chen and Vergon, 1981).

Carcinosarcomas appear to contain an intimate admixture of carcinomatous and sarcomatous elements, the relative proportions of which vary considerably (Sternberg *et al.*, 1954; Ober, 1959; Norris and Taylor, 1966b; Norris *et al.*, 1966; Chuang *et al.*, 1970; Kempson and Bari, 1970; Williamson and Christopherson, 1972; Barwick and LiVolsi, 1979; Östör and Rollason, 1995). These neoplasms are widely regarded as mixed neoplasms but tissue culture, molecular and immunocytochemical studies suggest that they are metaplastic carcinomas (George *et al.*, 1991; DeBrito *et al.*, 1993; Emoto *et al.*, 1993; Gorai *et al.*, 1993; Mayall *et al.*, 1994; Abeln *et al.*, 1997; Guarino *et al.*, 1998; Kounelis *et al.*, 1998; Szukala *et al.*, 1999) and it has been proposed that they be classed as sarcomatoid carcinomas (Colombi, 1993; Wick and Swanson, 1993). The scientific evidence for adopting this nomenclature is quite persuasive but many pathologists are reluctant to make this terminological change and retain, as we do here, the term carcinosarcoma.

Although sometimes anaplastic or very poorly differentiated (Fig. 11.11), the carcinomatous component of a carcinosarcoma is

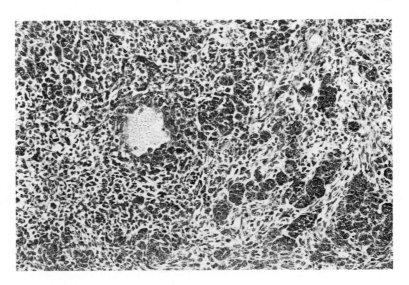

Figure 11.11 Carcinosarcoma. Poorly defined and poorly differentiated epithelial elements, to the right, are set in a sarcomatous stroma. It is difficult in a case such as this to distinguish the carcinomatous and sarcomatous components using morphological criteria alone: immunocytochemistry is often, but not invariably helpful in making the distinction. Haematoxylin and eosin.

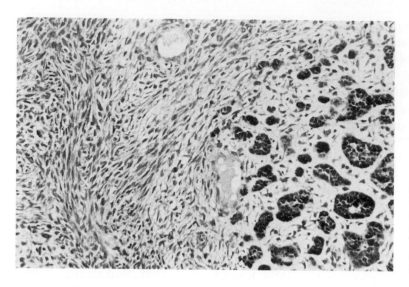

Figure 11.12 Carcinosarcoma. Well-differentiated glandular structures lined by an epithelium of uncertain type are seen on the right. The sarcomatous component in this area is largely undifferentiated. Haematoxylin and eosin.

often quite well differentiated and may show an endometrioid, serous papillary, mucinous, clear cell or indeterminate pattern (Fig. 11.12). Bland, metaplastic squamous epithelium is not uncommonly present within the acini of an endometrioid adenocarcinomatous element, while, occasionally, there is a mixture of adenocarcinoma and squamous cell carcinoma. In rare instances, the epithelial component is represented by a squamous cell carcinoma.

The non-epithelial component of a carcinosarcoma may resemble an endometrial stromal sarcoma, while, infrequently, a leiomyosarcomatous or fibrosarcomatous pattern predominates. Often, however, the appearances are those of a sarcoma of indeterminate type (Fig. 11.12) and, as Östör and Rollason (1995) have commented, 'there is little point in agonising over the exact type of stroma present as this has no influence on prognosis'. The non-epithelial component is usually highly cellular, commonly lacks the 'cambium' layer formation that characterizes mixed Müllerian tumours of lesser malignancy and almost invariably shows conspicuous pleomorphism, atypia and

mitotic activity. Bizarre tumour giant cells with grossly atypical nuclei are often present while mitotic figures number more than 20 per 10 high-power fields and are frequently of markedly aberrant form. Small, intracellular or extracellular, rounded, eosinophilic hyaline bodies have been noted in the stroma of mixed tumours of high-grade malignancy and are, in our experience, a common and characteristic feature (Clement and Scully, 1988): they often, but not invariably, stain positively for α-1-antitrypsin and α-1-antichymotrypsin (Marshall and Braye, 1985).

Heterologous components are present in about 50 per cent of carcinosarcomas, with malignant striated muscle, cartilage, bone and fat being the alien tissues most frequently encountered. Neuroectodermal or neuroendocrine differentiation may occasionally be apparent (Manivel *et al.*, 1986: Gersell *et al.*, 1989; Fukunaga *et al.*, 1996), while rhabdoid differentiation has also been noted in exceptional cases (Mount *et al.*, 1995; Baschinsky *et al.*, 1999). The commonest heterologous component is striated muscle, which is usually seen as scattered, occasionally aggregated,

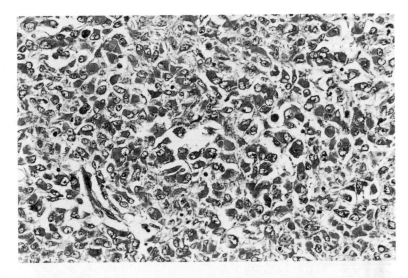

Figure 11.13 Carcinosarcoma with a heterologous component. Rhabdomyoblasts are present in the stroma of the neoplasm. The cells have abundant eosinophilic cytoplasm and eccentric nuclei. Cross-striations may be seen but are not always apparent. Haematoxylin and eosin.

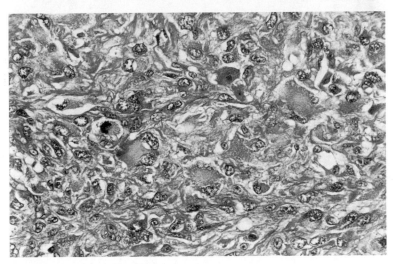

Figure 11.14 Carcinosarcoma with a heterologous component. Within the stroma of the neoplasm are large cells with irregular outlines and eccentric, sometimes multiple, nuclei. These are thought to be immature rhabdomyocytes. Haematoxylin and eosin.

rhabdomyoblasts (Fig. 11.13). These are typically 'strap' or 'tadpole' shaped and have cross-striations which may be apparent in haematoxylin and eosin stained sections but are more easily identified in PTAH stained preparations. Relatively large, plump, rounded or 'racquet-shaped' cells with abundant fibrillary or granular cytoplasm and atypical nuclei are also often seen in mixed tumours of high-grade malignancy (Fig. 11.14), commonly in association with clearly definable rhabdomyoblasts but sometimes in the absence of such cells. The practice of classing such cells also as rhabdomyoblasts has been deplored by some who would maintain that cells only merit this categorization if they show either cross-striations or electron microscopic evidence of skeletal muscle differentiation (Hendrickson and Kempson, 1980). We do, however, regard these racquet cells as rhabdomyoblasts and in

187

defence of our apparently relaxed approach to diagnostic criteria would maintain that cells with visible cross-striations are immature rhabdomyocytes rather than rhabdomyoblasts. Immunocytochemical staining for myoglobulin might be expected to resolve any difficulties in identifying cells of striated muscle type (Mukai *et al.*, 1980) but in our hands, this technique yields notably capricious results.

The second most common heterologous element in carcinosarcomas is cartilage, which usually takes the form of chondrosarcomatous foci with large, atypical nuclei (Fig. 11.15). Occasionally, however, the cartilaginous tissue is immature rather than overtly malignant (Fig. 11.16). Osteosarcomatous elements are uncommon while any fat present in these tumours usually results from

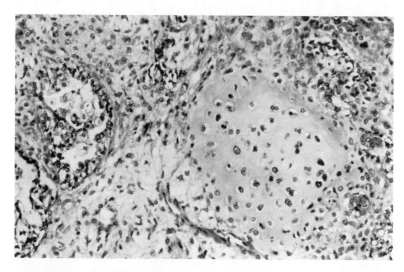

Figure 11.15 Carcinosarcoma with heterologous component. The glandular structures to the left are lined by clear cells similar to those seen in a clear cell adenocarcinoma. The cartilaginous area, to the right, shows pleomorphism and nuclear hyperchromatism. Haematoxylin and eosin.

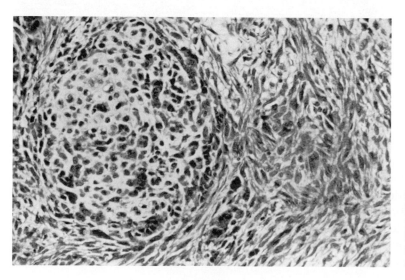

Figure 11.16 Carcinosarcoma with heterologous component. To the left, a focus of tissue resembling immature cartilage is set in an undifferentiated sarcomatous stroma. Haematoxylin and eosin.

degenerative changes rather than heterologous liposarcoma.

11.4.2 Differential diagnosis

Both the adenofibroma and the adenosarcoma can be mistaken for a simple endometrial or endocervical polyp. Simple polyps do not show papillary projections into clefts and cysts, lack any condensation of the stroma around the epithelial elements and differ from an adenosarcoma, though not an adenofibroma, in having a bland stroma. Atypical polypoid adenomyomas (Chapter 8) also enter into the differential diagnosis of adenofibromas and adenosarcomas but are distinguished by the leiomyomatous nature of their stroma and their lack of a cambium layer. Differentiation of an adenosarcoma from a pure endometrial stromal sarcoma with entrapped normal endometrial glands is based upon the lack of a cambium layer in the latter situation.

A carcinosarcoma has to be distinguished from a pure homologous or heterologous sarcoma and from an anaplastic carcinoma. The distinction from a pure sarcoma or carcinoma rests solely upon recognition of the biphasic pattern of a mixed tumour and this may not be possible in biopsy material, which can contain tissue from only one component of such a neoplasm. Even if both epithelial and non-epithelial elements are present in curettage material, they may be so intimately blended that their separate nature is not readily apparent. Under such circumstances, staining for intermediate filaments would be expected to be of considerable value since the carcinomatous areas express keratins and epithelial membrane antigen (EMA) and the sarcomatous tissues express desmin and/or vimentin. Unfortunately, while this staining pattern is usually found, the non-epithelial component may also stain positively for keratins and EMA, and the epithelial tissue often stains positively for vimentin (Bitterman

et al., 1988). Benign heterologous elements may be seen very occasionally in the stroma of an endometrial adenocarcinoma (Nogales *et al.*, 1982). Nevertheless, the presence of such elements in what is clearly seen on biopsy as a malignant tumour should raise a strong suspicion of a mixed neoplasm, as should the finding of bizarre cells with highly atypical nuclei.

Carcinosarcomas must also be distinguished from 'collision' tumours in which an adenocarcinoma and a sarcoma exist independently within the same uterus (Lam *et al.*, 1999): elements from both tumours may be present in a biopsy and this will, therefore, lead to confusion with a carcinosarcoma. A diagnosis of a collision tumour is, however, very much dependent upon gross and microscopic recognition of two separate and discrete neoplasms in the uterine cavity upon examination of a hysterectomy specimen. It is doubtful if a distinction can be made on morphological grounds between a collision tumour and a carcinosarcoma in biopsy material: the only possible clue is that while the mesenchymal component of a carcinosarcoma often stains positively (albeit patchily) for epithelial markers such as cytokeratins and EMA the mesenchymal element of a collision tumour is usually negative. A collision tumour characterized by the presence of independent endometrial carcinoma and rhabdoid tumour has been described (Gaertner *et al.*, 1999). Such a collision tumour could, and indeed almost certainly would, be diagnosed as a carcinosarcoma if elements from both neoplasms were present in biopsy material and the correct diagnosis would only be attained by examination of the hysterectomy specimen.

Occasionally, a carcinosarcoma which contains heterologous elements is confused with a teratoma; uterine teratomas are of extreme rarity (Chapter 12), occur usually in young patients rather than in elderly women and differ from mixed Müllerian tumours in their ectodermal and endodermal tissue content.

In the very unusual circumstances of a carcinosarcoma occurring in childhood or in young women (Amr *et al.*, 1986), it must be distinguished from an embryonal rhabdomyosarcoma (sarcoma botyroides) arising in the cervix or vagina but being present in curetted material. The distinction again depends upon demonstration of a biphasic pattern in the mixed tumour and this can be impossible if the biopsy contains only heterologous rhabdomyosarcomatous tissue.

11.4.3 Assessment of malignancy in mixed tumours

The pathologist encountering a mixed tumour must distinguish between the benign adenofibroma, the indolently malignant adenosarcoma and the highly aggressive carcinosarcoma. The distinction between an adenofibroma and an adenosarcoma can be difficult in biopsy material but cytological evidence of malignancy within the stromal component and the presence of heterologous elements point to a diagnosis of adenosarcoma. In doubtful cases, reliance has to be placed on the mitotic count in the neoplasm: tumours with less than 2 mitotic figures per 10 high-power fields behave as adenofibromas and those with 2 or more mitoses per 10 high-power fields behave, and are classified, as adenosarcomas (Mills *et al.*, 1981; Zaloudek and Norris, 1981). The distinction between an adenosarcoma and a carcinosarcoma usually presents few difficulties. Nevertheless, occasional neoplasms fall into a hinterland between these two clearly defined entities and here it is necessary once again to resort to mitotic counts, with neoplasms with 20 or more mitoses per 10 high-power fields being regarded as of high-grade malignancy.

There has been much debate about prognostic pathological features in carcinosarcomas, though it is now widely agreed that neither the presence nor the absence of heterologous elements is of prognostic importance and that vascular space invasion is an adverse prognostic factor (Gagne *et al.*, 1989; Larsen *et al.*, 1990; Silverberg *et al.*, 1990; Major *et al.*, 1993; George *et al.*, 1995). In one large study, the biological behaviour of these neoplasms depended principally on the histological type and grade of the carcinomatous element (Silverberg *et al.*, 1990). This would be in agreement both with current views of the nature of these neoplasms and with the fact that metastases are usually, though not invariably, purely carcinomatous in nature (Sreenan and Hart, 1995). Nevertheless, one subsequent study did find the grade of the sarcomatous element to be an important prognostic factor (Major *et al.*, 1993) and carcinosarcomas are certainly more aggressive tumours than are endometrial carcinomas, which are of the same type and grade as the epithelial component of a carcinosarcoma (George *et al.*, 1995).

REFERENCES

Abeln, E.C.A., Smit, V.T.H.B, Wessels, J.W., De Leeuw, W.J.F., Cornelisse, C.J., Fleuren, G.J. (1997) Molecular evidence for the conversion hypothesis of the origin of malignant mixed Müllerian tumours. *J. Pathol.* **183**, 424–31.

Altaras, M.M., Aviram, R., Cohen, I. *et al.* (1993) Role of prolonged stimulation of tamoxifen therapy in the etiology of endometrial sarcomas. *Gynecol. Oncol.* **49**, 255–8.

Amr, S.S., Tavassoli, F.A., Hassan, A.A., Issa, A.A., Maddnat, F.A. (1986) Mixed mesodermal tumor of the uterus in a 4-year old girl. *Int. J. Gynecol. Pathol.* **5**, 371–8.

Baggish, M.S., Woodruff, J.D. (1972) Uterine stromatosis: clinicopathologic features and hormone dependency. *Obstet. Gynecol.* **40**, 487–98.

Baker, R.J., Hildebrandt, R.H., Rouse, R.V., Hendrickson, M.R., Longacre, T.A. (1999) Inhibin and CD99 (MIC2) expression in uterine stromal neoplasms with sex cord-like elements. *Hum. Pathol.* **30**, 671–9.

Barwick, K.W., LiVolsi, V.A. (1979) Malignant mixed Müllerian tumors of the uterus: a clinicopathologic assessment in 34 cases. *Am. J. Surg. Pathol.* **3**, 125–35.

Baschinsky, D.Y., Niemann, T.H., Eaton, L.A., Frankel, W.L. (1999) Malignant mixed Müllerian tumor with rhabdoid features: a report of two cases and a review of the literature. *Gynecol. Oncol.* **73**, 145–50.

Binder, S., Nieberg, R., Cheng, L., Al-Jitawi, S. (1991) Histologic and immunohistochemical analysis of nine endometrial stromal tumors. *Int. J. Gynecol. Pathol.* **10**, 191–7.

Bitterman, P., Chun, B.K., Kurman, R.S. (1988) Uterine carcinosarcomas: a clinicopathologic and immunohistologic study providing evidence that these are biphasic carcinomas. *Mod. Pathol.* **1**, 10a.

Blom, R., Malmstrom, H., Guerrieri, C. (1999) Endometrial stromal sarcoma of the uterus: a clinicopathologic, DNA flow cytometic, p53, and mdm-2 analysis of 17 cases. *Int. J. Gynecol. Cancer* **9**, 98–104.

Bocklage, T., Lee, K.R., Belingson, H. (1992) Uterine Müllerian adenosarcoma following adenomyoma in a woman on tamoxifen therapy. *Gynecol. Oncol.* **44**, 104–9.

Bonazzi del Poggetto, C., Virtanen, I., Lehto, V-P, Wahlstrom, I., Saksela, E. (1983) Expression of intermediate filaments in ovarian and uterine tumors. *Int. J. Gynecol. Pathol.* **1**, 359–66.

Brown, D.C., Theaker, D.M., Banks, P.M., Catter, K.C., Mason, D.Y. (1987) Cytokeratin expression in smooth muscle tumours. *Histopathology* **11**, 477–86.

Chaiarle, R., Godio, L., Fusi, D., Soldata, T., Palestro, G. (1997) Pure alveolar rhabdomyosarcoma of the corpus uteri: description of a case with increased serum level of CA-125. *Gynecol. Oncol.* **66**, 320–3.

Chang, K.L., Crabtree, G.S., Lim-Tan, S.K., Kempson, R.L., Hendrickson, M.R. (1990) Primary uterine stromal neoplasms: a clinicopathologic study of 117 cases. *Am. J. Surg. Pathol.* **14**, 415–38.

Chen, K.T.K. (1985) Rhabdomyosarcomatous uterine adenosarcoma. *Int. J. Gynecol. Pathol.* **4**, 146–52.

Chen, K.T.K., Vergon, J.M. (1981) Carcinomesenchymoma of the uterus. *Am. J. Clin. Pathol.* **75**, 746–8.

Chuang, J.T., van Velden, D.J.J., Graham, J.B. (1970) Carcinosarcomas and mixed mesodermal tumor of the uterine corpus: review of 49 cases. *Obstet. Gynecol.* **35**, 769–80.

Chumas, J.C., Mann, W.J., Tseng, L. (1983) Malignant mixed Müllerian tumor of the endometrium in a young woman with polycystic ovaries. *Cancer* **52**, 1478–81.

Clarke, M.R. (1993) Uterine malignant mixed Müllerian tumor in a patient on long-term tamoxifen therapy for breast cancer. *Gynecol. Oncol.* **51**, 1478–81.

Clement, P.B. (1978) Chondrosarcoma of the uterus: report of a case and review of the literature. *Hum. Pathol.* **9**, 726–32.

Clement, P.B. (1989) Müllerian adenosarcoma of the uterus with sarcomatous overgrowth: a clinicopathological analysis of ten cases. *Am. J. Clin. Pathol.* **91**, 664–72.

Clement, P.B., Scully, R.E. (1974) Müllerian adenosarcoma of the uterus: a clinicopathologic analysis of ten cases of a distinct type of Müllerian mixed tumor. *Cancer* **34**, 1138–49.

Clement, P.B., Scully, R.E. (1976) Uterine tumors resembling ovarian sex-cord tumors. *Am. J. Clin. Pathol.* **69**, 276–83.

Clement, P.B., Scully, R.E. (1988) Uterine tumors with mixed epithelial and mesenchymal elements. *Semin. Diagn. Pathol.* **5**, 199–222.

Clement, P.B., Scully, R.E. (1989) Müllerian adenosarcoma of the uterus with sex cord-like elements: a clinicopathologic analysis of eight cases. *Am. J. Clin. Pathol.* **13**, 28–38.

Clement, P.B., Scully, R.E. (1990a) Müllerian adenofibroma of the uterus with invasion of myometrium and pelvic veins. *Int. J. Gynecol. Pathol.* **9**, 363–71.

Clement, P.B., Scully, R.E. (1990b) Müllerian adenosarcoma of the uterus: a clinicopathologic analysis of 100 cases with a review of the literature. *Hum. Pathol.* **21**, 363–81.

Clement, P.B., Scully, R.E. (1992) Endometrial stromal sarcomas of the uterus with extensive endometrioid glandular differentiation: a report of three cases that caused problems in differential diagnosis. *Int. J. Gynecol. Pathol.* **11**, 163–73.

Clement, P.B., Oliva, E., Young, R.H. (1996) Müllerian adenosarcoma of the uterine corpus associated with tamoxifen therapy: a report of six cases and a review of tamoxifen-associated endometrial lesions. *Int. J. Gynecol. Pathol.* **15**, 222–9.

Colombi, R.P. (1993) Sarcomatoid carcinomas of the female genital tract (malignant mixed Müllerian tumors). *Semin. Diagn. Pathol.* **10**, 169–75.

Crum, C.P., Rogers, B.H., Anderson, W. (1980) Osteosarcoma of the uterus: case report and review of the literature. *Gynecol. Oncol.* **9**, 256–68.

De Brito, A., Silverberg, S.G., Orenstein, J.M. (1993) Carcinosarcoma (malignant mixed Müllerian [mesodermal] tumor) of the female genital tract: immunohistochemical and ultrastructural analysis of 28 cases. *Hum. Pathol.* **24**, 132–42.

De Nictolas, M., Curatola, A., Tommasoni, S., Magiera, G. (1994) High grade endometrial stromal sarcoma; clinicopathologic and immunohistochemical study of a case. *Pathologica* **86**, 217–21.

Donkers, B., Kazzaz, B.A., Meimering, H. (1972) Rhabdomyosarcoma of the corpus uteri: report of two cases with review of the literature. *Am. J. Obstet. Gynecol.* **114**, 1025–30.

Emeto, M., Iwasaki, H., Kikuchi, M., Shirakawa, K. (1993) Characteristics of cloned cells of mixed Müllerian tumor of the human uterus: carcinoma cells showing myogenic differentiation in vitro. *Cancer* **71**, 3065–75.

Emoto, M., Iwasaki, H., Kawarabayashi, T. *et al.* (1994) Primary osteosarcoma of the uterus: report of a case with immunocytochemical analysis. *Gynecol. Oncol.* **54**, 385–8.

Engdahl, E., Wolfhagen, U. (1988) Carcinofibroma – a variant of the mixed Müllerian tumour. *Br. J. Obstet. Gynaecol.* **88**, 1151–5.

Evans, H. (1982) Endometrial stromal sarcoma and poorly differentiated endometrial sarcoma. *Cancer* **50**, 2170–82.

Evans, M.J., Langlois, N.E.I., Kitchener, H.C., Milller, I.D. (1995) Is there an association between long term tamoxifen treatment and the development of carcinosarcoma (malignant mixed Müllerian tumor) of the uterus? *Int. J. Gynecol. Cancer* **5**, 310–13.

Farhood, A., Abrams, J. (1991) Immunohistochemistry of endometrial stromal sarcoma. *Hum. Pathol.* **22**, 224–30.

Fekete, P.S., Vellios, F. (1984) The clinical and histologic spectrum of endometrial stromal neoplasms: a report of 41 cases. *Int. J. Gynecol. Pathol.* **3**, 198–212.

Fitko, R., Brainer, J., Schink, J.C., August, C.Z. (1990) Endometrial stromal sarcoma with rhabdoid differentiation. *Int. J. Gynecol. Pathol.* **9**, 379–81.

Fox, H., Harilal, K.R., Youell, A. (1979) Müllerian adenosarcoma of the uterine body: a report of nine cases. *Histopathology* **3**, 167–80.

Franquemont, D.W., Frierson, H. Jr, Mills, S.E. (1991) An immunohistochemical study of normal endometrial stroma and endometrial stromal neoplasms: evidence for smooth muscle differentiation. *Am. J. Surg. Pathol.* **15**, 861–70.

Fukunaga, N., Nomura, K., Endo, Y., Ushigome, S., Aizawa, S. (1996) Carcinosarcoma of the uterus with extensive neuroectodermal differentiation. *Histopathology* **29**, 565–70.

Gaertner, E.M., Farley, J.H., Taylor, R.R., Silver, S.A. (1999) Collision of uterine rhabdoid tumor and endometrioid adenocarcinoma: a case report and review of the literature. *Int. J. Gynecol. Pathol.* **18**, 396–401.

Gagne, E., Tetu, B., Blondeau, L. *et al.* (1989) Morphologic prognostic factors for malignant mixed Müllerian tumor of the uterus: a clinicopathologic study of 58 cases. *Mod. Pathol.* **2**, 433–8.

George, E., Manivel, J.C., Dehner, L.P., Wick, M.R. (1991) Malignant mixed Müllerian tumors: an immunohistochemical study of 47 cases, with histogenetic considerations and clinical correlation. *Hum. Pathol.* **22**, 215–23.

George, E., Lillemoe, T.J., Twigs, L.B., Perrone, T. (1995) Malignant mixed Müllerian tumor versus high grade endometrial carcinoma and aggressive variants of endometrial carcinoma: a comparative analysis of survival. *Int. J. Gynecol. Pathol.* **14**, 39–44.

Gersell, D.J., Duncan, D.A., Fulling, K.H. (1989) Malignant mixed Müllerian tumor of the uterus with neuroectodermal differentiation. *Int. J. Gynecol. Pathol.* **8**, 168–78.

Gorai, I., Doi, C., Minaguchi, H. (1993) Establishment and characterization of carcinosarcoma cell line of the human uterus. *Cancer* **71**, 775–86.

Grimalt, M., Arghelles, M., Ferenezy, A. (1975) Papillary cystadenofibroma of endometrium: a histochemical and ultrastructural study. *Cancer* **36**, 137–44.

Guarino, M., Giordano, F., Pallotti, F., Polizzotti, G., Tricomi, P., Cristofori, E. (1998) Malignant mixed Müllerian tumor of the uterus: features favouring its origin from a common cell clone and an epithelial-to-mesenchymal transformation mechanism of histogenesis. *Tumori* **84**, 391–7.

Hart, W.R., Craig, J.R. (1978) Rhabdomyosarcoma of the uterus. *Am. J. Clin. Pathol.* **70**, 217–23.

Hart, W.R., Yoonessi, M. (1977) Endometrial stromatosis of the uterus. *Obstet. Gynecol.* **49**, 393–403.

Hendrickson, M.R., Kempson, R.L. (1980) *Surgical Pathology of the Uterine Corpus*. Philadelphia: W.B. Saunders.

Hirschfield, L., Kahn, L.B., Chen, S., Winkler, B., Rosenberg, S. (1986) Müllerian adenosarcoma with ovarian sex cord-like differentiation: a light- and electron-microscopic study. *Cancer* **57**, 1197–1200.

Hitchcock, C.I., Norris, H.J. (1992) Flow cytometric analysis of endometrial stromal sarcoma. *Am. J. Clin. Pathol.* **97**, 267–71.

Holcomb, K., Francis, M., Ruis, J., Abulafia, O., Matthews, R.P., Lee, Y.C. (1999) Pleomorphic rhabdomyosarcoma of the uterus in a postmenopausal woman with elevated serum CA125. *Gynecol. Oncol.* **74**, 499–501.

Kaku, T., Silverberg, S.G., Major, F.J. *et al.* (1992) Adenosarcoma of the uterus: a Gynecologic Oncology Group clinicopathologic study of 31 cases. *Int. J. Gynecol. Pathol.* **11**, 75–88.

Katz, L., Merino, M.J., Sakamoto, H., Schwartz, P.F. (1987) Endometrial stromal sarcoma: a clinicopathologic study of 11 cases with determination of estrogen and progestin receptor levels in three tumors. *Gynecol. Oncol.* **26**, 87–97.

Kempson, R.L., Bari, W. (1970) Uterine sarcomas: classification, diagnosis and prognosis. *Hum. Pathol.* **1**, 331–49.

Kempson, R.L., Hendrickson, M.R. (1995) Pure mesenchymal neoplasms of the uterine corpus. In Fox, H. (ed.), *Haines and Taylor: Textbook of Obstetrical and Gynaecological Pathology*, 4th Edn. Edinburgh: Churchill Livingstone, 519–86.

Kim, Y.-H., Cho, H., Kyoem-Kim, H., Kim, I. (1996) Uterine endometrial stromal sarcoma with rhabdoid and smooth muscle differentiation. *J. Korean Med. Sci.* **61**, 142–6.

Kounelis, S., Jones, M.W., Papadaki, H., Bakker, A., Swalsky, P., Finkelstein, S.D. (1998) Carcinosarcomas (malignant mixed Müllerian tumors) of the female genital tract: comparative molecular analysis of epithelial and mesenchymal components. *Hum. Pathol.* **29**, 82–7.

Krishnamurthy, S., Jungbluth, A.A., Busam, K. J., Rosai, J. (1998) Uterine tumors resembling ovarian sex-cord tumors have an immunophenotype consistent with true sex cord differentiation. *Am. J. Surg. Pathol.* **22**, 1078–82.

Lam, K.Y., Khoo, U.-S., Cheung, A. (1999) Collision of endometrioid carcinoma and stromal sarcoma of the uterus: a report of two cases. *Int. J. Gynecol. Pathol.* **18**, 77–81.

Larsen, B., Silfversward, C., Nilsson, B., Petterson, F. (1990) Mixed Müllerian tumours of the uterus – prognostic factors: a clinical and histopathological study of 147 cases. *Radiother. Oncol.* **17**, 123–32.

Lillemoe, T.J., Perrone, T., Norris, H.J., Dehner, L.P. (1991) Myogenous phenotype of epithelial-like areas in endometrial stromal sarcomas. *Arch. Pathol. Lab. Med.* **115**, 215–19.

Major, F.J., Blessing, J.A., Silverberg, S.G. *et al.* (1993) Prognostic factors in early-stage uterine sarcoma: a Gynecologic Oncology Group Study. *Cancer* **71**, 1702–9.

Manivel, C., Wick, M.R., Sibley, R.K. (1986) Neuroendocrine differentiation in Müllerian neoplasms: an immunohistochemical study of a 'pure' endometrial small cell carcinoma and a mixed Müllerian tumor containing small cell carcinoma. *Am. J. Clin. Pathol.* **86**, 438–43.

Marshall, R.J., Braye, S.C. (1985) Alpha-l-antitrypsin, alpha-l-antichymotrypsin, actin, and myosin in uterine sarcomas. *Int. J. Gynecol. Pathol.* **4**, 346–54.

Martinelli, G., Pileri, S., Bazzochi, F., Serra, L. (1980) Müllerian adenosarcoma of the uterus: a report of 5 cases. *Tumori* **66**, 499–506.

Mayall, F., Rutty, K., Campbell, F., Goddard, H. (1994) *p53* immunostaining suggests that uterine carcinosarcomas are monoclonal. *Histopathology* **24**, 211–14.

McCluggage, W.G. (1999) Uterine tumours resembling ovarian sex cord tumours: immunohistochemical evidence for true sex cord differentiation. *Histopathology* **34**, 374–5.

McCluggage, W.G., Shah, V., Walsh, M.Y., Toner, P.G. (1993) Uterine tumour resembling ovarian sex cord tumour: evidence for smooth muscle differentiation. *Histopathology* **23**, 83–5.

McCluggage, W.G., Date, A., Bharucha, H., Toner, P.G. (1996) Endometrial stromal sarcoma with sex cord-like area and focal rhabdoid differentiation. *Histopathology* **29**, 369–74.

McCluggage, W.G., McManus, D.T., Lioe, T.F., Hill, C.M. (1997) Uterine carcinosarcoma in association with tamoxifen therapy. *Br. J. Obstet. Gynaecol.* **104**, 748–50.

McCluggage, W.G., Abdulkader, M., Price, J.H. *et al.* (2000) Uterine carcinosarcomas in patients receiving tamoxifen: a report of 19 cases. *Int. J. Gynecol. Cancer* **10**, 280–4.

Mills, S.E., Sugg, K.N., Mahnesmith, R.C. (1981) Endometrial adenosarcoma with pelvic involvement following uterine perforation. *Diag. Gynecol. Obstet.* **3**, 149–54.

Mount, S.L., Lee, K.R., Taatjes, D.J. (1995) Carcinosarcoma (malignant mixed Müllerian tumor) of the uterus with a rhabdoid tumor component: an immunohistochemical, ultrastructural, and immunoelectron microscopic case study. *Am. J. Clin. Pathol.* **103**, 235–9.

Mourits, M.J.E., Hollema, H., Willemsee, P.H.B. *et al.* (1998) Adenosarcoma of the uterus following tamoxifen treatment for breast cancer. *Int. J. Gynecol. Cancer* **8**, 168–71.

Mukai, K., Varela-Duran, J., Nochomouitz, L.F. (1980) The rhabdomyoblast in mixed Müllerian tumors of the uterus and ovary: an immunohistochemical study of myoglobin in 25 cases. *Am. J. Clin. Pathol.* **74**, 101–4.

Nogales, F.F., Gomez-Morales, M., Raymundo, C., Aguilar, D. (1982) Benign heterologous tissue components associated with endometrial carcinoma. *Int. J. Gynecol. Pathol.* **1**, 286–91.

Norris, H.J., Taylor, H.B. (1966a) Mesenchymal tumors of the uterus. I. A clinical and pathological study of 53 endometrial stromal tumors. *Cancer* **19**, 755–66.

Norris, H.J., Taylor, H.B. (1966b) Mesenchymal tumors of the uterus. III. A clinical and pathological study of thirty-one cases of carcinosarcoma. *Cancer* **19**, 1459–65.

Norris, H.J., Roth, E., Taylor, H.B. (1966) Mesenchymal tumors of the uterus. II. A clinical and pathological study of thirty-one mixed mesodermal tumors. *Obstet. Gynecol.* **28**, 57–63.

Norton, A.J., Thomas, J.A., Isaacson, P.C. (1987) Cytokeratin-specific monoclonal antibodies are reactive with tumours of smooth muscle derivation: an immunocytochemical and biochemical study using antibodies to intermediate filament cytoskeletal proteins. *Histopathology* **11**, 487–96.

Ober, W.B. (1959) Uterine sarcomas: histogenesis and taxonomy. *Ann. N.Y. Acad. Sci.* **75**, 568–85.

Oliva, E., Clement, P.B., Young, R.H., Scully, R.E. (1998) Mixed endometrial stromal and smooth muscle tumors of the uterus: a clinicopathologic study of 15 cases. *Am. J. Surg. Pathol.* **22**, 997–1005.

Oliva, E., Young, R.H., Clement, P.B., Scully, R.E. (1999) Myxoid and fibrous endometrial stromal tumors of the uterus: a report of 10 cases. *Int. J. Gynecol. Pathol.* **18**, 310–19.

Ordi, J., Stamatakos, M.D., Tavassoli, F.A. (1997) Pure pleomorphic rhabdomyosarcomas of the uterus. *Int. J. Gynecol. Pathol.* **16**, 369–77.

Östör, A.C., Fortune, D.W. (1980) Benign and low grade variants of mixed Müllerian tumours of the uterus. *Histopathology* **4**, 369–82.

Östör, A.G., Rollason, T.P. (1995) Mixed tumours of the uterus. In Fox, H. (ed.), *Haines and Taylor's Textbook of Obstetrical and Gynaecological Pathology,* 4th Edn. Edinburgh: Churchill Livingstone, 587–621.

Podczaski, E., Sees, J., Kaminski, P. *et al.* (1990) Rhabdomyosarcoma of the uterus in a postmenopausal patient. *Gynecol. Oncol.* **37**, 429–42.

Rosty, C., Genestie, C., Blondon, J., Le Charpentier, Y. (1998) Endometrial stromal tumor associated with rhabdoid phenotype and zones of 'sex cord-like' differentiation. *Ann. Pathol.* **18**, 133–6.

Seltzer, V.L., Levine, A., Spiegel, G., Rosenfeld, D., Coffey, E.L. (1990) Adenofibroma of the uterus: multiple recurrences following wide local excision. *Gynecol. Oncol.* **37**, 427–31.

Seoud, M.A., Johnson, J., Weed, J.C. Jr (1993) Gynecologic tumors in tamoxifen-treated women with breast cancer. *Obstet. Gynecol.* **82**, 165–9.

Siegal, C.P., Taylor, L.L., Nelson, K.G., Reddick, R.L., Frazelle, M.M., Siegried, J.M., Walton, L.A., Kaufman, D.G. (1983) Characterisation of a pure heterologous sarcoma of the uterus: rhabdomyosarcoma of the corpus. *Int. J. Gynecol. Pathol.* **2**, 303–15.

Silverberg, S.G., Kurman, R.J. (1992) *Tumors of the Uterine Corpus and Gestational Trophoblastic Disease. Atlas of Tumor Pathology,* 3rd Series, Fasicle 3. Washington, DC: Armed Forces Institute of Pathology.

Silverberg, S.G., Major, F.J., Blessing, J.A. *et al.* (1990) Carcinosarcoma (malignant mixed mesodermal tumor) of the uterus: a Gynecologic Oncology Group pathologic study of 203 cases. *Int. J. Gynecol. Pathol.* **9**, 1–19.

Solder, E., Huter, O., Müller-Holzner, E., Brezinka, C. (1995) Adenofibrom und Adenosarkom des Uterus bei jungen Frauen. *Geburts. Frauenheilk.* **55**, 118–20.

Sreenan, J.J., Hart, W.R. (1995) Carcinosarcomas of the female genital tract: a pathologic study of 29 metastatic tumors: further evidence for the dominant role of the epithelial component and the conversion theory of histogenesis. *Am. J. Surg. Pathol.* **19**, 666–74.

Sternberg, W.R., Clark, W.H., Smith, R.C. (1954) Malignant mixed Müllerian tumor (mixed mesodermal tumor of the uterus): a study of twenty-one cases. *Cancer* **7**, 704–24.

Szukala, S.A., Marks, J.R., Burchette, J.L., Elbendary, A.A., Krigman, H.R. (1999) Co-expression of *p53* by epithelial and stromal elements in carcinosarcomas of the female genital tract: an immunohistochemical study of 19 cases. *Int. J. Gynecol. Cancer* **9**, 131–6.

Tavassoli, F.A., Norris, H.J. (1981) Mesenchymal tumors of the uterus. VII. A clinico-pathological study of 60 endometrial stromal nodules. *Histopathology* **5**, 1–10.

Thompson, M., Husemeyer, R. (1981) Carcinofibroma – a variant of the mixed Müllerian tumour: a case report. *Br. J. Obstet. Gynaecol.* **88**, 1151–5.

Toki, T., Shimizu, M., Takagi, Y., Ashida, T., Konishi, I. (2002) CD10 is a marker for normal and neoplastic endometrial stromal cells. *Int. J. Gynecol. Pathol.* **21**, 41–7.

Vakiani, M., Mawad, J., Talerman, A. (1982) Heterologous sarcomas of the uterus. *Int. J. Gynecol. Pathol.* **1**, 211–19.

Vellios, F., Ng, A.B.P., Reagan, J.W. (1973) Papillary adenofibroma of the uterus: a benign mesodermal mixed tumor of Müllerian origin. *Am. J. Clin. Pathol.* **60**, 543–51.

Verschraegen, C.F., Vasuratna, A., Edwards, C. *et al.* (1998) Clinicopathologic analysis of Müllerian adenosarcoma: the M.D. Anderson Cancer Center experience. *Oncol. Rep.* **5**, 439–44.

Wick, M.R., Swanson, P.E. (1993) Carcinosarcomas: current perspectives and an historical review of nosological concepts. *Semin. Diagn. Pathol.* **10**, 118–27.

Williamson, E.O., Christopherson, W.M. (1972) Malignant mixed Müllerian tumors of the uterus. *Cancer* **29**, 585–92.

Yoonessi, M., Hart, W.R. (1977) Endometrial stromal sarcomas. *Cancer* **40**, 898–906.

Zaino, R.J. (1996) *Interpretation of Endometrial Biopsies and Curettings*. Philadelphia: Lippincott-Raven.

Zaloudek, C.J., Norris, H.J. (1981) Adenofibroma and adenosarcoma of the uterus: a clinicopathologic study of 35 cases. *Cancer* **48**, 354–66.

12 Non-Müllerian endometrial neoplasms

All the neoplasms described in this chapter are rare or, at best, uncommon in a uterine site. However, any may be encountered in curettings and all can give rise to considerable diagnostic confusion, especially if the pathologist is unaware that these tumours can occur in the uterus.

12.1 VASCULAR TUMOURS

12.1.1 Haemangiopericytoma

Uterine haemangiopericytomas (Fig. 12.1) can develop at any age. A proportion form polypoid masses within the uterine cavity and tissue from these tumours, which often cause complaints of abnormal vaginal bleeding, may thus appear in curettings (Greene and Gerbie, 1954; Silverberg *et al.*, 1971; Sooriyaarachchi *et al.*, 1978; Buscema *et al.*, 1987).

The typical histological picture is of multiple vascular channels set amidst, and surrounded by, tightly packed cells that may be arranged in trabeculae, nests or sheets. Characteristically, the tumour cells in some areas are disposed concentrically around the vascular channels in an 'onion-skin' pattern. The tumour cells are rounded, polygonal or spindle-shaped and have round or ovoid nuclei, a moderate amount of cytoplasm and ill-defined margins. The vascular channels range in size from small vessels of capillary calibre to wide sinusoids and form a ramifying network within the neoplasm. Very typically, the dividing sinusoidal channels tend to have a 'staghorn' appearance. The vessels are lined by a single layer of endothelial cells, which is often markedly attenuated. A reticulin stain shows that the vessels within the neoplasm are supported by a well-defined basal lamina and that reticulin fibres enmesh individual tumour cells to give a basket-weave appearance.

About 25 per cent of uterine haemangiopericytomas behave in a malignant fashion but attempts to define those with a poor prognosis in terms of the degree of cytological atypia and

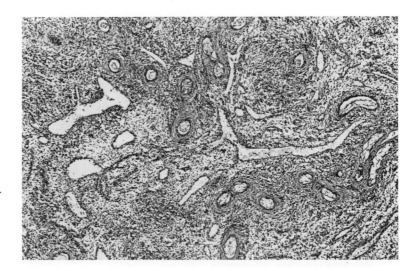

Figure 12.1 Haemangiopericytoma. The neoplasm has a cellular stroma in which can be identified the thin-walled, branching 'staghorn' vessels as well as thick-walled vessels. Haematoxylin and eosin.

pleomorphism, the presence of foci of necrosis and the number of mitotic figures have not proved successful for haemangiopericytomas at this site (Buscema *et al.*, 1987).

Uterine haemangiopericytomas resemble closely the pericytic type of endometrial stromal sarcoma of low-grade malignancy, to the extent that many workers have maintained that all apparent uterine haemangiopericytomas are in fact misdiagnosed endometrial stromal sarcomas (Kempson and Hendrickson, 1987). However, we accept uterine haemangiopericytomas as a distinct entity and maintain that they can be recognized, even in curettings, by their content of irregular sinusoidal vessels, particularly those showing a branching 'staghorn' pattern. The fact that stromal sarcomas stain positively for α-l-antitrypsin and α-antichymotrypsin (Chapter 11) may be of some value in discriminating between the two neoplasms, though it has to be admitted that information about the immunochemistry of haemangiopericytomas is scanty.

In some cases, no distinction can be drawn in biopsy material between a haemangiopericytoma and a low-grade endometrial sarcoma but since both tumours necessitate a hysterectomy, this diagnostic impasse is of no great practical importance.

12.1.2 Angiosarcoma

Uterine angiosarcomas are rare but aggressive neoplasms (Ongkasuwan *et al.*, 1982; Witkin *et al.*, 1987; Milne *et al.*, 1990; Quinonez *et al.*, 1991; Morrel *et al.*, 1993; Schammel and Tavassoli, 1998; Mendez *et al.*, 1999) that commonly form polypoid masses projecting into the uterine lumen. When encountered in curettings they may appear either as highly vascular neoplasms (Fig. 12.2) or as poorly differentiated tumours that may show papillary, solid or epithelioid patterns. If the tumour contains distinct vessels of irregular size and shape which communicate with each other to create an anastomosing vascular network the diagnostic problem becomes that of distinguishing an angiosarcoma from a haemangiopericytoma, endometrial stromal sarcoma or a highly vascular leiomyosarcoma. If the neoplasm is very poorly differentiated a quite different diagnostic problem is presented, namely its differentiation from a carcinoma, sarcoma or

197

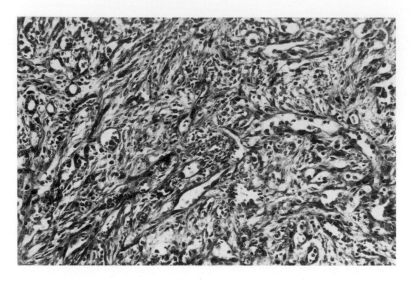

Figure 12.2 Angiosarcoma. The tumour consists of irregular, poorly developed, thin-walled vascular channels lined by large cells. Haematoxylin and eosin.

metastatic malignant melanoma. Recognition of a uterine angiosarcoma depends to a considerable extent upon an awareness that such neoplasms can occur at this site. Most doubts as to the nature of the neoplasm can be removed in some cases, but unfortunately not all, by showing positive staining of the tumour cells with either factor VIII or *Ulex europica*, it being preferable to use both stains. The neoplasms also stain positively for CD31 and CD34.

12.2   NEURAL TUMOURS

Both primitive neuroectodermal (Hendrickson and Scheithauer, 1986; Daya *et al.*, 1992; Molyneux *et al.*, 1992; Christensen *et al.*, 1994; Fraggetta *et al.*, 1997) and gliomatous neoplasms (Young *et al.*, 1981) of the endometrium may occur, their histogenesis being, to say the least, debatable. The primitive neuroectodermal tumours, which usually occur in elderly women, tend to show a predominantly neuroblastomatous, ependymal or medulloblastomatous pattern with focal glial or neuronal differentiation, while the only reported

gliomatous uterine tumour resembled a low-grade fibrillary astrocytoma (Fig. 12.3). Staining for glial fibrillary acidic protein, vimentin and neurone specific enolase has been generally positive in these exceedingly rare neoplasms.

Neoplastic glial tissue in an endometrial biopsy has to be differentiated from glial tissue that is present in the uterus as a fetal remnant. Fetal glial tissue commonly evokes a mild, local chronic inflammatory cell infiltrate and is often admixed with other fetal tissues, such as cartilage or bone, while a history of recent miscarriage, the presence of chorionic villi or decidual tissue and the bland nature of the glial tissue will all point to a diagnosis of fetal remnants. Immature neural tissue may, however, be simply one component of a uterine teratoma or, most exceptionally, can occur as a heterologous element in a carcinosarcoma. The finding in a biopsy of other mature tissue elements or of sarcomatous tissue will clearly be of value in establishing a correct diagnosis though, to confuse the issue further, cartilaginous differentiation has been described in one primitive neuroectodermal tumour. Neural tumours, uterine teratomas containing immature neural elements

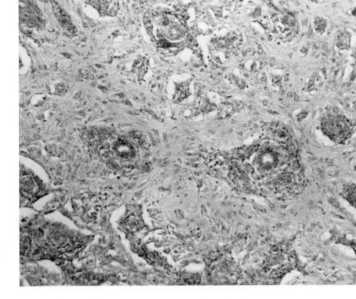

Figure 12.3 Glioma of the endometrium. The endometrial stroma is replaced by glial tissue, which envelops inactive endometrial glands. The specimen is from the uterus of a 15-year-old who presented with menorrhagia. Glial tissue formed a uterine mass and extensively infiltrated the myometrium. In these respects it differs from endometrial gliomatosis, which it resembles histologically (see Fig. 8.11). Photograph kindly supplied by Dr R.H. Younq, Boston.

and carcinosarcomas are all indications for hysterectomy and the pathologist should not therefore suffer severe anxiety about difficulties encountered in differentiating these conditions. Fetal remnants do not, however, necessitate hysterectomy and every effort has to be made to draw a distinction between a primary neural neoplasm and these residues of a previous pregnancy.

Paraganglioma can also occur, albeit with extreme rarity, in the endometrium (Young and Thrasher, 1982; Beham *et al.*, 1992). The appearances in a biopsy specimen are characteristic of such neoplasms, with tumour cells (containing abundant mildly eosinophilic cytoplasm and uniform vesicular nuclei) being arranged in nests that are limited by delicate fibrous septa containing prominent capillaries. In the only uterine paraganglioma that we have encountered (Fig. 12.4) the principal diagnostic difficulty was in distinguishing it from an epithelioid leiomyoma growing into the uterine cavity. As with many of the rare neoplasms discussed in this chapter, the

diagnosis is very dependent upon the pathologist being aware that tumours of this type can occur in the uterus. The definitive diagnosis of uterine paragangliomas may rest upon electron microscopic identification of their content of typical granules, this being one of the few instances in which electron microscopy of an endometrial biopsy is of value.

Endometrial tumours having the general characteristic of paragangliomas, but containing melanin granules, have also been described (Tavassoli, 1986); the true nature of these melanotic paragangliomas is uncertain.

12.3 TUMOURS OF FAT

Most, if not all, tumours reported as uterine lipomas are lipoleiomyomas with an unusually prominent lipomatous component (Dharkar *et al.*, 1981; Pounder, 1982; Krenning and De Goey, 1983). The majority of such neoplasms are purely intramyometrial but in occasional cases, the tumour protrudes into the uterine cavity and

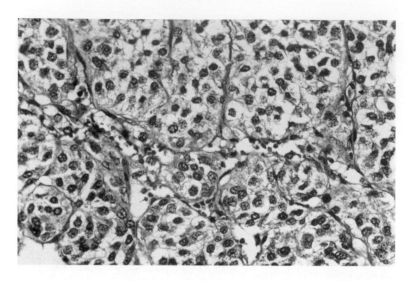

Figure 12.4 Non-chromaffin paraganglioma of the endometrium. The tumour forms the typical, clearly defined nests of polygonal or round cells with clear or rather granular cytoplasm and round to oval nuclei. Haematoxylin and eosin.

may thus be present in curettings. If, in a biopsy, mature fatty tissue is admixed with smooth muscle fibres, the diagnosis of a lipoleiomyoma will be fairly clear, but if purely fatty tissue is obtained, the pathologist must consider the possibility that the fat is of fetal origin or is a component of a uterine teratoma (Boateng *et al.*, 1985). A history of recent pregnancy, histological evidence of a gestation and the presence of other fetal tissues will all indicate a diagnosis of fetal remnants while fatty tissue from a teratoma will usually be admixed with other mature elements. Perhaps the most important point that the pathologist should bear in mind when encountering fat in curettings is the possibility that the curette has perforated the uterus and has obtained omental tissue.

12.4 MISCELLANEOUS SOFT TISSUE TUMOURS

Malignant fibrous histiocytomas (Chou *et al.*, 1985; Fujii *et al.*, 1987; Isaksen *et al.*, 1995; Salvaggi *et al.*, 1997), giant cell tumours (Kindblom and Seidal, 1981), malignant rhabdoid tumours (Cho *et al.*, 1989; Cattani *et al.*, 1992; Niemann *et al.*, 1994; Hsueh and Chang, 1996) and alveolar soft-part sarcomas (Gray *et al.*, 1986; Burch *et al.*, 1994; Radig *et al.*, 1998) have all been reported to occur in the uterus, with varying degrees of credibility. Biopsied tissue from such rare neoplasms may show diagnostically suggestive features, such as a storiform pattern, an alveolar arrangement of cells, typical rhabdoid cells with eccentric vesicular nuclei and prominent nucleoli together with cytoplasmic globular inclusions or the presence of osteoclast-like giant cells, but can also appear simply as a poorly differentiated sarcoma.

12.5 GERM CELL AND EMBRYONIC TUMOURS

There have been a number of reasonably convincing reports of uterine teratomas (Martin *et al.*, 1979; Ansah-Boateng *et al.*, 1985; Iwanaga *et al.*, 1993), usually of the mature cystic variety. Tissue in a biopsy from such a neoplasm must be distinguished from fetal remnants, from cartilaginous or osseous metaplasia of the endometrial stroma and from a mixed Müllerian neoplasm with heterologous components. Most uterine teratomas have been detected in women of reproductive age and hence the most difficult to eliminate of these diagnostic alternatives is that of fetal remnants (Ansah-Boateng *et al.*, 1985). The lack of a history of pregnancy, the absence of placental villi, decidua or hypersecretory endometrium together with the maturity of the teratomatous tissues and their haphazard relationship to each other will all suggest a teratoma rather than fetal remnants. Metaplastic cartilage or bone in the endometrial stroma can usually be seen to merge with stromal cells, while the absence of endometrial stromal sarcomatous tissue and of either benign or malignant Müllerian type glands will eliminate the possibility of a mixed Müllerian neoplasm with heterologous elements.

Yolk sac tumours do occur in the endometrium (Joseph *et al.*, 1990), though less commonly than in the vagina. They usually develop in children and can only be diagnosed in curettings if typical Schiller–Duval bodies are present.

Occasional Wilms' tumours (Bittencourt *et al.*, 1981; Comerci *et al.*, 1993; Benatar *et al.*, 1998) and a retinal anlage tumour (Schultz, 1957) of the uterus have been described; these neoplasms occurred in children or young adults and showed the typical appearances of such tumours as seen when encountered in more conventional sites.

12.6   BRENNER TUMOUR

A single, quite definite, example of a uterine Brenner tumour has been reported (Arhelger and Bogian, 1976). Any pathologist unfortunate enough to encounter a further example of a neoplasm of this type in a biopsy would have to take into account the cytological blandness of the neoplastic cells when attempting to distinguish the tumour from a metastasis from a transitional cell carcinoma of the bladder or malignant Brenner tumour of the ovary.

12.7   ADENOMATOID TUMOUR

The vast majority of uterine adenomatoid tumours, now generally accepted as being of mesothelial origin, lie within the myometrium but, very exceptionally, tissue from such a neoplasm can be found in curettings (Carlier *et al.*, 1986). In a biopsy, an adenomatoid tumour may appear as an infiltrating neoplasm and the presence of signet ring cells may well rouse a suspicion of metastatic adenocarcinoma. Adenomatoid tumours give positive reactions with Alcian blue and Hale's colloidal iron, this reactivity being abolished by hyaluronidase. The adenomatoid tumours generally stain positively for keratin but there have been conflicting reports concerning their staining reactions for carcinoembryonic antigen (CEA) and Factor VIII.

12.8   LYMPHOMA AND LEUKAEMIA

Infiltration of the endometrium by lymphomatous or leukaemic cells (Fig. 12.5) is not uncommon in women suffering from the advanced stages of these diseases. On rare occasions, however, lymphomas present initially as an endometrial lesion, some of these having been confined to, and apparently arisen primarily at, this site (Fox and More, 1965; Harris and Scully, 1984; Chorlton, 1987; Ferry and Young, 1991; Aozasa *et al.* 1993; Kawakami *et al.*, 1995; Latteri *et al.*, 1995; Meunier *et al.*, 1995; Cahill *et al.*, 1997). Lymphomas presenting as an

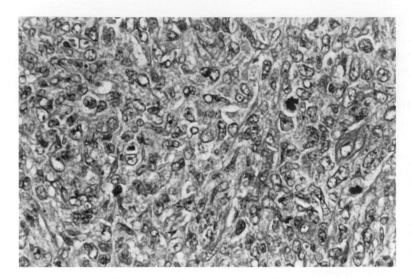

Figure 12.5 A non-Hodgkin's lymphomatous infiltrate in the uterus. The patient was a 58-year-old woman in whom severe menorrhagia necessitated hysterectomy. The uterus, Fallopian tubes and one ovary were found to be heavily infiltrated by neoplastic cells. Haematoxylin and eosin.

endometrial lesion are usually of the non-Hodgkin's B-cell type, though occasional instances of endometrial T-cell lymphoma (Masunaga *et al.* 1998) and of Hodgkin's disease (Hung and Kurtz, 1985) have been noted. Granulocytic sarcoma may also occur in the endometrium (Kapadia *et al.*, 1978; Huter *et al.*, 1996) while, very exceptionally, an endometrial lesion is the presenting feature of a chronic lymphatic leukaemia (Lucia *et al.*, 1952). Endometrial involvement in myelomatosis has also been described (Smith *et al.*, 1997).

Endometrial lymphomas usually present as polypoid masses which cause abnormal vaginal bleeding and from which tissue is readily obtained by curettage. The characteristic histological appearance is that of a morphologically malignant, rather monotonous infiltrate, usually diffuse but sometimes with a nodular pattern. Infrequently, the lymphomatous cells form cords and show an 'Indian file' pattern. Very typically, a lymphomatous infiltrate respects the normal endometrial structures, surrounding and infiltrating between, but not destroying, normal, endometrial glands.

Recognition of lymphomatous or leukaemic infiltration of the endometrium depends primarily upon a degree of awareness, by the pathologist, of such a possibility and the differential diagnosis includes a dense inflammatory infiltrate, a 'lymphoma-like lesion', stromal cell sarcoma, poorly differentiated carcinoma and metastatic carcinoma from an extragenital site. Carcinomas and sarcomas can often be distinguished from a lymphoma both in terms of their cytological features and their destructive, rather than infiltrative growth pattern but the distinction from a metastatic lobular carcinoma of the breast can be exceptionally difficult. Stains for mucin, may, however, help to resolve this diagnostic dilemma. Staining for vimentin, desmin, epithelial membrane antigen and common leucocyte antigen will usually resolve any diagnostic doubts about distinguishing a lymphoma from an epithelial or mesenchymal neoplasm but still leaves the pathologist with the problem of differentiating a lymphoma from a severe chronic endometritis and from a 'lymphoma-like lesion'. In most cases of endometritis with an unusually dense chronic inflammatory cell infiltrate there is often destruction of the glandular tissue, while the inflammatory nature of the infiltrate is usually revealed by the presence of ill-formed germinal centres, tingible body macrophages and by the recognition that the inflammatory cells show a polymorphic, rather than a monomorphic, pattern. Whether or not a severe endometritis differs fundamentally from the 'lymphoma-like lesions' described by Young *et al.* (1985) is perhaps a moot point but these reactive lymphoid lesions of the endometrium have a typical appearance characterized by a heterogeneous pattern of large lymphoid cells of various types admixed with plasma cells, mature lymphocytes, neutrophil polymorphonuclear cells and eosinophils. The large lymphoid cells contain numerous mitotic figures and although usually forming ill-defined focal aggregates may be diffusely distributed. The histological pattern of a lymphoma-like lesion does therefore differ significantly from that of a genuine lymphoma and this is fortunate as Young *et al.* (1985) found that immunoperoxidase stains were of little value in distinguishing between benign and malignant lymphoid infiltration of the endometrium.

It should be noted that the description of the gross and histological appearances of an endometrial lymphoma given above applies to high-grade B-cell lymphomas, which constitute nearly all reported instances of a lymphoma of the endometrium. van de Rijn *et al.* (1997) have, however, described three cases of apparently primary low-grade B-cell lymphoma of the endometrium. These were asymptomatic and did not form a lesion visible to the naked eye: histologically, the endometrium contained lymphoid nodules in which the nuclei were slightly enlarged and had an irregular contour. Recognition of the lymphomatous nature of these nodules rested upon showing (by immunohistochemistry) that they had a B-cell phenotype and by proving with polymerase chain reaction (PCR) that they were monoclonal. Recognition of a lesion of this nature and its distinction from a normal lymphoid aggregate in curettings would clearly be very difficult and would require a considerable degree of astute observation and diagnostic awareness.

12.9 METASTATIC TUMOUR

Uterine metastases from extragenital tumours are uncommon but pose a diagnostic trap for the unwary (Kaier and Holm-Jensen, 1972; Kumar and Hart, 1982; Kumar and Schneider, 1983; Bauer *et al.*, 1984). Although a majority of such metastases are confined to the myometrium approximately one-third involve the endometrium and will thus be apparent in endometrial curettings. The usual clinical presentation of a uterine metastasis is with abnormal vaginal bleeding or discharge and, while there is a history of previous removal of an extragenital tumour in three quarters of the patients, these symptoms represent the initial presentation of a primary extragenital neoplasm in 25 per cent of cases.

The primary tumours metastasizing most commonly to the uterus are, in descending order of frequency, carcinomas of the breast (particularly the lobular variety), colon, stomach and pancreas. Less commonly, metastases may arise from carcinomas of the kidney, bladder, gall bladder or thyroid whilst cutaneous malignant melanomas may also give rise to uterine metastases.

Metastatic tumours in endometrial curettings commonly present a characteristic and diagnostic appearance, with malignant cells infiltrating – singly, in cords or in clumps – normal endometrial stroma and surrounding normal endometrial glands. This appearance is

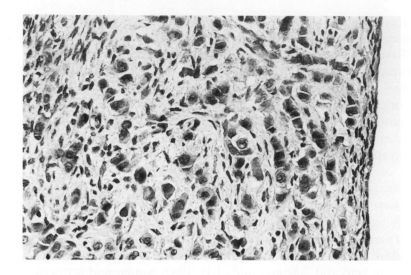

Figure 12.6 Lobular carcinoma of the breast metastatic to the endometrium. The neoplastic infiltrate is composed of small undifferentiated carcinoma cells with hyperchromatic nuclei and scanty cytoplasm arranged in Indian file. Haematoxylin and eosin.

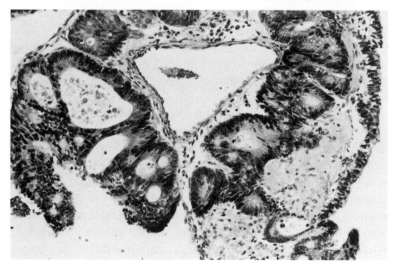

Figure 12.7 Colonic adenocarcinoma metastatic to the endometrium. The endometrium is infiltrated by a columnar cell, mucus-secreting adenocarcinoma. The patient, a 64-year-old woman, was known to have had a rectal carcinoma resected 9 months previously. She developed postmenopausal bleeding and curettage revealed fragments of carcinoma similar to that removed previously from the rectum. Haematoxylin and eosin.

seen particularly strikingly with metastatic lobular carcinoma of the breast (Fig. 12.6), which characteristically retains its 'Indian-file' pattern, and with metastatic signet ring cell carcinomas of the stomach or colon. The differential diagnosis in such cases is from an endometrial stromal sarcoma, a Müllerian adenosarcoma, and a malignant lymphoma. Distinction from an endometrial stromal sarcoma rests upon noting the absence of a rich

vascular background, the encompassing rather than the destruction, of endometrial glands, the cytological characteristics of the infiltrating cells (which bear little or no resemblance to those of a stromal sarcoma) and, in many cases, the presence of mucin. Differentiation of a metastatic neoplasm from a Müllerian adenosarcoma is dependent, again, on the cytological features, the usually atrophic nature of the encircled endometrial glands, the absence of a cambium layer and the presence of mucin. In the occasional difficult case, positive staining of the infiltrating cells for epithelial membrane antigens, keratins and, in the case of malignant melanoma, S-100 will usually resolve the diagnostic problem. The differential diagnosis from a lymphoma is discussed in Section 12.8.

Some metastases to the endometrium may not show this typical infiltrative pattern and can present as a neoplastic mass, which can be mistaken, in endometrial curettings, for a primary adenocarcinoma of the endometrium. This is particularly true for metastases from a colonic adenocarcinoma (Fig. 12.7), which can mimic a primary mucinous or signet-ring carcinoma of the endometrium, and from renal adenocarcinoma, which can closely resemble a clear cell carcinoma of the endometrium.

REFERENCES

Ansah-Boateng, Y.A., Wells, M., Poole, D.R. (1985) Co-existent immature teratoma of the uterus and endometrial carcinoma complicated by gliomatosis peritonei. *Gynaecol. Oncol.* **21**, 106–10.

Aozasa, K., Saeki, K., Ohsawa, M., Horiuchi, K., Mishima, K., Tajimoto, M. (1993) Malignant lymphoma of the uterus. *Cancer* **72**, 1958–64.

Arhelger, R.E., Bogian, J.J. (1976) Brenner tumor of the uterus. *Cancer* **38**, 1741–3.

Bauer, R.D., McCoy, C.P., Roberts, D.K., Fritz, G. (1984) Malignant melanoma metastatic to the endometrium. *Obstet. Gynecol.* **63**, 264–7.

Beham, A., Schmid, C., Fletcher, C.D., Aubock, L. and Pickel, H. (1992) Malignant paraganglioma of the uterus. *Virchows Arch. A – Pathol. Anat. Histopathol.* **420**, 453–7.

Benatar, B., Wright, C., Freinkel, A.L., Cooper, K. (1998) Primary extrarenal Wilms' tumor of the uterus presenting as a cervical polyp. *Int. J. Gynecol. Pathol.* **17**, 277–80.

Bittencourt, A.L., Britto, J.F., Fonseca, L.E. (1981) Wilm's tumor of the uterus: the first report in the literature. *Cancer* **47**, 2496–9.

Burch, D.J., Hitchcock, A., Masson, G.M. (1994) Alveolar soft part sarcoma of the uterus: case report and review of the literature. *Gynecol. Oncol.* **54**, 91–4.

Buscema, J., Klein, V., Rotmensch, J., Rosenhein, N., Woodruff, J.D. (1987) Uterine hemangiopericytoma. *Obstet. Gynecol.* **69**, 104–8.

Cahill, L.A., Stastny, J.F., Frable, W.J. (1997) Primary lymphoma of the uterus. A report of two cases diagnosed on cervicovaginal smears. *Acta Cytol.* **41**, 522–8.

Carlier, M.T., Dardick, I., Lagace, A.F., Steeram, V. (1986) Adenomatoid tumor of uterus: presentation in endometrial curettings. *Int. J. Gynecol. Pathol.* **5**, 69–74.

Cattani, M.G., Viale, G., Santini, D., Martinelli, G.N. (1992) Malignant rhabdoid tumor of the uterus: an immunohistochemical and ultrastructural study. *Virchows Archiv A Pathol. Anat.* **420**, 4590–62.

Cho, R.K., Rosenhein, N.B., Epstein, J.L (1989) Malignant rhabdoid tumor of the uterus. *Int. J. Gynecol. Pathol.* **8**, 381–7.

Chorlton, I. (1987) Malignant lymphoma of the female genital tract and ovaries. In Fox, H. (ed.), *Haines and Taylor: Obstetrical and Gynaecological Pathology*, 3rd edn. Edinburgh: Churchill Livingstone, 737–62.

Chou, S.T., Fortune, D., Beischer, N.A. *et al.* (1985) Primary malignant fibrous histiocytoma of the uterus – ultrastructural and immunocytochemical studies of two cases. *Pathology* **17**, 36–40.

Christensen, B., Schmidt, U., Schindler, A. (1994) Primitive neuroectodermal tumor of the uterus; a monophasic differentiated Müllerian tumor? *Zentralb. Gynäk.* **116**, 577–80.

Comerci, J.T., Denehey, T., Gregori, C.A., Breen, J.L. (1993) Wilms' tumor of the uterus: a case report. *J. Reprod. Med.* **38**, 829–32.

Daya, D., Lukka, H., Clement, P. (1992) Primitive neuroectodermal tumors of the uterus: a report of four cases. *Hum. Pathol.* **23**, 1120–9.

Dharkar, D.D., Kraft, J.R., Gangaoharem, D. (1981) Uterine lipomas. *Arch. Pathol. Lab. Med.* **105**, 43–5.

Ferry, J., Young, R.E. (1991) Malignant lymphoma, pseudolymphoma, and hematopoietic disorders of the female genital tract. *Pathol. Annu.* **26**, 227–63.

Fox, H., More, J.R.S. (1965) Primary malignant lymphoma of the uterus. *J. Clin. Pathol.* **18**, 724–8.

Fraggetta, F., Magro, G., Vasquez, E. (1997) Primitive neuroectodermal tumour of the uterus with focal cartilaginous differentiation. *Histopathology* **30**, 483–5.

Fujii, S., Kanzaki, H., Konishi, I., Yamabe, H., Okamura, H., Mori, T. (1987) Malignant fibrous histiocytoma of the uterus. *Gynecol. Oncol.* **26**, 319–30.

Gray, D.G., Glick, A.D., Kurtin, P.J., Jones, H.W. (1986) Alveolar soft part sarcoma of the uterus. *Hum. Pathol.* **17**, 297–300.

Greene, R.R., Gerbie, A.B. (1954) Hemangiopericytoma of the uterus. *Obstet. Gynecol.* **3**, 150–61.

Harris, N.L., Scully, R.E. (1984) Malignant lymphoma and granulocytic sarcoma of the uterus and vagina: a clinicopathologic analysis of 27 cases. *Cancer* **53**, 2530–45.

Hendrickson, M.R., Scheithauer, B.W. (1986) Primitive neuroectodermal tumor of the endometrium: report of two cases, one with electron microscopic observations. *Int. J. Gynecol. Pathol.* **5**, 249–59.

Hsueh, S., Chang, T.-C. (1996) Malignant rhabdoid tumor of the uterine corpus. *Gynecol. Oncol.* **61**, 142–6.

Hung, L.H., Kurtz, D.M. (1985) Hodgkin's disease of the endometrium. *Arch. Pathol. Lab. Med.* **109**, 762–4.

Huter, O., Brezinka, C., Nachbaur, D., Schwaighofer, H., Lang, A., Niederwieser, D. (1996) Successful treatment of primary extramedullary leukemia (EML) of the uterus with radical surgery, chemotherapy, autologous bone marrow transplantation (BMT) and prophylactic local irradiation. *Bone Marrow Transplant.* **18**, 663–4.

Isaksen, C.V., Lindboe, C.F., Hagen, B. (1995) Malignant fibrous histiocytoma of the uterus: some immuno-histochemical and ultrastructural observations. *Acta Obstet. Gynecol. Scand.* **74**, 224–6.

Iwanaga, S., Shimada, A., Hasuo, Y. *et al.* (1993) Immature teratoma of the uterine fundus. *Korume Med. J.* **40**, 153–8.

Joseph, M., Fellows, F., Hearn, S. (1990) Primary endo-dermal sinus tumor of the endometrium. *Cancer* **65**, 297–302.

Kaier, W., Holm-Jensen, S. (1972) Metastases to the uterus. *Acta Pathol. Microbiol. Scand.* **80**, 835–40.

Kapadia, S.B., Krause, J.R., Kanbour, A.I., Hartsock, R.J. (1978) Granulocytic sarcoma of the uterus. *Cancer* **41**, 687–91.

Kawakami, S., Togashi, K., Kojima, N., Morikawa, K., Mori, T., Konishi, J. (1995) MR appearance of malignant lymphoma of the uterus. *J. Comput. Assist. Tomogr.* **19**, 238–42.

Kempson, R.L., Hendrickson, M.R. (1987) Pure mesen-chymal tumours of the uterine corpus. In Fox, H. (ed.), *Haines and Taylor: Obstetrical and Gynaecological Pathology*, 3rd edn. Edinburgh: Churchill Livingstone, 411–56.

Kindblom, L.G., Seidal, T. (1981) Malignant giant cell tumour of the uterus. *Acta Path. Microbiol. Scand. Sect. A* **89**, 179–84.

Krenning, R.A., De Goey, W.B. (1983) Uterine lipomas: review of the literature. *Clin. Exp. Obstet. Gynecol.* **10**, 91–4.

Kumar, A., Schneider, V. (1983) Metastases to the uterus from extrapelvic primary tumors. *Int. J. Gynecol. Pathol.* **2**, 134–40.

Kumar, N.B., Hart, W.R. (1982) Metastases to the uterine corpus from extragenital cancers: a clinicopathologic study of 63 cases. *Cancer* **50**, 2163–9.

Latteri, M.A., Cipolla, C., Gebbia, V., Lampasona, G., Amato, C., Gebbia, N. (1995) Primary extranodal non-Hodgkin lymphomas of the uterus and breast: report of three cases. *Eur. J. Surg. Oncol.* **21**, 432–4.

Lucia, S.P., Mills, H., Lowenhaupt, E., Hunt, M.L. (1952) Visceral involvement in primary neoplastic diseases of the reticuloendothelial system. *Cancer* **5**, 1193–200.

Martin, E., Scholes, J., Richart, R.M., Fenoglio, C.M. (1979) Benign cystic teratoma of the uterus. *Am. J. Obstet. Gynecol.* **135**, 429–31.

Masunaga, A., Abe, M., Tsujii E. *et al.* (1998) Primary uterine T-cell lymphoma. *Int. J. Gynecol. Pathol.* **17**, 376–9.

Mendez, L.E., Joy, S., Angioli, R. *et al.* (1999) Primary uterine angiosarcoma. *Gynecol. Oncol.* **75**, 272–6.

Meunier, B., Leveque, J., Fliper, F. *et al.* (1995) Non-Hodgkin malignant lymphomas of the uterus: report of two cases and review of the literature. *J. Gynecol. Obstet. Biol. Reprod. Paris* **24**, 260–3.

Milne, D.S., Hinshaw, K., Malcolm, A.J., Hilton, P. (1990) Primary angiosarcoma of the uterus: a case report. *Histopathology* **16**, 203–5.

Molyneux, A.J., Deen, S., Sundaresan, V. (1992) Primitive neuroectodermal tumour of the uterus. *Histopathology* **21**, 584–5.

Morrel, B., Mulder, A.F., Chadha, S., Tjokrowardojo, A.J., Wijnen, J.A. (1993) Angiosarcoma of the uterus follow-ing radiotherapy for squamous cell carcinoma of the cervix. *Eur. J. Obstet. Gynecol. Reprod. Biol.* **49**, 193–7.

Niemann, T.H., Goetz, S.P., Benda, J.A., Cohen, M.B. (1994) Malignant rhabdoid tumor of the uterus: report of a case with findings in a cervical smear. *Diagn. Cytopathol.* **10**, 54–9.

Ongkasuwan, C., Taylor, J.E., Tang, C.K., Prempree, T. (1982) Angiosarcomas of the uterus and ovary. *Cancer* **49**, 1469–75.

Pounder, D.J. (1982) Fatty tumours of the uterus. *J. Clin. Pathol.* **35**, 1380–3.

Quinonez, G.E., Paraskevas, M.P., Diocee, M.S. and Lorimer, S.M. (1991) Angiosarcoma of the uterus: a case report. *Am. J. Obstet. Gynecol.* **164**, 90–2.

Radig, K., Buhtz, P., Roessner, A. (1998) Alveolar soft part sarcoma of the uterine corpus Report of two cases and review of the literature. *Pathol. Res. Pract.* **194**, 59–63.

van de Rijn, M., Kamel, O.W., Chang, P.P., Lee, A., Warnke, R.A., Salhany, K.E. (1997) Primary low-grade endometrial B-cell lymphoma. *Am. J. Surg. Pathol.* **21**, 187–94.

Salvaggi, L., Di-Vagno, G., Maorano, E. *et al.* (1997) Giant malignant fibrous histiocytoma of the uterus. *Arch Gynecol. Obstet.* **259**, 197–200.

Schammel, P., Tavassoli, F.A. (1998) Uterine angiosarcoma: a morphologic and immunohistochemical study of four cases. *Am. J. Surg. Pathol.* **22**, 2246–50.

Schultz, D.M. (1957) A malignant melanotic neoplasm of the uterus, resembling the 'retinal anlage' tumor. *Am. J. Clin. Pathol.* **28**, 524–33.

Silverberg, S.G., Wilson, M.A., Board, J.A. (1971) Hemangiopericytoma of the uterus: an ultrastructural study. *Am. J. Obstet. Gynecol.* **110**, 397–404.

Smith, N.L., Baird, D.B., Strausbauch, P.H. (1997) Endometrial involvement by multiple myeloma. *Int. J. Gynecol. Pathol.* **16**, 173–5.

Sooriyaarachchi, G.S., Ramirez, G., Roley, E.L. (1978) Hemangiopericytoma of the uterus: report of a case with a comprehensive review of the literature. *J. Surg. Oncol.* **10**, 399–408.

Tavassoli, F.A. (1986) Melanotic paraganglioma of the uterus. *Cancer* **58**, 942–8.

Witkin, G.B., Askin, F.B., Geratz, J.D., Reddick, R.L. (1987) Angiosarcoma of the uterus: a light microscopic, immunohistochemical and ultrastructural study. *Int. J. Gynecol. Pathol.* **6**, 176–84.

Young, R.H., Harris, N.L., Scully, R.E. (1985) Lymphoma-like lesions of the lower female genital tract: a report of 16 cases. *Int. J. Gynecol. Pathol.* **4**, 289–99.

Young, R.H., Klienman, G.M., Scully, R.E. (1981) Glioma of the uterus: report of a case with comments on histogenesis. *Am. J. Surg. Pathol.* **5**, 695–9.

Young, T.W., Thrasher, T.V. (1982) Non-chromaffin paraganglioma of the uterus: a case report. *Arch. Pathol. Lab. Med.* **106**, 608–9.

13 The endometrium in normal and abnormal pregnancy

A high proportion of curettings received in most pathology laboratories are from women who are, or have very recently been, pregnant and it is important therefore that the pathologist be conversant with the normal pattern of pregnancy-induced changes in the endometrium. Knowledge of the processes of implantation and placentation is also of value in interpreting those biopsies that include the implantation site (the placental site reaction).

It is recognized that the endometrium of a woman with a very early normal pregnancy is rarely deliberately sampled. Occasional biopsies will, however, be received from unsuspected early pregnancies, these, ironically, often having been taken for investigation of infertility. Usually, curettage during or immediately after pregnancy is, apart from therapeutic termination of pregnancy, undertaken because the gestation has not followed a normal course, being ectopically situated, ending prematurely in miscarriage or being attended by post-partum complications.

In some centres, post-partum placental bed biopsies will also be received. These are taken principally for an assessment of the adequacy and extent of conversion of spiral arteries into uteroplacental vessels and are of great value in the study of pregnancies complicated by pre-eclampsia or fetal intrauterine growth retardation. However, biopsies of this type lie outside the remit of this text and those wishing to pursue further this important topic are referred to several excellent reviews (Robertson *et al.*, 1986; Pijnenborg *et al.*, 1991).

13.1 PREGNANCY-INDUCED CHANGES IN THE ENDOMETRIUM

If conception occurs during the course of a normal menstrual cycle, the blastocyst will begin to implant in the endometrium at about the 9th post-ovulatory day, i.e. during the mid-secretory phase of the cycle. Secretion of

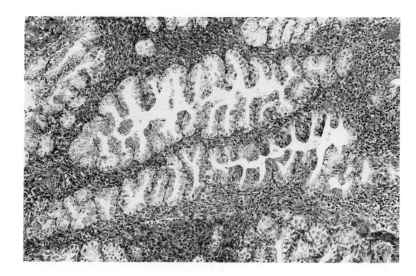

Figure 13.1 Hypersecretory endometrium of pregnancy. The glandular serrations are particularly prominent, almost forming papillae, and the glandular epithelium is secretory. Haematoxylin and eosin.

human chorionic gonadotrophin (hCG) from the blastocyst prevents decay of the corpus luteum and thus progesterone levels fail to decline and progesterone-induced changes in the endometrium persist. Hence, an endometrial biopsy taken between the 25th and 28th days of a cycle in which conception has occurred will show a well-marked predecidual change, together with considerable residual oedema in the stroma, well-developed spiral arterioles and continuing secretory activity in the endometrial glands (Mazur *et al.*, 1989). If implantation is successful, unabated secretory activity will continue in the endometrial glands and within a few weeks a hypersecretory pattern will emerge (Fig. 13.1), with the glandular epithelium becoming increasingly vacuolated and thrown into pseudopapillary folds. Towards the end of the first trimester, this hypersecretory pattern will begin to regress and the glands subsequently become inactive and involuted. In many but by no means all cases, a focal Arias-Stella change will be present within the endometrium of the gravid woman, this phenomenon usually not becoming apparent until after the fifth week of pregnancy. This is characterized

by excessively convoluted glands, the epithelial cells of which have abundant clear cytoplasm, extensively vacuolated by glycogen, and nuclei showing variable degrees of pleomorphism, hyperchromasia and atypia (Fig. 13.2). Irregular stratification and papillary tufting, or infolding, of the epithelial cells are characteristic features. Mitotic figures are present in a small proportion of Arias-Stella reactions and, rarely, these may have a tripolar form (Arias-Stella, 1994). An Arias-Stella change during pregnancy is thought to be due to the action of hCG and, possibly, progesterone on the endometrium and, as such, its presence simply indicates that trophoblastic tissue is present either in an intrauterine or ectopic site and either as a component of a normal pregnancy or as part of a hydatidiform mole or choriocarcinoma. It should be noted, however, that while an Arias-Stella reaction is highly suggestive of pregnancy it can also occasionally occur in non-gravid women, particularly those receiving exogenous progestagens or gonadotrophins (Huettner and Gersel, 1994). The focal nature of this hormonally induced change is a curious, currently unexplained, fact. There is a theoretical possibility

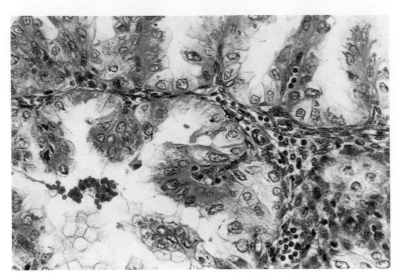

Figure 13.2 Arias-Stella change. The glandular epithelium exhibits hypersecretory features and the nuclei have lost their polarity. The epithelium forms small tufts which protrude into the glandular lumina. Note the absence of epithelial mitoses and the normal distribution of the nuclear chromatin. Haematoxylin and eosin.

that an Arias-Stella reaction in a curettage specimen could be confused with a clear cell adenocarcinoma: the age of the patient and the setting of the atypical glands in a decidualized stroma should serve to dispel this possibility.

Eleven examples of an unusual, and rare, endometrial glandular proliferation in early pregnancy, unrelated to the Arias-Stella reaction, have been described by Genest *et al.* (1995). This is a focal abnormality involving anything from 2 to 50 glands and is characterized by enlargement of the glands, retention of the normal smooth contour of the glands, mild to severe cellular stratification, architectural complexity ranging from the formation of accessory lumina to the development of an intraglandular cribriform pattern and intraglandular laminated calcifications. Mitotic figures are seen in this lesion but there is no nuclear atypia; the overall appearances resemble those seen in an intraductal hyperplasia of the breast. The authors felt it was probable that this unusual lesion is a benign self-limited glandular proliferation or metaplasia related to pregnancy but, as they comment, the natural history of this lesion is not yet fully understood

and careful follow up of the patients should be advised.

A further pregnancy-related change in the endometrial glands that can occur either in association with, or independently of, an Arias-Stella reaction is the development of optically clear nuclei (Mazur *et al.*, 1983). These are found in 7–10 per cent of first trimester pregnancies and persist to term. This nuclear change appears to result from an accumulation (for unknown reasons) of biotin (Yokoyama *et al.*, 1993; Sickel and di Sant'Agnese, 1994).

The predecidual stromal cells present towards the end of a cycle in which fertilization has occurred soon become converted into true decidual cells, increasing in size, with pale nuclei and prominent nucleoli, abundant cytoplasm and sharply defined borders. As the stromal oedema regresses, these cells form solid sheets that are progressively infiltrated by large granulated lymphocytes whose function is uncertain (Bulmer *et al.*, 1987).

Immunohistochemical changes in the endometrium thought to be characteristic of the pregnant state have been described. Thus, it has been claimed that S-100 is expressed in the endometrial glands during the first 12 weeks of gestation but in no other circumstances (Nakamura *et al.*, 1989; Agrawal and Singh, 1991) and that vimentin expression in the glands is inhibited during gestation (Norwitz *et al.*, 1991). The validity and specificity of these claims require further evaluation.

13.2 PLACENTATION AND THE DEVELOPMENT OF THE PLACENTAL SITE REACTION

Soon after implantation, probably between the 15th and 20th post-ovulatory days, the developing fetal placenta is separated from the decidua by the trophoblastic shell into which anchoring villi are inserted via their distal cytotrophoblastic cell columns. Extravillous cytotrophoblastic cells from the tips of the anchoring villi penetrate the trophoblastic shell and stream out to colonize the decidua and adjacent myometrium of the placental bed. These cells form the interstitial extravillous cytotrophoblastic cell population (also sometimes referred to as intermediate trophoblastic cells). The extent of the invasion of the placental bed by cytotrophoblastic cells has been seriously underestimated in the past and many of the cells that at first appear to be decidual are trophoblastic (Pijnenborg *et al.*, 1980). As pregnancy progresses many of the infiltrating interstitial cytotrophoblastic cells regress while those remaining tend increasingly to fuse and form multinucleated, syncytiotrophoblastic-like cells which are particularly aggregated at the junction of the endometrium and myometrium.

Extravillous cytotrophoblastic cells also stream into the lumens of the intradecidual portions of the spiral arteries of the placental bed where they often form intraluminal cellular plugs. These intravascular cytotrophoblastic cells destroy and replace the endothelial cells of the invaded vessels and then infiltrate the media, with resulting destruction of the medial elastic and muscular tissue (Brosens *et al.*, 1967). The arterial wall becomes replaced by fibrinoid material that is derived partly from fibrinogen in the maternal blood and partly from proteins secreted by the trophoblastic cells. At a later stage of gestation, between weeks 14 and 16, there is a resurgence of intravascular trophoblastic migration, with a second wave of cells moving down into the intramyometrial segments of the spiral arteries. Within the intramyometrial portion of these vessels, the same process that occurs in their intradecidual portion is repeated (i.e. replacement of the endothelium, invasion and destruction of the medial musculo-elastic tissue and fibrinoid change in the vessel wall). The end result of this trophoblastic invasion and attack upon the vessels of the placental bed is that the thick-walled muscular spiral arteries are converted into flaccid, sac-like uteroplacental vessels which can passively dilate in order to accommodate the greatly augmented blood flow through this vascular system, which is required as pregnancy progresses.

The practical aspect of this process of trophoblastic invasion of the placental bed and the vessels contained is the 'placental site reaction', which is often seen in biopsies from gravid uteri. In biopsies from first trimester pregnancies, the placental site reaction will be apparent as mononuclear and multinucleated trophoblastic cells infiltrating the decidua (Fig. 13.3) with trophoblastic cells within intradecidual spiral arteries (Fig. 13.4) both in their lumina and in their walls, the vessels invaded showing fibrinoid necrosis. In biopsies from term pregnancies, the placental site reaction is apparent mainly as multinucleated syncytiotrophoblastic-like cells within the placental bed; no trophoblastic cells will be apparent at this stage in the widely dilated uteroplacental vessels.

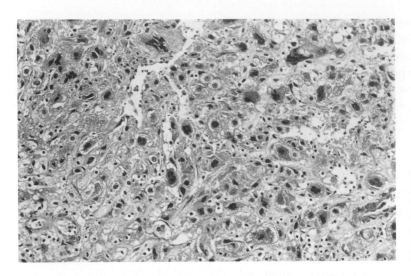

Figure 13.3 Placental site reaction in the first trimester. Interstitial cytotrophoblast cells are seen infiltrating the decidua. Some of the cells have become converted to syncytial placental bed giant cells. Haematoxylin and eosin.

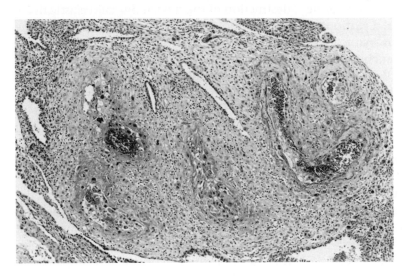

Figure 13.4 Placental bed in the first trimester. The decidual spiral arteries contain cytotrophoblast both in their lumens and in their walls. The vessels are dilated and fibrinoid material has been laid down in the walls. Haematoxylin and eosin.

The trophoblastic site reaction may be difficult in some cases to identify because the invading trophoblastic cells can closely resemble those of the decidua. The trophoblastic cells do, however, differ from decidual cells in giving a somewhat erratic positive staining reaction for human placental lactogen (hPL) and a consistently positive reaction for cytokeratins (Khong *et al.*, 1994).

Five points need to be stressed. Firstly, the placental site reaction is the morphological hallmark of successful placentation. It is a physiological process and the term 'syncytial endometritis', which is sometimes applied to the placental site reaction, is totally inappropriate. Secondly, a placental site reaction is the only absolute indicator of an intrauterine pregnancy for placental villi and fetal tissue within the uterus could be derived from an intrauterine rupture of a tubal pregnancy. Thirdly, the degree of prominence of the placental site reaction at term varies considerably; a very marked placental site reaction can be confused with a placental site trophoblastic tumour (the differentiation of these conditions is discussed in Chapter 14). Fourthly, the trophoblast of the placental site can become aggregated to form a placental site nodule (see Chapter 14) that can persist for many years after a pregnancy. Finally, the process of placentation results, for reasons that are far from clear, in focal necrosis of the decidua of the placental bed. This change is not seen in the decidua capsularis or in the decidua vera away from the placental bed. The necrotic areas are infiltrated by polymorphonuclear leucocytes and this change should be recognized in the placental bed as a physiological phenomenon and not classed as a 'deciduitis'.

13.3 ENDOMETRIAL BIOPSY IN ECTOPIC PREGNANCY

Endometrial biopsies are often received from women with an ectopic pregnancy, with curettage usually being performed for what is erroneously thought to be an incomplete miscarriage of an intrauterine gestation. Less commonly, the endometrium is biopsied as part of the investigation of a woman with pelvic pain or an adnexal mass while, rather rarely, confirmation is sought that the endometrial morphology is in accord with a clinical diagnosis of ectopic pregnancy.

The appearances of the endometrium from a woman with an ectopic pregnancy will depend upon whether the fetus or embryo is alive or dead and, if dead, the time interval that has elapsed between fetal demise and endometrial sampling. An ectopic pregnancy is, in all respects other than the site of nidation, a normal gestation (Randall *et al.*, 1987; Fox, 1997a); hCG is produced by the ectopic trophoblast and there is a normally functioning corpus luteum of pregnancy. If the ectopically sited fetus is still alive at the time of biopsy the endometrium will usually show the changes characteristic of the pregnant state with decidualization of the stroma and hypersecretory changes in the glands. Occasionally, however, the endometrium shows no pregnancy-related changes and a normal secretory or proliferative pattern is found (Ollendorf *et al.*, 1987). A focal Arias-Stella change is present in 60–70 per cent of cases (Bernhardt *et al.*, 1966) though, as already remarked, this change does not specifically indicate an extrauterine gestation. The decidualized endometrium from a woman with an ectopic pregnancy has a characteristically 'clean' appearance (Fig. 13.5) without any of the decidual necrosis and inflammatory cell infiltration that characterizes an intrauterine gestation (Robertson, 1981). No placental villi, extraplacental fetal membranes or fetal tissues will be seen and, even more importantly, no evidence will be found of a placental site reaction; there will be a complete absence of any trophoblastic infiltration of the decidua, no trophoblastic invasion of the spiral arteries and no evident transformation of spiral arteries into uteroplacental vessels.

Following death of an ectopically sited fetus, the entire uterine lining may be sloughed off as a decidual cast; this shows the typically 'clean' appearance noted above. More commonly, the decidua disintegrates and is irregularly shed. A biopsy taken at this stage shows a crumbling decidua with areas of haemorrhage, necrosis and inflammation. Appearances similar to these are often found after miscarriage of an intrauterine pregnancy and hence it is under these circumstances that an assiduous search for placental villi or a placental site

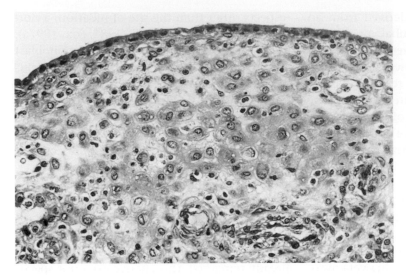

Figure 13.5 'Clean decidua' from a patient with an ectopic pregnancy. There is no placental site reaction in the uterus and the decidua, while exhibiting the features associated with pregnancy, is devoid of inflammation and necrosis. Spiral arteries in such cases become well-muscularized but show no evidence of transformation to uteroplacental vessels. Haematoxylin and eosin.

reaction is mandatory. If, as is not uncommonly the case, there are relatively few residual placental site cells, their detection may be made easier by the use of stains for hPL and cytokeratins (Kaspar *et al.*, 1991; Sorenson *et al.*, 1991). If there has been a prolonged interval between fetal death and endometrial biopsy the decidua may have been completely shed and replaced by a proliferative endometrium which, because the first two cycles after an ectopic pregnancy tend to be anovulatory, may show a picture of a prolonged proliferative phase or an early simple hyperplasia (Robertson, 1981).

Many potential pitfalls await those studying endometrial biopsies from possible cases of ectopic pregnancy and it is wise to avoid dogmatic statements. The appearance of an endometrial biopsy may be compatible with, and indeed highly suggestive of, an ectopic pregnancy but are never diagnostic of an extrauterine gestation. The finding of 'clean' decidua lacking a placental site reaction, together with an absence of placental villi and fetal parts, is suggestive of an ectopic pregnancy. However, an identical appearance can occasionally be seen in biopsies following miscarriage of an intrauterine gestation, particularly if the biopsy contains only tissue from the decidua capsularis or the decidua basalis away from the placental site. Conversely, an intrauterine pregnancy should not be diagnosed solely on the basis of finding decidual tissue showing focal necrosis and inflammation. To sustain a diagnosis of an intrauterine pregnancy it is necessary to identify placental tissue, fetal parts or a placental site reaction within the curetted tissue. Only a placental site reaction in an endometrial biopsy specimen is an absolute proof of an intrauterine gestation since, on rare occasions, a tubal pregnancy may rupture into the uterine cavity, with subsequent retrieval of placental tissue on curettage (Gruber *et al.*, 1997). Under these circumstances, a uterine placental implantation site will be absent and a report of this being present in association with an ectopic pregnancy will almost certainly represent a misidentification of a placental site nodule (Gruber *et al.*, 1997).

Finally, it must always be borne in mind that a woman may have concurrent intrauterine and ectopic gestations (heterotopic pregnancies). While such pregnancies are still rare, their incidence appears to be rising, probably because they occur with increased frequency following the use of ovulatory agents and assisted reproductive techniques (Glassner *et al.*, 1990; Goldman *et al.*, 1992; Svare *et al.*, 1993). Hence, histological proof of an intrauterine pregnancy in a woman who is thought, on clinical grounds, to have an ectopic gestation does not completely negate the clinical diagnosis.

13.4 ENDOMETRIAL BIOPSY IN SPONTANEOUS MISCARRIAGE

Approximately 15 per cent of established pregnancies spontaneously miscarry; curettage is commonly performed in such cases, usually because the miscarriage is thought to be incomplete with retention of 'products of conception'. Curettage under these circumstances is therefore primarily for therapeutic rather than diagnostic purposes but the material obtained is usually submitted for pathological examination, partly for confirmation that an intrauterine pregnancy has actually been present and partly to exclude any possibility of gestational trophoblastic disease.

The material received from a miscarriage can range from a complete fetus and placenta to a few fragments of necrotic decidual tissue. If a fetus is present, this should, with parental consent, be submitted for a 'mini-autopsy', the details of which are fully provided elsewhere (Berry, 1980). In the majority of cases, however, a recognizable fetus is not macroscopically evident and the curetted material consists of a mixture of blood clot, partly necrotic decidual tissue, fragments of pregnancy-type endometrium and first trimester-type placental villi.

Under these circumstances, there will be no difficulty in confirming that a gestation has been present. If placental villi are absent, which is not uncommon, a search should be made for a placental site reaction, identification of which provides unequivocal evidence of a recent intrauterine pregnancy. If neither placental villi nor a placental site reaction are detected, the pathologist will be unable to confirm a recent uterine gestation and should comment on the possibility of an ectopic pregnancy, this being particularly the case if hypersecretory endometrium is also present. The pathologist should never accept the presence of decidual tissue unaccompanied by trophoblast as confirmation of a pregnancy, since the changes in the stroma evoked by exogenous progestagens can mimic closely those of true decidua.

The pathologist should also be very cautious of making a diagnosis of a 'septic miscarriage'. As already remarked, patchy decidual necrosis, with an inflammatory cell infiltrate, is a physiological phenomenon and the degree of inflammation in a miscarriage may be further increased as a response to tissue breakdown and the presence of a dead fetus. The possibility of a septic miscarriage should therefore only be raised if there is a very marked inflammatory cell infiltrate, involving not only the decidua but also the hypersecretory glands and stroma of the endometrium well away from the placental site.

If trophoblastic tissue is present in curettage material received from a miscarriage, it is necessary to exclude gestational trophoblastic disease (Chapter 14). It is, in most cases, relatively easy to exclude a complete hydatidiform mole but difficulties can be encountered in making a distinction between a partial hydatidiform mole and a hydropic abortus (Howat *et al.*, 1993). The term 'hydropic abortion' is applied to the presence of swollen, avascular villi, which are rarely, if ever, sufficiently distended

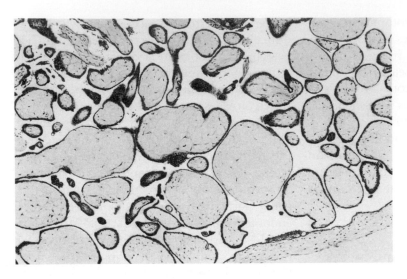

Figure 13.6 Hydropic change in placenta from a miscarriage. The villi are swollen and rounded while their trophoblastic mantle is attenuated. There are no fetal vessels. Haematoxylin and eosin.

to be macroscopically visible. These villi very rarely show central cavitation, have a smooth, rounded contour, are usually admixed with others of normal size (but often showing stromal fibrosis) and have a covering mantle of trophoblast that is commonly markedly attenuated (Fig. 13.6). The rounded villi of a hydropic abortus usually differ markedly from the irregularly shaped villi of a partial mole. However, it is often suggested that the differential diagnosis between a hydropic abortion and a partial hydatidiform mole rests upon the presence of trophoblastic hyperplasia in the latter, which is theoretically in marked contrast to the attenuation of the villous trophoblast in a hydropic abortion. In reality, there is often little or no trophoblastic hyperplasia in a partial mole and differential diagnosis rests upon the recognition of an abnormal pattern of villous trophoblastic growth in a partial mole: circumferential or multifocal trophoblastic growth is characteristically seen in partial moles, while in non-molar pregnancies trophoblastic growth is at one pole or along one side of a villus (Fox, 1997b).

Having confirmed the presence of a recent intrauterine gestation and having excluded trophoblastic disease, the pathologist may feel that no further diagnostic information can be derived from examination of curettings from spontaneous miscarriages and this is, indeed, largely true. There have, however, been many claims that it is possible to correlate villous histology in material from miscarriages either with specific chromosomal abnormalities or, less ambitiously, with an abnormal as opposed to a normal fetal karyotype. Prospective studies have, however, shown with considerable clarity that villous morphology is an insensitive and inaccurate indicator of fetal chromosomal abnormality (Fox, 1997c). Rushton (1988) has maintained that the appearance of the placental villi in material from miscarriages may be of some value in defining the cause of the failure of the pregnancy. In general terms the placental villi from miscarriages may be hydropic, may be non-hydropic but show changes that have occurred as a consequence of fetal death (i.e. stromal fibrosis and sclerosis of the fetal vessels; Fig. 13.7) or be well vascularized and

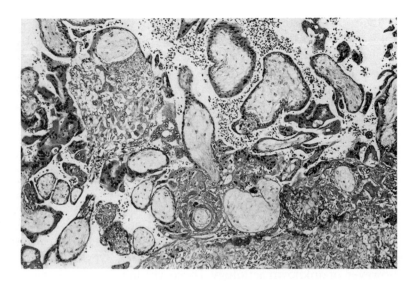

Figure 13.7 Spontaneous miscarriage. The stroma in many of the villi has undergone fibrosis secondary to fetal death. There is also sclerosis of many of the fetal vessels. Haematoxylin and eosin.

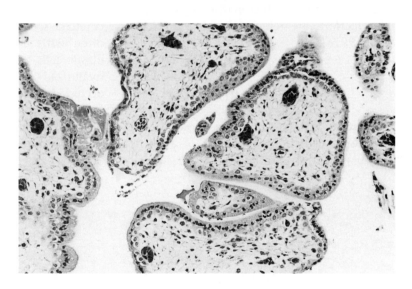

Figure 13.8 Normal first trimester placental villi. The villi contain a small number of fetal blood vessels in which red blood cells can be seen. Their stroma is immature and the covering trophoblast is composed of two clearly discernible layers, the inner cytotrophoblastic layer and the outer syncytial layer. Haematoxylin and eosin.

have a fully normal first trimester pattern (Fig. 13.8). Rushton argued that widespread hydropic change indicates that fetal demise occurred at an early stage of pregnancy, the most probable cause of this being a gross fetal malformation or a fetal chromosomal abnormality. If, in contrast, the placental villi are well vascularized and show a normal first trimester pattern it is probable that miscarriage occurred because of an abnormal fetal environment owing to factors such as uterine malformations or maternal immune disease. If the placental villi show only the post-mortem changes of stromal fibrosis and obliteration of the fetal vessels, then the pregnancy failure is more likely to be due to intrinsic fetal abnormality than to a fault in the fetal environment, though this is less certain than is the case with

217

a hydropic abortus. Rushton's reasoning is impeccable but prospective studies have not shown that application of his classification is of any value in distinguishing between sporadic and recurrent miscarriages and have failed to show any correlation with the outcome of subsequent pregnancies (Houwert-de-Jong *et al.*, 1990).

Finally, the pathologist should examine the placental tissue from a miscarriage for evidence of a villitis. Maternal infections, such as toxoplasmosis, rubella or listeriosis are a recognized, but rare, cause of miscarriage and infections such as these can produce specific and diagnostic changes in the villi. Most cases of villitis are, however, of unknown aetiology. Those wishing a full account of the histopathology of placental infections are referred to a recent review (Fox, 1997c).

13.5 POSTPARTUM BLEEDING

Postpartum bleeding is often thought to be commonly caused by retention of a portion of the placenta within the uterus. Curettage in such cases occasionally reveals a mixture of blood clot and fibrotic placental villi (the so-called 'placental polyp') (Fig. 13.9), but this is the exception rather than the rule. In some instances of postpartum bleeding, there may be evidence of low-grade uterine infection (Gibbs *et al.*, 1975) but in the vast majority of cases postpartum bleeding appears to result from inadequate or delayed involution of the placental bed (Robertson, 1981). The mechanism of uterine involution following pregnancy is not well understood but the major factors limiting blood loss from the placental site after delivery are spasm and thrombosis of the uteroplacental vessels; following thrombotic occlusion of these vessels, they collapse and undergo rapid involution. In cases of delayed involution, curettage specimens contain hyalinized decidua, often with a population of 'ghost' trophoblastic cells, in which are set distended, partly hyalinized vessels that are incompletely occluded by thrombus (Fig. 13.10) and occasionally contain residual endovascular trophoblast (Andrew *et al.*, 1989). Very often both fresh and old thrombi are seen in the vessels and the presence of these suggests that

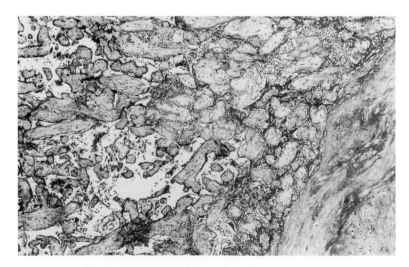

Figure 13.9 A fragment of retained third trimester placental tissue, a 'placental polyp' from a patient who complained of postpartum haemorrhage. Many of the villi are ghost-like and closely packed. Haematoxylin and eosin.

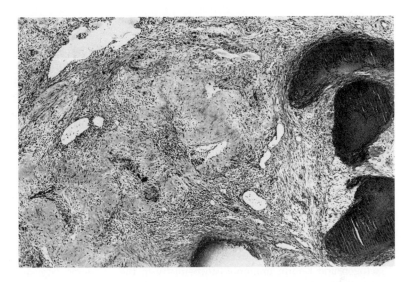

Figure 13.10 Subinvolution of the placental bed in a patient who had had a spontaneous miscarriage some weeks previously. The uteroplacental vessels to the left show the features of early involution with recanalization of their thrombosed lumina. The vessels to the right remain widely patent and their lumina contain fresh blood clot. Haematoxylin and eosin.

adequate thrombotic occlusion of the utero-placental vessels was not attained at delivery, leading to postpartum bleeding.

REFERENCES

Agrawal, N., Singh, U.R. (1992) Immunoreactivity with S-100 protein as an indicator of pregnancy. *Ind. J. Med. Res.* **96**, 24–6.

Andrew, A.C., Bulmer, J.N., Wells, M., Morrison, L., Buckley, C.H. (1989) Subinvolution of the uteroplacental arteries in the human placental bed. *Histopathology* **15**, 395–405.

Arias-Stella, J. (1994) Normal and abnormal mitoses in the atypical endometrial change associated with chorionic tissue effect. *Am. J. Surg. Pathol.* **18**, 694–701.

Bernhardt, R.N., Bruns, P.D., Druse, V.E. (1966) Atypical endometrium associated with ectopic pregnancies. *Obstet. Gynecol.* **28**, 849–53.

Berry, C.O. (1980) The examination of embryonic and fetal material in diagnostic histopathology laboratories. *J. Clin. Pathol.* **38**, 317–26.

Brosens, I., Robertson, W.B., Dixon, H.C. (1967) The physiological response of the vessels of the placental bed in normal pregnancy. *J. Pathol. Bacteriol.* **93**, 569–79.

Bulmer, J.N., Hollings, D., Ritson, A. (1987) Immuno-cytochemical evidence that endometrial stromal granulocytes are granulated lymphocytes. *J. Pathol.* **153**, 281–8.

Fox, H. (1997a) The pathology of ectopic pregnancy. In: Grudzinzkas, J.G., O'Brien, P.M.S. (eds), *Problems in Early Pregnancy: Advances in Diagnosis and Management.* London: RCOG Press, 77–96.

Fox, H. (1997b) Differential diagnosis of hydatidiform moles. *Gen. Diag. Pathol.* **143**, 109–17.

Fox, H. (1997c) *Pathology of the Placenta*, 2nd edn. London: W.B. Saunders.

Genest, D.R., Brodsky, G., Lage, J.A. (1995) Localized endometrial proliferations associated with pregnancy: clinical and histopathologic features of 11 cases. *Hum. Pathol.* **26**, 1233–40.

Gibbs, R.S., O'Dell, I.N., MacGregor, R.R., Schwarz, R.H., Morton, H. (1975) Puerperal endometritis: a prospective microbiologic study. *Am. J. Obstet. Gynecol.* **121**, 919–25.

Glassner, M.J., Aron, E., Eskin, B.A. (1990) Ovulation induction with clomiphene and the rise in heterotopic pregnancies: a report of two cases. *J. Reprod. Med.* **35**, 175–8.

Goldman, G.A., Fisch, B., Ovadia, J., Tadir, Y. (1992) Heterotopic pregnancy after assisted reproductive technologies. *Obstet. Gynecol. Surv.* **47**, 217–21.

Gruber, K., Gelven, P.L., Austin, R.M. (1997) Chorionic villi or trophoblastic tissue in uterine samples of four women with ectopic pregnancies. *Int. J. Gynecol. Pathol.* **16**, 28–32.

Huettner, P.C., Gersell, D.J. (1994) Arias-Stella reaction in nonpregnant women: a clinicopathologic study of nine cases. *Int. J. Gynecol. Pathol.* **13**, 241–7.

Houwert-de-Jong, M.H., Bruinse, H.W., Eskes, T.K.A.B. *et al.* (1990) Early recurrent miscarriage: histology of conception products. *Br. J. Obstet. Gynaecol.* **97**, 533–5.

Howat, A.J., Beck, S., Fox, H. *et al.* (1993) Can pathologists reliably diagnose molar pregnancy? *J. Clin. Pathol.* **46**, 599–602.

Kaspar, H.G., To, D., Dinh, T.V. (1991) Clinical use of immunoperoxidase markers in excluding ectopic gestation. *Obstet. Gynecol.* **78**, 433–7.

Khong, T.G., Stewart, C., Mott, C., Chambers, H., Staples, A. (1994) The usefulness of human placental lactogen and keratin immunohistochemistry in the assessment of tissue from purported intrauterine pregnancies. *Am. J. Clin. Pathol.* **102**, 72–5.

Mazur, M.T., Hendrickson, M.R., Kempson, R.L. (1983) Optically clear nuclei: an alteration of endometrial epithelium in the presence of trophoblast. *Am. J. Surg. Pathol.* **7**, 415–23.

Mazur, M.T., Duncan, D.A., Younger, J.B. (1989) Endometrial biopsy in the cycle of conception: histologic and lectin histochemical evaluation. *Fertil. Steril.* **51**, 764–7.

Nakamura, Y., Moritsuka, Y., Ohta, Y. *et al.* (1989) S-100 protein in glands within the decidua and cervical glands during early pregnancy. *Hum. Pathol.* **20**, 1204–9.

Norwitz, E.R., Fernandez-Shaw, S., Barlow, D.H., Starkey, P.M. (1991) Expression of intermediate filaments in endometrial glands with the onset of pregnancy and in endometriosis. *Hum. Reprod.* **6**, 1470–3.

Ollendorf, D.A., Feigin, M.D., Barzilai, M., Ben-Noon, I., Gerbie, A.B. (1987) The value of curettage in the diagnosis of ectopic pregnancy. *Am. J. Obstet. Gynecol.* **151**, 71–2.

Pijnenborg, R., Dixon, C., Robertson, W.B., Brosens, I. (1980) Trophoblastic invasion of human decidua from 8 to 18 weeks of pregnancy. *Placenta* **1**, 3–19.

Pijnenborg, R., Anthony, J., Davey, D.A. *et al.* (1991) Placental bed spiral arteries in hypertensive disorders of pregnancy. *Br. J. Obstet. Gynaecol.* **98**, 6648–55.

Randall, S., Buckley, C.H., Fox, H. (1987) Placentation in the Fallopian tube. *Int. J. Gynecol. Pathol.* **6**, 132–9.

Robertson, W.B. (1981) *The Endometrium.* London: Butterworths.

Robertson, W.B., Khong, T.Y., Brosens, I., DeWolf, F., Sheppard, B.L., Bonnar, J. (1986) Placental bed biopsy: a review from three European centres. *Am. J. Obstet. Gynecol.* **155**, 401–12.

Rushton, D.I. (1988) Placental pathology in spontaneous miscarriage. In: Beard, R.W., Sharpe, F. (eds), *Early Pregnancy Loss: Mechanisms and Treatment.* London: Springer-Verlag, 149–57.

Sickel, J.Z., di Sant'Agnese, P.A. (1994) Anomalous immunostaining of optically clear nuclei in gestational endometrium: a potential pitfall in the diagnosis of herpes virus infection. *Arch. Pathol. Lab. Med.* **118**, 831–3.

Sorensen, F.B., Marcussen, N., Daugaard, H.O., Kristiansen, J.D., Moller, J., Ingeslev, H.J. (1991) Immunohistochemical demonstration of intermediate trophoblast in the diagnosis of uterine versus ectopic pregnancy – a retrospective survey and results of a prospective trial. *Br. J. Obstet. Gynaecol.* **98**, 463–9.

Svare, J., Norrup, P., Grove-Thomsen, S. *et al.* (1993) Heterotopic pregnancies after *in-vitro* fertilization and embryo transfer – a Danish survey. *Hum. Reprod.* **8**, 116–18.

Yoyoyama, S., Kashima, K., Inoue, S., Daa, T., Kakayama, L., Moriuchi, A. (1993) Biotin-containing intranuclear inclusions in endometrial glands during gestation and puerperium. *Am. J. Clin. Pathol.* **99**, 13–17.

14 Gestational trophoblastic disease

The term 'gestational trophoblastic disease' encompasses hydatidiform moles, choriocarcinoma and placental site trophoblastic tumour, all of which are defined in strictly morphological terms (Table 14.1). A diagnosis of 'persistent trophoblastic disease' is made when plasma hCG levels remain elevated or increase after evacuation of a mole, and this term does not, therefore, indicate or presuppose any specific histopathological findings. Many patients with persistent trophoblastic disease are treated, empirically, but successfully, with chemotherapy without any attempt being made to establish a morphological diagnosis and, in this respect, the role of the pathologist in the management of trophoblastic disease has been much diminished. Some women with persistent trophoblastic disease are, however, subjected to curettage and interpretation of these biopsies is notoriously difficult. Other problems for the pathologist are the distinction between partial moles, complete moles and hydropic miscarriages, the diagnosis of choriocarcinoma in women presenting with vaginal bleeding and the distinction between an exaggerated placental site reaction and a placental site trophoblastic tumour. These problems are at their

Table 14.1 Histopathological classification of gestational trophoblastic disease

Hydatidiform mole
   Complete
   Partial
Invasive hydatidiform mole
Choriocarcinoma
   Placental site trophoblastic tumour
Trophoblastic lesions, miscellaneous
   Exaggerated placental site
   Placental site nodule
   Epithelioid trophoblastic tumour
   Unclassified trophoblastic lesion

most acute in curettage or suction material and it is largely because of this that trophoblastic disease is considered in this volume.

14.1 HYDATIDIFORM MOLE

Hydatidiform moles of all types are a form of abnormal pregnancy and not, as is often implied, neoplasms, as the ability of molar tissue to invade and to metastasize to extrauterine sites is shared by normal placental trophoblast. Within the last few decades, a distinction has been drawn between complete and partial hydatidiform moles. Both forms of mole can progress to an invasive mole or to persistent trophoblastic disease, and each can be followed by the development of a choriocarcinoma, although the risk of such complications is very much lower after partial moles than it is after complete moles (Bagshawe *et al.*, 1990; Rice *et al.*, 1990; Gardner and Lage, 1992).

14.1.1 Complete hydatidiform mole

Most complete moles are diploid and, of these, about 90 per cent have a 46XX chromosomal constitution, the remainder being 46XY (Fox, 1997). In all cases the genome is of wholly paternal (androgenetic) origin and in the vast majority of XX moles there appears to be fertilization of an 'empty' ovum by a single haploid sperm, which then duplicates without cytokinesis (Jacobs *et al.*, 1980): such moles are classed as monospermic or homozygous. All XY moles and a small proportion of XX moles appear to be the result of fertilization of an 'empty' ovum by two haploid sperms which then fuse and replicate (Surti *et al.*, 1982): these are classed as dispermic or heterozygous moles. Flow cytometry has shown that a proportion of complete moles are tetraploid (Fukunaga *et al.*, 1995) but the exact incidence of these is still uncertain and their pathogenesis is unknown.

In a complete hydatidiform mole there is generalized vesicular distension of the villi, the entire villous population being involved to a greater or lesser extent. The vesicular villi are usually evident to the naked eye in material retrieved by curettage but tend to be collapsed, and not grossly visible, in tissue obtained by suction. Histologically (Fig. 14.1), the distension of the villi, which is of variable degree,

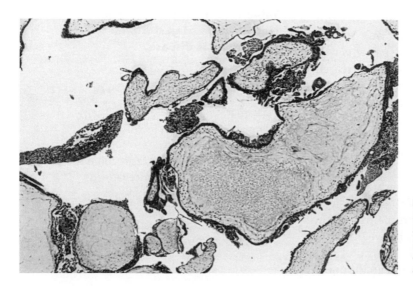

Figure 14.1 Complete hydatidiform mole. The villi are abnormally large, show an abnormal pattern of trophoblastic proliferation and lack fetal vessels. Haematoxylin and eosin.

is seen to be caused by an accumulation of fluid in the villous stroma and there is commonly central cavitation (cistern formation). It is usually maintained that fetal tissues are not found in association with a complete mole. Nevertheless, while villous stromal vessels are usually absent, attenuated vestiges of such vessels are apparent in a small minority of cases and in occasional complete moles there may be quite well-formed fetal vessels containing nucleated red blood cells; amniotic tissue may also occasionally be seen (Paradinas *et al.*, 1997). A characteristic feature is the presence of stromal nuclear debris (Paradinas, 1994; Paradinas *et al.*, 1996). All moles show, by definition, some degree of atypical trophoblastic proliferation, although this is not necessarily present in all the villi, some of which may have a flattened trophoblastic mantle. Most villi do, however, show trophoblastic proliferation, and this may be circumferential, focal or multifocal (Figs 14.2 and 14.3) and of slight, moderate or marked degree (Figs 14.4–14.6). It should be noted that similarly marked or even greater trophoblastic proliferation than that encountered in a mole may be seen not only in villi

from a normal first-trimester pregnancy but also in villi from cases of fetal trisomy (Redline *et al.*, 1998). In the normal placenta, however, proliferating trophoblast is always at one pole or along one side of the villus (Fig. 14.7) and never shows the focal or circumferential pattern characteristic of a mole. Variable nuclear atypia is invariably present in proliferating trophoblast, though this is commonly no more marked than the atypia often seen in normal first-trimester placentas. There are no morphological features that allow histological distinction to be made between diploid and tetraploid complete moles (Bewtra *et al.*, 1997).

This classical description of complete hydatidiform moles is based on cases that have been diagnosed clinically. With the increasing use of ultrasound, complete moles are, however, now being diagnosed at an earlier stage of gestation than previously (Jauniaux and Nicolaides, 1997; Mosher *et al.*, 1998). In these early lesions, vesicular villi are often not visible to the naked eye and histologically there may be coexisting vesicular and non-vesicular villi: those villi that are not vesicular are often branching (Fig. 14.8) and have a polypoid or

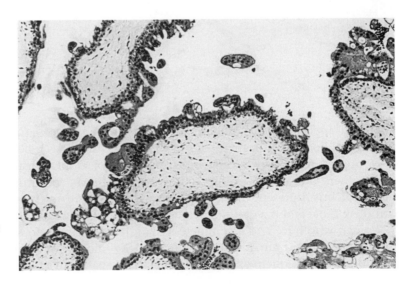

Figure 14.2 Complete hydatidiform mole. The central villus shows an abnormal pattern of trophoblastic proliferation. Haematoxylin and eosin.

223

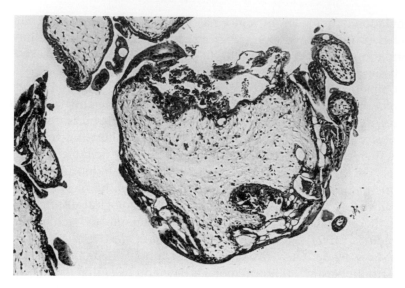

Figure 14.3 Complete hydatidiform mole. There is a circumferential pattern of trophoblastic proliferation. Haematoxylin and eosin.

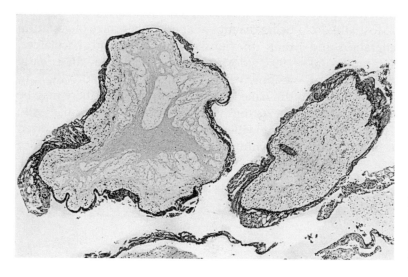

Figure 14.4 Complete hydatidiform mole showing only a minor degree of trophoblastic proliferation. Haematoxylin and eosin.

lobulated appearance (Paradinas, 1994). Fetal vessels will be present in many of the villi and these are set in a somewhat mucoid stroma in which there are a few spindly cells: stromal nuclear debris is present in the villi of an early complete mole and is a defining feature.

Women who have had a complete hydatidiform mole have a small but definite risk of developing a subsequent choriocarcinoma, and it has been suggested that the magnitude of this risk can be estimated by grading the degree of trophoblastic proliferation, the possibility of an eventual choriocarcinoma increasing progressively with the degree of trophoblastic proliferation and atypia (Hertig and Sheldon, 1947). We do not grade complete hydatidiform moles and indeed would actively dissuade pathologists from attempting to grade these

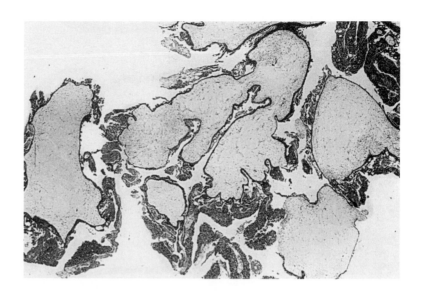

Figure 14.5 Complete hydatidiform mole showing a moderate degree of trophoblastic proliferation. Haematoxylin and eosin.

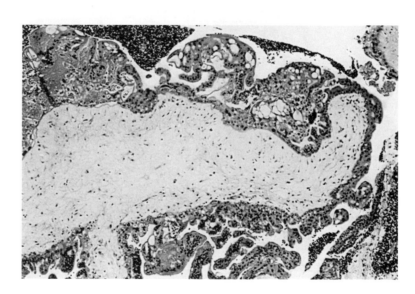

Figure 14.6 Complete hydatidiform mole showing a marked degree of trophoblastic proliferation. Haematoxylin and eosin.

lesions. We take this attitude for the following reasons:

1. More recent studies have shown that the degree of trophoblastic proliferation is of little or no prognostic value (Genest *et al.*, 1991);
2. The practice of prognostic grading may lead to the unjustified use of prophylactic chemotherapy in some patients and to unwarranted neglect of others;
3. Grading has become obsolete since the introduction of radioimmunoassay for hCG; it is mandatory that all patients who have had a complete mole be followed up by serial hCG estimations, irrespective of the histological findings in the mole.

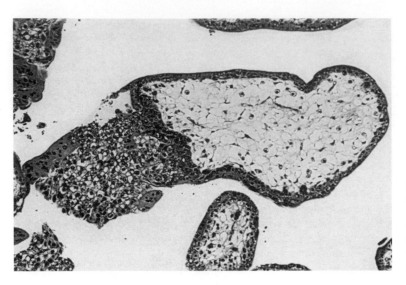

Figure 14.7 A normal first-trimester placental villus showing the typical polar trophoblastic growth, which is quite distinct from the circumferential or multifocal trophoblastic proliferation of a molar pregnancy. Haematoxylin and eosin.

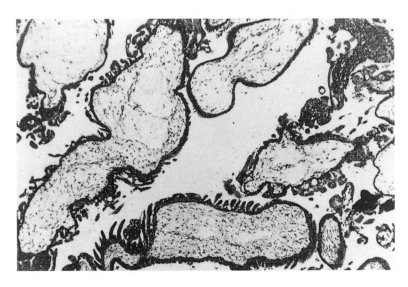

Figure 14.8 A polypoid villus from a very early complete hydatidiform mole. Haematoxylin and eosin. Courtesy of Professor F.J. Paradinas.

14.1.2 Partial hydatidiform mole

This term is applied to a mole in which only a small proportion of the villi show vesicular change associated with trophoblastic proliferation. The vast majority of partial hydatidiform moles have a triploid karyotype, usually 69XXY but occasionally 69XXX or 69XYY (Lawler *et al.,* 1982); very occasional partial moles have been associated with a trisomy or a 46XX karyotype (Elston, 1995). Not all placentas from fetal triploidies take the form of a partial mole and it is now clear that, if the additional chromosomal load is of paternal origin, a partial mole will result, while if the extra chromosomal material is derived from the mother, the gestation will be non-molar (Jacobs *et al.,* 1982; Jauniaux, 1999).

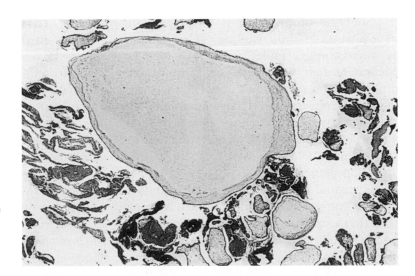

Figure 14.9 A partial hydatidiform mole. The field shows the typical mixture of small villi of normal configuration and a large vesicular villus. Haematoxylin and eosin.

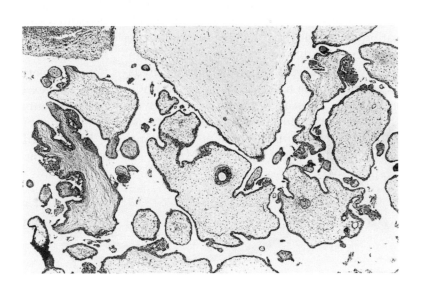

Figure 14.10 A partial hydatidiform mole showing the 'fjord-like' irregular contour of the villi. Haematoxylin and eosin.

A fetus is commonly present in a partial hydatidiform mole, and hence fetal tissue may be seen in curetted material. Histologically, villi showing vesicular change are scattered amidst a villous population of normal size (Fig. 14.9). Fetal vessels, not infrequently containing erythrocytes, are often seen both in the villi of normal calibre and in the distended villi. The vesicular villi are rarely as large as are those seen in a complete mole, frequently show central cistern formation and, very characteristically, have an irregular, deeply indented outline (the Norwegian fjord or coast of Ireland appearance) (Fig. 14.10). Cross-sectional cutting of these deep indentations results in the presence of 'trophoblastic inclusions' within the villous stroma, which can be round and cystic or solid. A degree of abnormal

227

trophoblastic proliferation is always present in at least some of the vesicular villi, which is, as with complete moles, focal, multifocal or circumferential: the degree of trophoblastic proliferation is usually not only less than that seen in complete moles but sometimes less than that encountered in normal first-trimester placentas (Fig. 14.11). The proliferating trophoblast frequently has a somewhat vacuolated or 'lacy' appearance.

The natural history of partial hydatidiform moles is still not fully defined, though it is now clear that a small proportion can progress to an invasive mole and to persistent trophoblastic disease (Goto *et al.*, 1993). Choriocarcinoma has been reported as following a partial mole (Bagshawe *et al.*, 1990; Gardner and Lage, 1992) but it is not known if the risk of such a complication is any higher than is that following a normal pregnancy. It is currently recommended that all patients with a partial hydatidiform mole be followed up by serial β-hCG estimations in exactly the same way as are those who have had a complete mole, although with a much shorter period of surveillance after normalization of the β-hCG levels.

14.1.3 Differential diagnosis of molar pregnancy

Because all women with molar disease are subjected to follow-up, the distinction in biopsy material between partial and complete moles is a useful but not a vital one to make. In practice, it is relatively easy to distinguish between a classical complete mole and a partial mole on morphological grounds alone. However, difficulties do arise when an early complete mole is encountered since, under these circumstances, neither the finding of villous fetal vessels nor an admixture of vesicular and non-vesicular villi is of any distinguishing value: greater stress has to be placed on the lobulated or polypoid appearance of the villi and the presence of stromal nuclear debris in complete moles (Paradinas, 1994). If it is felt that a precise diagnosis is required in truly doubtful cases of molar disease, this can usually be achieved with flow cytometry as the complete moles have, with rare exceptions, a diploid or tetraploid DNA content and the partial moles a triploid DNA content (Lage and Bagg, 1996).

The distinction between a hydatidiform mole and a hydropic miscarriage is one of considerable

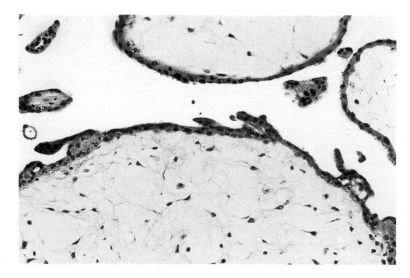

Figure 14.11 A partial hydatidiform mole showing the minimal trophoblastic proliferation seen in many such pregnancies. Haematoxylin and eosin.

practical importance, for on this rests the decision as to whether a woman requires surveillance or not. It is usually quite easy to distinguish between a complete mole and a hydropic miscarriage, though this is not invariably the case (Conran *et al.*, 1993), but serious difficulties may be encountered in making a distinction between a partial mole and a hydropic miscarriage. The criterion for making this distinction is the contrast between the highly irregular vesicular villi with central cistern formation and focal trophoblastic hyperplasia seen in the partial mole and the rounded villi, lacking cisternal change and showing no abnormal trophoblastic proliferation, in a hydropic miscarriage. It has to be admitted, however, that while on paper it appears relatively easy to distinguish a partial mole from a hydropic miscarriage, there are in practice very considerable inter-observer differences in making this differential diagnosis (Howat *et al.*, 1993). Flow cytometry is of some help but it must be borne in mind that some non-molar hydropic miscarriages also have a triploid DNA content (Lage *et al.*, 1992).

An uncommon, but difficult, diagnostic problem may occur if curettage material is received from a twin pregnancy in which one twin has a normal placenta and the other is a complete hydatidiform mole, the difficulty being that the admixture of vesicular and non-vesicular villi may suggest a diagnosis of a partial mole. Under such circumstances it may be possible to discern that the vesicular villi have the features of a complete rather than a partial mole but an absolute diagnosis depends upon showing that all the villi are diploid and that, while some are biparental, others are androgenetic (van de Kaa *et al.*, 1995).

14.1.4 Invasive hydatidiform mole
An invasive mole is one in which vesicular villi invade the myometrium or its blood vessels. By implication, this term also applies to cases of extrauterine molar 'metastasis'.

Except under unusual circumstances, when curetted tissue contains fragments of myometrium invaded by molar villi, an invasive mole cannot be diagnosed in biopsy material. The mere presence in curettings of residual molar villi after evacuation of a mole does not justify a diagnosis of invasive mole; under these circumstances, a comment should be made that the findings are compatible with persistent trophoblastic disease.

14.2 CHORIOCARCINOMA

A choriocarcinoma may occur after a normal pregnancy, a spontaneous miscarriage or a hydatidiform mole, with 50 per cent of cases being preceded by a molar gestation. Classically, nodules of choriocarcinoma show extensive central necrosis with only a thin peripheral rim of viable tumour tissue – a feature reflecting the lack of an intrinsic tumour vasculature and one that results in curettage specimens from cases of choriocarcinoma often containing only necrotic tissue. Viable tumour has a characteristically bilaminar structure that recapitulates the appearance of the trophoblast of the implanting blastocyst (Fig. 14.12), the central cores of cytotrophoblastic cells being covered by rims or caps of syncytiotrophoblast. Atypia and mitotic activity are seen but are often no more marked than is the case in the trophoblast of a normal blastocyst. Appearances such as these are rarely, if ever, seen in curettage material and the biopsy diagnosis of a choriocarcinoma presents considerable practical difficulties. Curettage to confirm a possible diagnosis of choriocarcinoma is usually undertaken when vaginal bleeding occurs following either a non-molar or a molar gestation and is still sometimes performed in patients

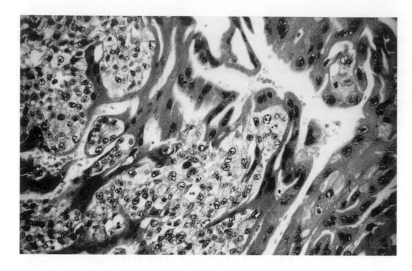

Figure 14.12 A choriocarcinoma showing the typical biphasic pattern of solid cores of cytotrophoblastic cells capped by a rim of syncytiotrophoblast. Haematoxylin and eosin.

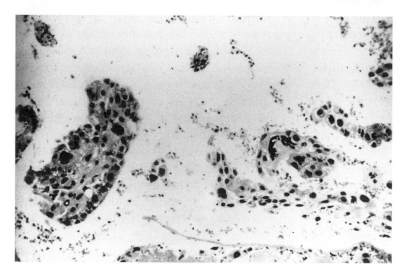

Figure 14.13 'Simple' trophoblast in curettings obtained because of persistent bleeding after evacuation of a hydatidiform mole. There is no clear differentiation into cytotrophoblast and syncytiotrophoblast. Haematoxylin and eosin.

with persistent trophoblastic disease. A logical approach to the interpretation of the findings in such curettings has been proposed by Elston (1987). If the curettings contain trophoblastic tissue, this can be divided into three categories: (1) villous trophoblast, (2) simple or suspicious non-villous trophoblast or (3) non-villous trophoblast diagnostic of choriocarcinoma.

The term 'villous trophoblast' indicates that placental villi, either of normal or molar type,

are present in the curettings. The term 'simple non-villous trophoblast' refers to small fragments of pyknotic trophoblastic cells with no clear distinction into cytotrophoblast and syncytiotrophoblast (Fig. 14.13), while 'suspicious non-villous trophoblast' indicates the presence of trophoblastic tissue showing a bilaminar arrangement of cytotrophoblast and syncytiotrophoblast but without evidence of tissue invasion (Fig. 14.14). The expression 'non-villous

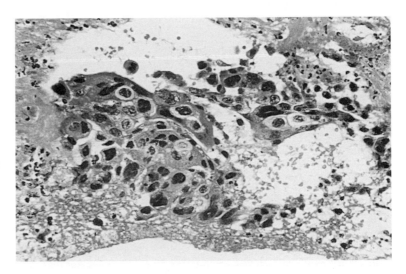

Figure 14.14 'Suspicious' trophoblast seen in curettings from a woman who continued to bleed after evacuation of a hydatidiform mole. There is a biphasic pattern of cytotrophoblast and syncytiotrophoblast but no evidence is seen of tissue invasion. Haematoxylin and eosin.

trophoblast diagnostic of choriocarcinoma' is used only when the curettings contain myometrial fragments that are being invaded by bilaminar trophoblast.

Interpretation of the significance of these findings depends upon knowledge of the nature of the antecedent pregnancy. If the preceding pregnancy was a molar gestation, then the finding of villous trophoblast, simple non-villous trophoblast or suspicious non-villous trophoblast indicates a diagnosis of persistent trophoblastic disease and the patient will require continuing follow-up. If the previous gestation was a normal pregnancy or a spontaneous miscarriage, then the presence of villous trophoblast indicates retained products of conception. In contrast, the finding of non-villous trophoblast of either simple or suspicious type after a non-molar pregnancy is an almost certain indication of choriocarcinoma and immediate full investigation should be instigated.

Two points must be stressed: a diagnosis of choriocarcinoma should never be made if villi are present in curettings and a pathologist cannot evaluate the significance of non-villous trophoblast in curettings without an adequate history that details the nature of the previous pregnancy.

14.3 PLACENTAL SITE TROPHOBLASTIC TUMOUR

Most neoplasms of this type follow a normal term pregnancy and, while the clinical picture is very variable, about 50 per cent of patients present with amenorrhoea or irregular bleeding (Elston, 1995; How *et al.*, 1995). This tumour is derived from the interstitial extravillous cytotrophoblastic cells of the placental bed; the lesion was originally regarded as an exaggerated placental site reaction or as a pseudotumour but is now recognized to be neoplastic (Young and Scully, 1984). A placental site trophoblastic tumour forms a mass involving the endometrium and myometrium and is composed predominantly of mononuclear, polygonal cytotrophoblastic-like cells that infiltrate between and dissect the myometrial fibres (Fig. 14.15) as cords or sheets; spindling of cells is sometimes seen. Coagulative necrosis and haemorrhage are often present

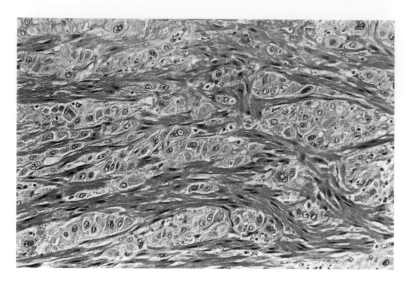

Figure 14.15 A placental site trophoblastic tumour. The neoplastic cells resemble extravillous cytotrophoblast and are infiltrating between myometrial muscle fibres: there is a notable lack of haemorrhage and necrosis. Haematoxylin and eosin.

but are sometimes notably absent. Although the classical bimorphic pattern of a choriocarcinoma is not seen, a number of irregularly distributed multinucleate cells are usually present. The cytotrophoblastic-like cells that predominate in these neoplasms tend to stain positively for human placental lactogen (hPL) rather than hCG (Kurman *et al.*, 1984). These tumours also stain positively for the melanoma cell adhesion molecule Mel-CAM (Shih and Kurman, 1998a). Fibrinoid necrosis of vessel walls and deposition of fibrinoid material around tumour cells is very commonly present, while tumour cells are present within the blood vessels in most, but not all, cases; entrapped vessels often show fibrinoid necrosis. The endometrium adjacent to the neoplastic cells may have a pseudodecidual appearance. Most placental site trophoblastic tumours appear to be benign but between 10 and 15 per cent behave in a malignant fashion (Young *et al.*, 1988).

The diagnosis of a placental site trophoblastic tumour in curettings is far from easy (Baergen and Rutgers, 1997), the major difficulty being in attempting to distinguish between a neoplasm of this type and an exaggerated, but non-neoplastic, placental site reaction. One of the most useful criteria in making this differential diagnosis is the clinical history, since the greater the time interval between the previous pregnancy and curettings, the more likely is it that infiltrating cytotrophoblastic cells are neoplastic in nature. Findings suggestive of an exaggerated placental site reaction include the presence of true decidua and placental villi, the presence of a relatively large number of multinucleated trophoblastic cells and an absence of mitotic figures. In contrast, features indicating a diagnosis of placental site trophoblastic tumour are the presence of sheets or confluent masses of cytotrophoblastic cells, a paucity of multinucleated cells and the presence of mitotic figures. The higher Ki-67 index of a placental site tumour may also help in differentiation from an exaggerated placental site reaction (Shih and Kurman, 1998a).

The distinction between a placental site tumour and a choriocarcinoma in curettings can also prove difficult, but a preponderance of cytotrophoblast, a relative or absolute absence of syncytiotrophoblast, a haphazard juxtaposition of cytotrophoblast and any multi-nucleated cells that may be present all point to a diagnosis of placental site trophoblastic tumour. In equivocal cases staining for hPL and hCG may help to resolve the dilemma, as the true choriocarcinoma shows extensive positive staining for hCG and the placental site tumour tends to stain predominantly for hPL and only focally for hCG. A positive staining for Mel-CAM also characterizes a placental site tropho-blastic tumour, since choriocarcinomas stain negatively for this marker (Shih and Kurman, 1998a).

Occasionally, a placental site tumour in curettage material may be confused with a poorly differentiated endometrial adenocarci-noma, a squamous cell carcinoma of the cervix, a clear cell carcinoma or an epithelioid leiomyo-sarcoma. The positive staining of a placental site tumour for cytokeratins, inhibin-α, hPL and hCG, together with the negative staining for vimentin and actin will almost invariably resolve such diagnostic difficulties.

Assessment of the degree of malignancy of a placental site trophoblastic tumour is difficult, largely because criteria for distinguishing benign from malignant placental site tropho-blastic tumours have not yet been firmly established. It has been claimed that tumours with a mitotic count of less than two per 10 high-power fields behave in a benign fashion (Young and Scully, 1984) but occasional neoplasms with this count have pursued a highly malig-nant course (Eckstein et al., 1982; Fukunaga and Ushigome, 1993; Chang et al., 1999). There is little doubt that a placental site tro-phoblastic tumour with a high mitotic count should be considered as being at least poten-tially malignant but a false sense of security should not be engendered by a low mitotic count. Whether or not the degree of atypia in the neoplasm is of prognostic importance is currently undecided.

14.4 PLACENTAL SITE NODULE

These are trophoblast-containing nodules that are retained within the uterus after the termination of a pregnancy and may be single or multiple (Young et al., 1988, 1990; Huettner and Gersell, 1994; Baergen and Rutgers, 1997). It was thought that the pla-cental site nodule is derived from the tropho-blast of the placental bed but Shih et al. (1999) have suggested that the trophoblastic cells in the nodules resemble those of the chorion laeve. Placental site nodules are asympto-matic but are detected as an incidental find-ing, months or years after a pregnancy, either in a hysterectomy specimen or in biopsy material. They are small, well circumscribed, oval, elongated or rounded and are typi-cally eosinophilic and prominently hyalinized (Fig. 14.16). Within the nodule are embed-ded extravillous trophoblastic cells, which can occur singly or in cords: the trophoblastic cells commonly show degenerative changes, such as cytoplasmic vacuolation and nuclear chro-matin condensation, but may appear well pre-served. Multinucleated cells are sometimes seen but mitotic figures are absent or scanty. There are often small pseudopods projecting from the nodules into the surrounding tissues: these consist of extravillous trophoblastic cells admixed with eosinophilic fibrinoid material and may give a misleading impression of a squamous cell carcinoma. The nodules stain positively for cytokeratins, epithelial mem-brane antigen and placental alkaline phos-phatase: there is focal positivity for hPL in most cases and weak focal positivity for hCG in a minority of cases.

The placental site nodule is distinguished from a placental site tumour by its small size, circumscription, lack of infiltration, hyalinized nature, low cellularity and lack of mitotic figures.

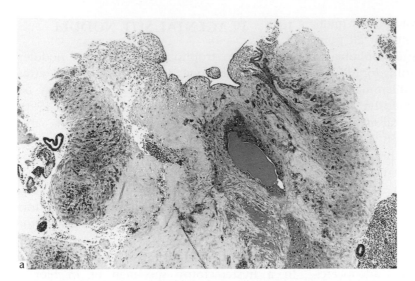

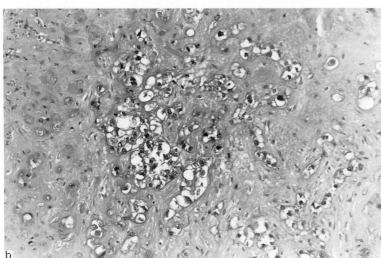

Figure 14.16 **(a)** A placental site nodule. This is sharply localized and extensively hyalinized. As commonly occurs, the nodule has partly shelled out of the surrounding endometrium. **(b)** Extravillous trophoblastic cells, some of which are vacuolated, are embedded in the hyalinized material. Haematoxylin and eosin.

14.5 EPITHELIOID TROPHOBLASTIC TUMOUR

This is a recently introduced entity (Shih and Kurman, 1998b), which has not yet been fully delineated: it has been suggested that it is the malignant counterpart of a placental site nodule (Shih *et al.*, 1999). The clinical features and gross appearances of this neoplasm are very similar to those of a placental site trophoblastic tumour. Histologically, mononuclear trophoblastic cells form nests, cords and solid masses. The tumours grow in a nodular expansile fashion and lack the infiltrative growth pattern of a placental site trophoblastic tumour. There is often a surrounding lymphocytic infiltrate and the cords and nests are intimately associated with eosinophilic fibrillary hyaline-like material and necrotic debris. Mitotic figures are usually sparse. The cells stain positively for epithelial markers, inhibin-α and, in a patchy focal fashion, hPL, hCG and Mel-CAM.

This tumour is distinguished from a placental site trophoblastic tumour by its non-infiltrative nodular growth pattern, the presence of hyaline and necrotic debris and the patchy, as opposed to diffuse, staining for hCG, hPL and Mel-CAM.

Distinction from a squamous cell carcinoma, which is often difficult on purely histological grounds, rests upon the positive staining for trophoblastic markers, including inhibin.

The clinical course of the epithelioid trophoblastic tumour is not yet fully defined but appears to be very similar to that of the placental site trophoblastic tumour with 10–15 per cent of cases pursuing a malignant course: there appear to be no histological features to allow for the identification of those neoplasms that will behave in a malignant fashion.

REFERENCES

Baergen, R.N., Rutgers, J.L. (1997) Trophoblastic lesions of the placental site. *Gen. Diagn. Pathol.* **143**, 143–58.

Bagshawe, K.D., Lawler, S.D., Paradinas, F.J., Dent, J., Brown, P., Boxer, G.M. (1990) Gestational trophoblastic tumours following initial diagnosis of partial hydatidiform mole. *Lancet* **335**, 1074–6.

Bewtra, C., Frankforter, S., Marcus, J.N. (1997) Clinicopathologic differences between diploid and tetraploid complete hydatidiform moles. *Int. J. Gynecol. Pathol.* **16**, 239–44.

Chang, Y.L., Chang, T.C., Hsueh, S. *et al.* (1999) Prognostic factors and treatment for placental site trophoblastic tumor – report of 3 cases and analysis of 88 cases. *Gynecol. Oncol.* **73**, 216–22.

Conran, R.M., Hitchcock, G.L., Popek, E.J. *et al.* (1993) Diagnostic considerations in molar gestations. *Hum. Pathol.* **24**, 41–8.

Eckstein, R.P., Paradinas, F.J., Bagshawe, K.D. (1982) Placental site trophoblastic tumour (trophoblastic pseudotumour): a study of four cases requiring hysterectomy including one fatal case. *Histopathology* **6**, 221–6.

Elston, C.W. (1995) Gestational trophoblastic disease. In Fox, H. (ed.), *Haines and Taylor: Textbook of Obstetrical and Gynaecological Pathology*, 4th Edn. Edinburgh: Churchill Livingstone, 1597–640.

Fox, H. (1997) *Pathology of the Placenta*, 2nd Edn. London: W.B. Saunders.

Fukunaga, M., Ushigome, S. (1993) Metastasizing placental site trophoblastic tumor: an immunohistochemical and flow cytometric study of two cases. *Am. J. Surg. Pathol.* **17**, 1003–10.

Fukunaga, M., Ushigome, S., Endo, Y. (1995) Incidence of hyatidiform mole in a Tokyo hospital: a 5 year (1989 to 1993) prospective morphological and flow cytometric study. *Hum. Pathol.* **26**, 758–64.

Gardner, H.A.R., Lage, J.M. (1992) Choriocarcinoma following a partial mole: a case report. *Hum. Pathol.* **23**, 467–71.

Genest, D.G., Laborde, O., Berkowitz, R.S., Goldstein, D.P., Bernstein, M.R., Lage, J.M. (1991) A clinico-pathologic study of 153 cases of complete hydatidiform mole (1980–1990): histologic grade lacks prognostic significance. *Obstet. Gynecol.* **78**, 402–9.

Goto, S., Yamada, A., Ishizuka, T., Tomoda, Y. (1993) Development of postmolar trophoblastic disease after partial molar pregnancy. *Gynecol. Oncol.* **48**, 165–70.

Hertig, A.T., Sheldon, W.H. (1947) Hydatidiform mole: a pathologico-clinical correlation of 200 cases. *Am. J. Obstet. Gynecol.* **53**, 1–36.

How, J., Scurry, J., Grant, P. *et al.* (1995) Placental site tumor: report of three cases and review of the literature. *Int. J. Gynecol. Cancer* **5**, 241–9.

Howat, A.J., Beck, S., Fox, H. *et al.* (1993) Can histopathologists reliably diagnose molar pregnancy? *J. Clin. Pathol.* **46**, 599–602.

Huettner, P., Gersell, D. (1994) Placental site nodule: a clinicopathologic study of 38 cases. *Int. J. Gynecol. Pathol.* **13**, 191–8.

Jacobs, P.A., Wilson, C.M., Sprenkle, J.A., Rosenhein, N.B., Migeon, B.R. (1980) Mechanism of origin of complete hydatidiform moles. *Nature* **286**, 714–16.

Jacobs, P.A., Szulman, A.E., Funkmouska, J., Maatsura, J.S., Wilson, C.C. (1982) Human triploidy: relationship between parental origin of the additional haploid complement and development of partial hydatidiform mole. *Ann. Hum. Genet.* **46**, 223–31.

Jauniaux, E. (1999) Partial moles: from postnatal to prenatal diagnosis. *Placenta* **20**, 379–88.

Jauniaux, E., Nicolaides, K.H. (1997) Early ultrasound diagnosis and follow-up of molar pregnancies. *Ultrasound Obstet. Gynaecol.* **9**, 17–21.

van de Kaa, C.A., Robben, J.C.M., Hopman, A.H.N., Hanselaar, A.G.J.M., Vooijs, G.P. (1995) Complete hydatidiform mole in twin pregnancy: differentiation from partial mole with interphase cytogenetic and DNA cytometric analysis on paraffin embedded tissues. *Histopathology* **26**, 123–9.

Kurman, R.J., Young, R.H., Norris, H.J., Lawrence, W.D., Scully, R.E. (1984) Immunocytochemical localization of placental lactogen and chorionic gonadotrophin in the normal placenta and trophoblastic tumors with emphasis on intermediate trophoblast and the placental site trophoblastic tumor. *Int. J. Gynecol. Pathol.* **3**, 101–21.

Lage, J.M., Bagg, A. (1996) Hydatidiform moles: DNA flow cytometry, image analysis and selected topics in molecular biology. *Histopathology* **28**, 379–82.

Lage, J.M., Mark, S.D., Roberts, D.J., Goldstein, D.P., Bernstein, M.R., Berkowitz, R.S. (1992) A flow cytometric study of 137 fresh hydropic placentas: correlation between types of hydatidiform moles and nuclear DNA ploidy. *Obstet. Gynecol.* **79**, 403–10.

Lawler, S.D., Fisher, R.A., Pickthall, V.J., Povey, S., Evans, M.W. (1982) Genetic studies on hydatidiform moles. I. The origin of partial moles. *Cancer Genet. Cytogenet.* **5**, 309–20.

Mosher, R., Goldstein, D.P., Berkowitz, R., Genest, D.R. (1998) Complete hydatidiform mole: comparison of clinicopathologic features, current and past. *J. Reprod. Med.* **43**, 21–7.

Paradinas, F.J. (1994) The histological diagnosis of hydatidiform moles. *Curr. Diag. Pathol.* **1**, 24–31.

Paradinas, F.J., Browne, P., Fisher, R.A., Foskett, M., Bagshawe, K.D., Newlands, E. (1996) A clinical, histological and flow cytometric study of 149 complete moles, 146 partial moles and 107 non-molar hydropic abortions. *Histopathology* **28**, 101–9.

Paradinas, F.J., Fisher, R.A., Browne, P., Newlands, E.S. (1997) Diploid hydatidiform moles with fetal red blood cells in molar villi. 1. Pathology, incidence and prognosis. *J. Pathol.* **181**, 183–8.

Redline, R.W., Hassold, T., Zaragoza, M. (1998) Determinants of villous trophoblastic hyperplasia in spontaneous abortions. *Mod. Pathol.* **11**, 762–8.

Rice, L.W., Berkowitz, R.S., Lage, J.M., Goldstein, D.P., Bernstein, M.E. (1990) Persistent gestational trophoblastic tumor after partial hydatidiform mole. *Gynecol. Oncol.* **36**, 358–62.

Shih, I.-M., Kurman, R.J. (1998a) Assessment of proliferation activity in the differential diagnosis of placental site trophoblastic lesions and choriocarcinoma – a double immunohistochemical staining technique using Ki-67 and Mel-CAM antibodies. *Human Pathol.* **28**, 27–33.

Shih, I.-M., Kurman, R.J. (1998b) Epithelioid trophoblastic tumor: a neoplasm distinct from choriocarcinoma and placental site trophoblastic tumor simulating carcinoma. *Am. J. Surg. Pathol.* **22**, 1393–403.

Shih, I.-M, Seidman, J.D., Kurman, R.J. (1999) Placental site nodule and characterization of distinctive types of intermediate trophoblast. *Hum. Pathol.* **30**, 687–94.

Surti, U., Szulman, A.E., O'Brien, S. (1982) Dispermic origin and clinical outcome of three complete hydatidiform moles with 46XY karyotype. *Am. J. Obstet. Gynecol.* **144**, 84–7.

Young, R.H., Scully, R.E. (1984) Placental site trophoblastic tumor: current status. *Clin. Obstet. Gynecol.* **27**, 248–58.

Young, R.H., Kurman, R.J., Scully, R.E. (1988) Proliferations and tumors of the placental site. *Semin. Diagn. Pathol.* **5**, 223–37.

Young, R.H., Kurman, R.J., Scully, R.E. (1990) Placental site nodules and plaques: a clinicopathologic analysis of 20 cases. *Am. J. Surg. Pathol.* **15**, 1001–9.

15 Endometrial biopsy in specific circumstances

In the preceding chapters of this book, endometrial biopsies have been discussed in terms of specific pathological lesions of the endometrium, such as inflammation, hyperplasia or neoplasia. In daily practice, however, most endometrial biopsies received in the laboratory are accompanied by clinical information that is couched in terms of the patient's symptoms rather than in terms of a suggested pathological lesion. Thus, the request form usually specifies complaints, for example, 'infertility' or 'postmenopausal bleeding' without suggesting a specific diagnosis, such as chronic endometritis or endometrial adenocarcinoma. It may also describe problems that have occurred during the procedure (Fig. 15.1). In this chapter, therefore, we consider the approach to endometrial biopsies in women with particular symptoms, acknowledging that we are, to a considerable extent, reiterating information already remarked upon in relationship to specific pathological processes.

During the reproductive years of a woman's life, the most common indications for endometrial biopsy are abnormal uterine bleeding and infertility: curettage is also performed frequently for complications of pregnancy, sometimes for diagnostic purposes but often for therapeutic reasons. In the peri- and post-menopausal years, the principal indication for biopsy is abnormal uterine bleeding whilst curettage is sometimes undertaken to exclude an endometrial abnormality in women being treated for unrelated gynaecological disorders, such as uterine prolapse. It is sometimes stated that endometrial biopsy for dysfunctional uterine bleeding is indicated only in women of more than 40 years. This view has been challenged by Ash *et al.* (1996) who are of the opinion that biopsy is indicated in any woman who has a history of menstrual cycle irregularity and dysfunctional uterine bleeding whatever her age (see below).

237

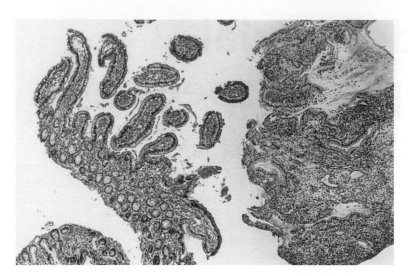

Figure 15.1 Small intestinal mucosa and endocervical tissue in an endometrial biopsy: the surgeon thought that uterine perforation had occurred during the procedure. Haematoxylin and eosin.

15.1 ABNORMAL BLEEDING DURING THE REPRODUCTIVE YEARS

Uterine bleeding may be abnormal in respect to its frequency, duration, quantity or the age at which it occurs and may take several clinical forms. Although the menstrual disturbance cannot always be exactly correlated with the underlying pathological process, the clinical features will often supply a clue to the possible nature of the abnormality. In practice, however, the pathologist should be aware that a term such as menorrhagia might be used on a histopathological request form in a rather general manner to refer to any type of abnormal or excessive bleeding. Care has also to be taken to distinguish between single episodes of heavy bleeding, which may be the result, for example, of recent pregnancy and those episodes which persist or recur and for which a potentially more serious underlying cause should be sought.

15.1.1 Amenorrhoea
15.1.1.1 Primary amenorrhoea

Primary amenorrhoea rarely necessitates biopsy of the endometrium, since investigations are largely concerned with the identification of a genital tract, chromosomal or endocrinological abnormality. However, in those rare cases in which biopsy is undertaken, we have seen both inactive, atrophic endometrium (Fig. 3.22) and inactive endometrium with a shallow, rather poorly developed functionalis, the appearances depending upon the degree of oestrogenic deprivation (Fig. 3.24).

15.1.1.2 Secondary amenorrhoea

Secondary amenorrhoea (amenorrhoea preceded by spontaneous menstruation) may be the result of conditions, which are physiological, such as those that often occur in the postmenarchal (but still adolescent) girl, pregnancy (which surprisingly is not always suspected by the patient), lactation and the menopause, or those which occur at inappropriate times

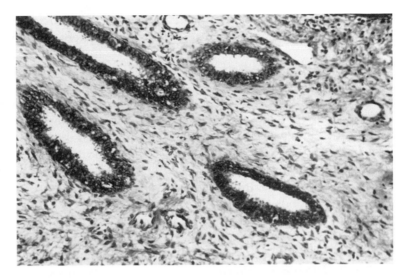

Figure 15.2 Asherman's syndrome. The endometrial stroma is fibrous and the glands narrow and inactive. At subsequent hysterectomy, more normal proliferative endometrium was identified elsewhere in the uterine cavity. Haematoxylin and eosin.

and are the consequence of a pathological process.

Secondary amenorrhoea, which is the consequence of a pathological process, occurs in patients with developing or established ovarian failure due to a variety of causes (severe systemic illness, and lesions in the cerebral cortex, hypothalamus, pituitary or ovary) or, less commonly, is due to abnormalities in the uterus itself. This symptom is, therefore, common to women with a wide variety of clinical disorders but, when the amenorrhoea is the consequence of ovarian failure, the appearance of the endometrium is similar whatever the underlying abnormality: the endometrial biopsy resembles that seen in the postmenopausal woman (see Chapters 2 and 3).

Very rarely, secondary amenorrhoea, or, more commonly, oligomenorrhoea, is the consequence of endometrial damage due to tuberculosis (Tindall, 1987), radiation (although amenorrhoea in these circumstances is usually secondary to ovarian failure) or Asherman's syndrome. Asherman's syndrome, also known as intrauterine synechiae, fibrotic endometritis or traumatic hypomenorrhoea–amenorrhoea, is characterized by the presence of adhesions between the surfaces of the uterine cavity, which are usually a consequence of curettage after miscarriage, particularly in the presence of sepsis. They may also, rarely, follow myomectomy (Giatras *et al.*, 1999), Caesarean section, transcervical endometrial resection (McCulloch *et al.*, 1995) or schistosomiasis (Krolikowski *et al.*, 1995). The uterine curettings in Asherman's syndrome are typically scanty and composed of endometrium completely or partly lacking evidence of normal cyclical changes, with fibrosed or even ossified, scarred stroma and sparse, inactive glands which may be cystically dilated (Fig. 15.2). The endometrial scarring and adhesions in Asherman's syndrome may be quite focal, and particularly when the scarring is limited to the isthmic area of the uterus, the complete amenorrhoea and the limited extent of the endometrial damage suggests that factors other than scarring are relevant to the amenorrhoea. The presence of Asherman's syndrome does not preclude the development of endometrial carcinoma (Sandridge *et al.*, 1994).

15.1.2   Scanty bleeding

15.1.2.1   Hypomenorrhoea

This is, by definition, the occurrence of menstrual periods that last less than 2 days. The cause is nearly always constitutional and, in these cases, the endometrial biopsy will almost certainly be normal in appearance for the stated day of the cycle. In some patients, however, scanty periods may presage the onset of amenorrhoea and in that case, the abnormalities described above may be seen.

15.1.2.2   Oligomenorrhoea

Infrequent, and often irregular, periods may, rarely, occur in women that are normally fertile but are more commonly encountered in patients with an ovulatory defect and this symptom is therefore of more significance than simple hypomenorrhoea.

In the patient with constitutional oligomenorrhoea, the variations in cycle length appear to be due entirely to prolongation or arrest of the pre-ovulatory phase, the secretory phase remaining remarkably constant at 14 days. The appearance of the endometrium will vary, therefore, according to the stage in the cycle at which the biopsy has been taken. During the follicular phase, a picture of weak or normal proliferative activity or, in some cases, a picture of prolonged proliferation is seen and maturation will appear to be retarded if related only to the date of the last menstrual period. Once ovulation has occurred, the appearance of the secretory endometrium is consistent with the date of ovulation unless the patient also has a luteal phase insufficiency.

More significantly, infrequent menstruation may also be an indication of developing ovarian failure or of the polycystic ovary syndrome and the appearance of the endometrium under these circumstances is very variable. In the patient with ovarian failure, this may range from the inactive, postmenopausal appearance associated with low oestrogen production through varying degrees of hyperplasia in the patient with polycystic ovary syndrome, who has a hyperoestrogenic state associated with non-ovulatory follicular development, to a normal appearance if the patient has recently had a normal cycle.

15.1.3   Excessive bleeding

In this text, we are concerned only with those abnormalities of bleeding that originate within the uterine body and not those which arise in the tubes, lower genital tract or cervix or are the result of abnormalities of haemostasis. It should be mentioned, however, that defects in local haemostatic mechanisms are a common and important cause of excessive bleeding from a morphologically normal uterus (Sheppard, 1984). The single most common cause of abnormal uterine bleeding during the reproductive years is pregnancy, or more precisely, abnormalities of pregnancy, in particular threatened or inevitable miscarriage or ectopic gestation.

In many other patients, however, examination of the endometrium reveals no abnormality, because the cause of the abnormal bleeding lies elsewhere. There may be abnormalities outside the uterus, e.g. pelvic infection or endometriosis, or within the myometrium or vasculature of the uterus: there may be defects in haemostatic mechanisms, endocrine abnormalities or psychiatric disorders. The bleeding may also have its origin in the vagina or cervix and thus, not be abnormal uterine bleeding in the strict meaning of the term.

In those women in whom an endometrial abnormality is observed, the fault may lie in the hypothalamic–pituitary–ovarian axis and thus the endometrial changes reflect abnormalities of ovarian hormone secretion while in others there may be an intrinsic endometrial lesion.

In women with dysfunctional uterine bleeding, there is less than 1 per cent chance of an endometrial abnormality when the cycle is regular but abnormalities are found in 14.3 per cent of women in whom the cycle is irregular (Ash *et al.*, 1996). In the same group of women, the authors found that menstrual cycle irregularity ($P = 0.0001$), age ≥ 40 years ($P = 0.022$) and hypertension ($P = 0.058$) were independently significant risk factors for abnormal endometrial histology.

15.1.3.1 Menorrhagia

Heavy periods occur most frequently when there is an increase in the surface area of the endometrium, e.g. in patients with submucous leiomyomas, adenomyosis, uterine polyps (Fig. 8.14) or uterus didelphis or bicornis (Tindall, 1987). In such cases, the endometrium may be entirely normal or there may be evidence of thinning of the endometrium where it overlies a leiomyoma (Fig. 1.6) or where it is ulcerated and/or inflamed at the tip of a polypoidal submucous leiomyoma. In patients with uterus bicornis, it is important to recognize that the samples obtained from the two halves of the uterus may not be identical, e.g. there may be a pregnancy in one horn while curettings from the second horn may strongly suggest the possibility of an ectopic gestation.

Menorrhagia occurs in a proportion of intrauterine contraceptive devices (IUCD) users and endometrial biopsy may reveal the full range of histological features described in Chapter 6, it may also be indicative of luteal phase insufficiency (see Chapter 4) but this condition more commonly causes occasional heavy periods rather than persistent menorrhagia.

When menorrhagia is the consequence of faults in the haemostatic mechanisms, there may be no morphological abnormality but it must be remembered that bleeding can be a consequence of a neoplastic process in the haemopoietic tissues: thus there may be, for example, a leukaemic infiltrate of the endometrium. In patients with congestive cardiac failure, haemorrhagic infarction of the endometrium (uterine apoplexy) may result in heavy vaginal bleeding (Daly and Balogh, 1968).

Occasionally, the endometrial biopsy in women with menorrhagia reveals an abnormality the significance of which may be difficult to evaluate. Two of these are illustrated in Figs 15.3 and 15.4.

15.1.3.2 Polymenorrhoea

Periods that are regular but occur more frequently than every 22 days are due to a short follicular phase and are the consequence either of disturbances in the hypothalamic–pituitary–ovarian axis, or of alterations in ovarian function secondary to pelvic infection or endometriosis: polymenorrhoea may occur for a short time when ovulation returns following pregnancy.

The appearance of the endometrium is usually normal in relation to the date of ovulation but appears accelerated if related only to the date of the last menstrual period.

15.1.3.3 Polymenorrhagia

This is a combination of frequent and heavy bleeding, which is usually the consequence of uterine or ovarian dysfunction and is seen particularly in patients with pelvic infection. There may be no abnormality in the endometrial biopsy or there may be an inflammatory cell infiltrate composed predominantly of haemosiderin-laden macrophages with scanty plasma cells and lymphocytes (Fig. 7.4). It is debatable whether the inflammation is the cause of the excessive bleeding or is its consequence. The sparse nature of the inflammation in most cases and the absence of any disturbance in the hormonal response suggest that,

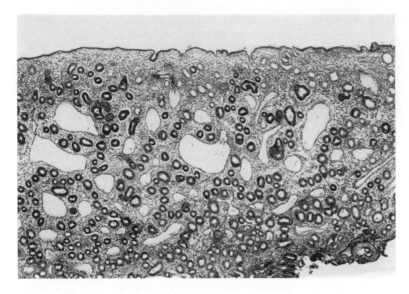

Figure 15.3 Lymphangiectasia in the endometrium of a woman with menorrhagia. The significance of this finding was never satisfactorily explained but may have been a complication of the leiomyomas that were present in the uterus. Haematoxylin and eosin.

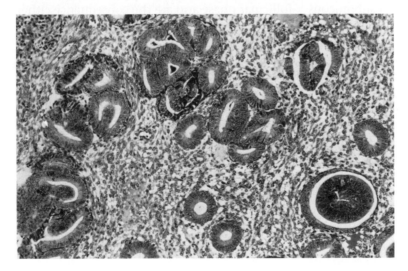

Figure 15.4 The endometrium in a patient with menorrhagia. Apparent crowding of the glands in this example was thought to result from traumatic loss of stroma during curettage. Note also the 'gland within gland' appearance at the lower right: this too is an artefact. Haematoxylin and eosin.

in most cases, it is the result of the repeated tissue breakdown rather than its cause.

15.1.3.4 Metrorrhagia

This is continuous or intermittent non-cyclical bleeding and includes intermenstrual and post-menopausal bleeding. It has a wide variety of causes, varying from disturbances of ovarian function, for example, anovulatory cycles and luteal phase insufficiency, to intrauterine neo-plastic processes or the demise of an intrauter-ine or ectopic gestation. While careful timing of the biopsy is usually recommended when evalu-ating the endometrium in infertile patients, biopsy as soon as possible is more appropriate in patients with metrorrhagia as there is nothing to gain by delaying the procedure and, indeed, further loss of tissue may hamper diagnosis.

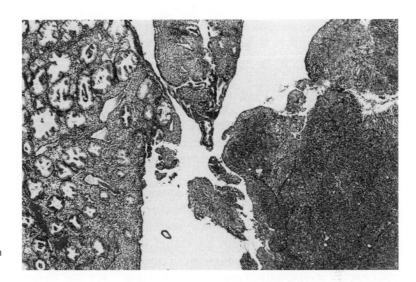

Figure 15.5 Fragments of cervical squamous carcinoma in an endometrial curetting. To the left there is normal secretory endometrium and to the right, non-keratinizing, large cell squamous carcinoma. Haematoxylin and eosin.

The appearance of the endometrium in patients with anovulatory cycles is very variable. The sample may be scanty, particularly if bleeding has been prolonged, and show little or no proliferative activity in a poorly formed shallow functionalis with evidence of stromal crumbling and interstitial haemorrhage. This is typical of the perimenopausal anovulatory state with low or fluctuating oestrogen levels in which oestrogen secretion has been sufficient to stimulate the endometrium and permit oestrogen withdrawal bleeding but has been insufficient for the development of a normal functionalis.

In women with polycystic ovary syndrome, or in perimenarchal or perimenopausal women, in whom there is follicular development without ovulation, it is more usual to find some degree of hyperplasia, most commonly a simple hyperplasia and very much less commonly, an atypical hyperplasia or even carcinoma (see Chapter 9). The history is typically that of a period of amenorrhoea followed by spotting, which terminates in a heavy prolonged bleed 'metropathia haemorrhagica'. A similar range of endometrial appearances is seen in the patient with an oestrogen-secreting neoplasm and in women who have been given unopposed oestrogen therapy at the menopause (see Chapter 5). In those women in whom there is evidence of a hyperplastic process, progestagen therapy or induction of ovulation may be followed by re-examination of the endometrium and in the majority of cases it will have reverted to normal. There is a small group of patients, however, in whom atypical hyperplasia was originally recognized and in whom, following progestagen therapy, there is a persistence of multifocal atypical features (Fig. 5.15). Some of these women may eventually require hysterectomy because of their failure to respond to progestagen and, in a very small number, carcinoma may supervene. Youth is no guarantee of safety from the development of carcinoma and while it is not common in the premenopausal woman, the possibility should always be borne in mind.

Intermenstrual bleeding often has a cause outside the uterine cavity, e.g. carcinoma of the cervix, and, indeed, fragments of such neoplasms are sometimes found in curettings (Fig. 15.5). It may also have less sinister causes.

Among these are ovulation bleeding, when the endometrial biopsy is normal, luteal phase insufficiency, characteristically occurring as premenstrual spotting (see Chapter 4), the presence of endometrial or isthmic polyps and, in some women, the use of steroid contraceptives, although in the latter case the bleeding is not so much intermenstrual as inter-hormone withdrawal bleeding. The endometrial biopsy appearances are described in Chapter 5.

Both premenstrual spotting and prolonged periods are characteristic of luteal phase insufficiency, the former being due to the premature demise of the corpus luteum associated with partial breakdown of the endometrium prior to the onset of menstruation and the latter to prolonged shedding of the endometrium (see Chapter 4).

The appearance of the endometrial biopsy in miscarriage and in ectopic pregnancy is discussed in Chapter 13 and endometrial neoplasms – stromal, epithelial or mixed – which may, rarely, be associated with abnormal bleeding in the reproductive years are fully covered in Chapters 10 and 11.

15.2   ABNORMAL PERIMENOPAUSAL OR POSTMENOPAUSAL BLEEDING

At the menopause, prior to the complete cessation of menstruation, the majority of women experience a gradual reduction in the amount and frequency of menstruation over a period of months or, less commonly, years. Less frequently, but equally normally, there may, without warning, be an abrupt cessation of menstrual loss. Biopsy of the endometrium is rarely carried out in these women, but when it is, the appearance is generally unremarkable and varies according to the patient's hormonal status at the time of biopsy.

In contrast, heavy perimenopausal bleeding is never normal and women experiencing excessive bleeding frequently undergo biopsy (Vakiani *et al.*, 1996).

15.2.1   Perimenopausal bleeding

The appearance of the endometrium varies greatly. Many of the more important features are described in the earlier section of this chapter dealing with the various forms of excessive bleeding. These will only be summarized here.

A shallow, poorly developed, weakly proliferative or inactive endometrium is characteristic of the patient with diminishing ovarian function and low oestrogen levels. These biopsies are frequently technically unsatisfactory, because they are so small and fragmented, and it may be possible to do no more than exclude the presence of a neoplasm on the material supplied. Such biopsies often show evidence of spontaneous stromal crumbling, breakdown and interstitial haemorrhage simultaneously with weak proliferative activity: the assumption is often made that oestrogenic stimulation has been insufficient to maintain endometrial growth.

Simple hyperplasia is characteristic of the patient with ovulatory failure in whom follicular development persists but the absence of follicular maturation and the failure of progesterone secretion allows unopposed oestrogenic activity. Biopsies in these cases are usually voluminous. It is important to exclude the presence of neoplasia or atypical hyperplasia.

Irregular shedding due to abnormal persistence of the corpus luteum is responsible for some cases of perimenopausal bleeding, and other facets of luteal phase insufficiency are not uncommon, the features being as described in Chapter 4.

Carcinoma is not common before the menopause but does occur, and should always be suspected in women with perimenopausal or postmenopausal bleeding. Indeed, the presence of a carcinoma may well mask the development of the menopause as menstrual bleeding is replaced by bleeding associated with the neoplastic process. Stromal sarcomas, though less common than carcinomas, are more likely to occur in younger women and may therefore be identified not only in the perimenopausal patient but also in the woman of reproductive age.

Simple polyps and adenomyomatous polyps are commonly encountered and the pathologist should always be aware of the possibility that the bleeding may have its origin in a cervical neoplasm. Great care should be taken to examine any cervical fragments included in the biopsy (Fig. 15.5).

15.2.2 Postmenopausal bleeding

With increasing age, postmenopausal bleeding tends to become less common but, simultaneously, the chance that it is the result of endometrial carcinoma increases (Gredmark *et al.*, 1995). Indeed, postmenopausal bleeding should always be regarded as due to the presence of a neoplasm until otherwise proven. Most commonly, the tumour is an adenocarcinoma and these tumours are fully described in Chapter 10. Postmenopausal bleeding may also occur in a patient with metastatic carcinoma of the endometrium and the finding of multifocal tumour or carcinoma of unusual morphology should always raise this possibility in the mind of the pathologist. A metastatic tumour is likely to have had a primary origin in the breast, ovary or large intestine (Figs 12.6 and 12.7).

In many women with postmenopausal bleeding, curettings reveal inactive endometrium showing no proliferative activity but glandular epithelial stratification, suggesting persistent though very low levels of oestrogenic stimulation. Particularly in the early months or years of the postmenopausal state, a proliferative endometrium of unremarkable appearance is seen; such a finding becomes progressively less common with time from the menopause.

Even long after the menopause, the endometrium retains the capacity to respond to oestrogenic stimulation and, therefore, if oestrogen is present, a proliferative or hyperplastic picture may be induced. This occurs in women using topical vaginal or vulval oestrogen creams, or receiving unopposed oestrogen replacement therapy. It also occurs in a small proportion of women receiving tamoxifen therapy for the treatment of breast carcinoma and in patients with an oestrogen-secreting ovarian neoplasm or a luteinized follicular cyst. This last abnormality has been described as occurring up to 7 years after the menopause. Frequently, women presenting with postmenopausal bleeding have been given progestagen therapy before the endometrial biopsy is carried out and, if the oestrogen has induced progesterone receptors, stromal pseudodecidualization and glandular secretion may be apparent.

In some patients with typical senile, cystic atrophy, the cystic tissue becomes polypoidal and the removal of such polyps is usually followed by cessation of bleeding despite the absence of histological evidence of tissue breakdown in the polyp (Fig. 15.6).

Postmenopausal bleeding or blood-stained discharge may also occur in women with endometrial inflammation (see Chapter 7). This is usually non-specific and may be associated with a pyometra or, rarely, utero-colonic fistula resulting from diverticular disease of the large bowel. The endometrial biopsy may contain acute purulent material, non-specific granulation tissue, atrophic endometrium heavily infiltrated by histiocytes and lymphocytes together with metaplastic squamous epithelium in which there may or may not be cytological

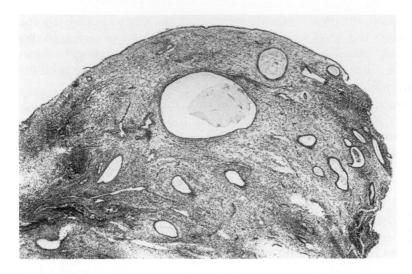

Figure 15.6 A polyp from a woman with postmenopausal bleeding. It is composed of inactive, rather atrophic endometrium in which many of the glands are cystically dilated. This is the appearance of senile cystic atrophy. Haematoxylin and eosin.

atypia. Postmenopausal bleeding may also complicate tuberculosis (see Section 7.2.3.1) or malakoplakia (see Section 7.1.2.2) and, in both cases, the curettings usually permit a specific diagnosis.

Thus, endometrial biopsies from women with postmenopausal bleeding may reveal an adenocarcinoma, show evidence of continuing oestrogenic stimulation, indicate an inflammatory process or demonstrate polypoidal senile cystic change. The fact remains, however, that in a proportion of women complaining of postmenopausal bleeding, the findings in the endometrial biopsy will reveal no morphological basis for this symptom.

15.3 ENDOMETRIAL BIOPSY IN THE INFERTILE PATIENT

Endometrial biopsies from infertile women are now infrequently taken but those that are, tend often to be rather small, having been taken with the intention of causing as little damage or disturbance to the endometrium as possible. They therefore require more than usual care in their handling, orientation and interpretation if the pitfalls of interpreting small biopsies are to be avoided.

Endometrial biopsy with accurate dating of the endometrium is still regarded as the most reliable test in the investigation of infertility (Annos *et al.*, 1980; Rosenfeld *et al.*, 1980). This depends heavily upon both close cooperation between the clinician and the pathologist, and the accuracy of the clinical information. It is important that, whenever possible, the appearance of the endometrium should be related to the date of ovulation and not to the date of the last menstrual period because of the variation in the length of the follicular phase. Where the date of ovulation is not known with accuracy, there are two alternatives: the date on which mittelschmerz occurred might be ascertained or the usual cycle length and duration of the menstrual period may be used as a basis for estimating the probable date of ovulation.

In the majority of infertile women, the morphology of the endometrial biopsy is normal and the appearance is approximately appropriate for the day of the cycle. This is the case when, as so often happens, the cause of the infertility lies outside the uterus, e.g. in women with the unruptured follicle syndrome in whom the pattern of hormonal secretion is normal but in whom the failure of ovum release precludes fertilization. In other cases, however, biopsy reveals an abnormality that may be due to a primary endometrial disorder or may be secondary to ovarian dysfunction. It has been reported, in a series from Turkey, that as many as one-fifth of the endometrial biopsies taken in the investigation of infertility showed evidence of luteal phase insufficiency (Sahmay *et al.*, 1995). Generally, infertility due to ovarian dysfunction is often associated with menstrual disturbances or amenorrhoea, while, clinically, endometrial abnormalities may be unsuspected.

15.3.1   Endometrial abnormalities

Acute endometrial inflammation is not usually regarded as a cause of infertility but may be indicative of infection elsewhere in the genital tract, which may be the basis of infertility, for example, in the cervix or Fallopian tubes. On the other hand, both non-specific and specific chronic endometritis are well recognized as a cause of infertility and, in certain circumstances, of recurrent miscarriage.

In interpreting inflammation in the biopsy from an infertile patient, care should be taken to distinguish between a focal inflammatory process, such as that seen on the surface of a polyp or submucous leiomyoma, where the inflammation may be irrelevant in relation to the infertility, and inflammation which affects the entire endometrium and is more likely to be of significance. Although leiomyomas are present in 3–5 per cent of infertile women, they are rarely submucous or apparent on endometrial biopsy: the relationship between infertility and their presence is uncertain.

Endometrial tuberculosis is now rarely seen in the UK but its association with infertility is well recognized: it is, however, the accompanying tubal disease that is the cause of the infertility and not the endometrial disease which is usually superficial, transient and rarely well established (see Section 7.2.3.1). Clearly, any woman who is so ill with tuberculosis that she becomes amenorrhoeic will be infertile and endometrial disease will, in the absence of regular shedding, show evidence of caseation.

Even in the absence of active inflammation, post-inflammatory fibrosis, particularly that seen in Asherman's syndrome, may cause infertility: the biopsy appearances are discussed on p. 239.

In a small proportion of women with long-standing primary or secondary infertility, there may be no evidence of active endometrial inflammation, the cyclical changes are appropriate for the hormonal status, secretory transformation is uniform and adequate and microbiological cultures are negative but many of the glands contain epithelial cells and macrophages in the absence of any other evidence of inflammation (Fig. 15.7). The full aetiology and significance of this condition is unknown but it is a recurrent finding in patients with unexplained infertility. In a small number of cases, it has been observed in women with cystic fibrosis and in low-grade infection.

15.3.2   Ovarian dysfunction

In infertile patients with oligomenorrhoea or amenorrhoea the endometrium may be shallow, poorly grown and either lacking in mitotic activity or exhibiting only weak proliferative activity, the appearance suggesting anovulation with low oestrogen levels, or there may be endometrial hyperplasia, suggesting anovulation with elevated or persistent oestrogen secretion. The latter is more likely to be associated with infrequent heavy bleeds interspersed with irregular spotting.

In some women, despite the presence of ovarian dysfunction, there may be little or no menstrual disturbance. Ovulation may occur

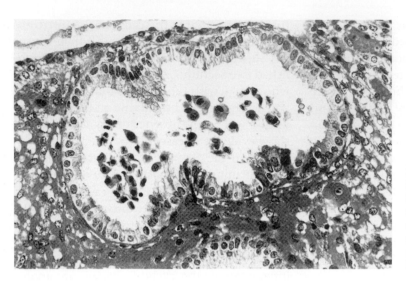

Figure 15.7 Endometrial biopsy from a patient with unexplained infertility. The secretory gland contains a cluster of histiocytes and epithelial cells: there is no evidence of active inflammation and secretory changes are uniform and adequate. Haematoxylin and eosin.

but the patient may have a short luteal phase, and hence frequent menstruation: luteal phase insufficiency may, however, be unsuspected until the biopsy reveals evidence of a secretory abnormality (the features of which are described in Chapter 4). It should not be assumed, however, that the infertility is necessarily the consequence of luteal phase insufficiency as the abnormality would have to be present in most cycles before it could be regarded as having any clinical significance. Care should also be exercised to prevent over-diagnosis of luteal phase abnormalities, particularly in the rather superficial biopsy typically received from the infertile patient. In the late secretory phase, when a well-developed superficial compact layer has formed, the glands in this part of the endometrium are often rather narrow and they may misleadingly suggest, to the unwary, a secretory defect (Fig. 3.17).

Rarely, ovarian hormone production is normal but the endometrium fails to show the appropriate cyclical changes because of insensitivity to the hormones.

REFERENCES

Annos, T., Thompson, I.E., Taymor, M.L. (1980) Luteal phase deficiency and infertility: difficulties encountered in diagnosis and treatment. *Obstet. Gynecol.* **55**, 705–10.

Ash, S.J., Farrell, S.A., Flowerdew, G. (1996) Endometrial biopsy in DUB. *J. Reprod. Med.* **41**, 892–6.

Daly, J.J., Balogh Jr, K. (1968) Hemorrhagic necrosis of the senile endometrium ('apoplexia uteri'): relation to superficial hemorrhagic necrosis of the bowel. *N. Engl. J. Med.* **278**, 709–11.

Giatras, K., Berkeley, A.S., Noyes, N., Licciardi, F., Lolis, D., Grifo, J.A. (1999) Fertility after hysteroscopic resection of submucous myomas. *J. Am. Assoc. Gynecol. Laparosc.* **6**, 155–8.

Gredmark, T., Kvint, S., Havel, G., Mattsson, L.A. (1995) Histopathological findings in women with postmenopausal bleeding. *Br. J. Obstet. Gynaecol.* **102**, 133–6.

Krolikowski, A., Janowski, K., Larsen, J.V. (1995) Asherman syndrome caused by schistosomiasis. *Obstet. Gynecol.* **85**, 898–9.

McCulloch, T.A., Wagner, B., Duffy, S., Barik, S., Smith, J.H. (1995) The pathology of hysterectomy specimens following trans-cervical resection of the endometrium. *Histopathology* **27**, 541–7.

Rosenfeld, D.L., Chodow, S., Bronson, R.A. (1980) Diagnosis of luteal phase inadequacy. *Obstet. Gynecol.* **56**, 193–6.

Sheppard, B.L., Chodow, S., Bronson, R.A. (1984) The pathology of dysfunctional uterine bleeding. *Clinics Obstet. Gynaecol.* **11**, 227–36.

Sandridge, D.A., Councell, R.B., Thorp, J.M. (1994) Endometrial carcinoma arising within extensive intrauterine synechiae. *Eur. J. Obstet. Gynecol. Reprod. Biol.* **56**, 147–9.

Sahmay, S., Oral, E., Saridogan, E., Senturk, L., Atasu, T. (1995) Endometrial biopsy findings in infertility: analysis of 12,949 cases. *Int. J. Fertil. Menopausal. Stud.* **40**, 316–21.

Tindall, V.R. (1987) *Jeffcoate's Principles of Gynaecology.* London: Butterworth, 512.

Vakiani, M., Vavilis, D., Agorastos, T., Stamatopoulos, P., Assimaki, A., Bontis, J. (1996) Histopathological findings of the endometrium in patients with dysfunctional uterine bleeding. *Clin. Exp. Obstet. Gynecol.* **23**, 236–9.

Index

Note: Page numbers in *italic* refer to figures